Genetics - Research and Issues

Rare Disorders Research Progress

nova
Medicine & Health
New York

Genetics - Research and Issues

Transcriptomics and Their Importance
Sarah Naiyer, PhD (Editor)
Khalid Hussain Bhat, PhD (Editor)
2022. ISBN: 979-8-88697-044-9 (Softcover)
2022. ISBN: 979-8-88697-203-0 (eBook)

Genetic Instability and Some Unusual Radiobiological Effects
Ekaterina S. Evstratova, Vladislav G. Petin, Andrey D. Kaprin and Petr V. Shegai (Editors)
2022. ISBN: 978-1-68507-886-7 (Hardcover)
2022. ISBN: 979-8-88697-007-4 (eBook)

More information about this series can be found at
https://novapublishers.com/product-category/series/genetics-research-and-issues/

Rare Disorders Research Progress

Meningiomas: From Diagnosis to Treatment
Richard A. Prayson, MD, MEd (Editor)
2022. ISBN: 978-1-68507-715-0 (Softcover)
2022. ISBN: 978-1-68507-807-2 (eBook)

Nerve Sheath Tumors: Signs, Symptoms and Treatment
Richard A. Prayson, MD, MEd (Editor)
2020. ISBN: 978-1-53617-366-6 (Softcover)
2020. ISBN: 978-1-53617-367-3 (eBook)

More information about this series can be found at
https://novapublishers.com/product-category/series/rare-disorders-research-progress/

Shazlin Shaharudin
Hisham Atan Edinur
and Nor Fazila Che Mat
Editors

Genetic Disorders and Rare Diseases

Current Updates

nova
Medicine & Health
New York

https://doi.org/10.52305/WNGG1520

NOTICE TO THE READER

The Publisher has taken reasonable care in the preparation of this book but makes no expressed or implied warranty of any kind and assumes no responsibility for any errors or omissions. No liability is assumed for incidental or consequential damages in connection with or arising out of information contained in this book. The Publisher shall not be liable for any special, consequential, or exemplary damages resulting, in whole or in part, from the readers' use of, or reliance upon, this material. Any parts of this book based on government reports are so indicated and copyright is claimed for those parts to the extent applicable to compilations of such works.

Independent verification should be sought for any data, advice or recommendations contained in this book. In addition, no responsibility is assumed by the Publisher for any injury and/or damage to persons or property arising from any methods, products, instructions, ideas or otherwise contained in this publication.

This publication is designed to provide accurate and authoritative information with regards to the subject matter covered herein. It is sold with the clear understanding that the Publisher is not engaged in rendering legal or any other professional services. If legal or any other expert assistance is required, the services of a competent person should be sought. FROM A DECLARATION OF PARTICIPANTS JOINTLY ADOPTED BY A COMMITTEE OF THE AMERICAN BAR ASSOCIATION AND A COMMITTEE OF PUBLISHERS.

Library of Congress Cataloging-in-Publication Data
Names: Shaharudin, Shazlin, editor. | Atan Edinur, Hisham, editor. | Fazila Che Mat, Nor, editor.
Title: Genetic disorders and rare diseases: current updates / Shazlin Shaharudin, Hisham Atan Edinur and Nor Fazila Che Mat, editors, School of Health Sciences, Universiti Sains Malaysia, Kota Bharu, Kelantan, Malaysia.
Identifiers: LCCN 2023030018 (print) | LCCN 2023030019 (ebook) | ISBN 9798886979534 (print) | ISBN 9798891130319 (adobe pdf)
Subjects: LCSH: Genetic disorders. | Genetic disorders--Diagnosis. | Genetic disorders--Treatment.
Classification: LCC RB155.5 .G45454 2023 (print) | LCC RB155.5 (ebook) | DDC 616/.042--dc23/eng/20230724
LC record available at https://lccn.loc.gov/2023030018
LC ebook record available at https://lccn.loc.gov/2023030019

Published by Nova Science Publishers, Inc. † New York

Contents

Preface

Genetic disorders are diseases caused by mutation in gene(s) or due to chromosomal disorder. They can be passed down to the offspring and manifested at birth, or triggered by lifestyle habits, such as smoking and exposure to specific substances in the environment. Some genetic disorders are very rare and mostly limited by demography, and therefore, will often be under-diagnosed. Although most genetic diseases are rare, but not all rare diseases are caused by genetic disorders. Rare diseases may also be caused by pathogens, immune deficiencies and cancer. Due to limited information and lack of access to treatment, the management of rare diseases is frequently complicated. Up to December 2020, a total of 470 rare diseases have been registered and recognised by the Ministry of Health, Malaysia. This book highlights some of the genetic disorders and their resulting rare diseases that have been reported in Malaysia, including their prevalence, molecular mechanism and pathogenesis, besides discussing their diagnosis, treatment and prevention methods.

Shazlin Shaharudin
Hisham Atan Edinur
Nor Fazila Che Mat
March 2023

Acknowledgments

Genetic Disorders & Rare Diseases: Current Updates consists of 13 chapters, written by the academic staff and postgraduate students at various universities and research institutions in Malaysia. They include Universiti Sains Malaysia, University of Nottingham Malaysia, Universiti Sains Islam Malaysia, Universiti Sultan Zainal Abidin, Universiti Kuala Lumpur-Royal College of Medicine Perak, Universiti Teknologi MARA Sungai Buloh, UCSI University, International Medical University, AIMST University, Universiti Kebangsaan Malaysia, MyGenome Sdn Bhd and National Institute of Health, Ministry of Health Malaysia. The compilation of this book is a success thanks to the extraordinary support provided by the management of these institutions through research funding, use of laboratory facilities, and administrative services. Images and illustrations are either created by the authors or adopted with permission from their sources.

We are grateful to the reviewers for sharing their expertise and insight to enhance the contents of this book: Ana Masara Ahmad Mokhtar, Azalina Zainuddin, Hazwani Ahmad Yusof@Hanafi, Hermizi Hapidin, Marjanu Hikmah Elias, Maryam Azlan, Nik Norliza Nik Hassan, Nur Asyilla Che Jalil, Nur Hasnah Ma'amor, Mohd Nizam Zahary, Mohd Nor Azim Ab Patar, Sabreena Safuan, Tee Get Bee@Yvonne, and Zatilfarihiah Easdi.

Chapter 1

Osteosarcopenic Obesity: A Comprehensive Guide to Prevention and Management

Nurdiana Zainol Abidin*
Department of Community Health, Advanced Medical and Dental Institute, Universiti Sains Malaysia, Pulau Pinang, Malaysia;
School of Biosciences, Faculty of Science and Engineering, University of Nottingham Malaysia, Jalan Broga, Semenyih, Selangor, Malaysia

Abstract

Osteosarcopenic obesity (OSO) is a cluster of three chronic and multi-factorial conditions that often co-occur: obesity, sarcopenia and osteoporosis. It is a relatively new term, but is gaining attention due to the increased risk of adverse health outcomes. Recent research suggested that OSO is common in the elderly, especially among those with obesity and sarcopenia, and is associated with increased risk of mortality. Additionally, it has also been linked to increased risk of disability, falls and fracture. There is increasing evidence to suggest that lifestyle intervention, including physical activity, healthy dietary intake and vitamin D supplementation may improve OSO outcomes. This chapter will discuss the pathophysiology of OSO, including its genetic predisposition, the impact of nutrition on the development and progression of OSO, as well as the role of physical activity in managing the condition. Additionally, the methods of diagnosing OSO are also discussed. This chapter also goes through the most recent research on OSO disorder, its many health effects, the impact of psychosocial factors and the effectiveness of interventions. It highlights the various

* Corresponding Author's Email: nurdianaabidin@usm.my.

In: Genetic Disorders and Rare Diseases
Editors: Shazlin Shaharudin, Hisham Atan Edinur and Nor Fazila Che Mat
ISBN: 979-8-88697-953-4

underlying co-morbidities that may cause or exacerbate OSO, such as low-grade chronic inflammation and chronic stress. It concludes by discussing knowledge gaps in OSO and proposes several dietary and exercise regimens that may be tailored to each person's needs to prevent or manage the condition.

Keywords: musculoskeletal, obesity, osteoporosis, osteosarcopenia, sarcopenia

Introduction

An individual exhibiting a combination of obesity with low bone and muscle mass is referred to as having osteosarcopenic obesity (OSO) (Ma et al., 2020; Ilich et al., 2016a; Ormsbee et al., 2014; Cooper et al., 2013). OSO is seen as the most severe impairment related to bone, muscle, and fat that is caused by ageing (Pang et al., 2021, Nasabian et al., 2017). Other forms of this disorder include osteopenic obesity (OO) and sarcopenic obesity (SO), which is judged not only by its clinical definitions, but also by the amount of fat infiltrated in the muscle tissues and its influence on the bones. Eventually, both conditions (OO and SO) may progress and result in OSO.

At present, there is limited knowledge about the cause, prevalence and long-term implications of OSO in older adults. One of the key characteristics of OSO is the interrelated nature of the disorder, ranging from its cellular connections to the weakening of musculoskeletal structures. In the past, osteoporosis, sarcopenia, and obesity were usually treated in isolation, with little research done into how they interacted. Nevertheless, multiple studies have indicated that bone, muscle, and fat are closely intertwined (Vaidya, 2014; Migliaccio et al., 2014). There is growing evidence that these disorders share similar pathophysiology (Ormsbee et al., 2014). Research suggests that sarcopenia and osteoporosis have similar risk factors, such as genetics, endocrine and mechanical function. Furthermore, a relationship between bone, and muscle has been established, which is not only mechanical in nature but also metabolic. This has resulted in 'osteosarcopenia' being acknowledged as a single entity (Hirschfeld et al., 2017). Studies are still in the nascent stages and there is a long way to go before causal relationships between aging, hormonal changes (e.g., a significant dip in anabolic hormone levels), and an increase in total and/or abdominal fat leading to increased expression of pro-inflammatory cytokines can be established. These processes cause both muscle and bone tissues to be reduced through a range of ways, which eventually influence clinical outcomes, such as an increased likelihood of falls and fractures (Ormsbee et al., 2014). It is suggested that recognising OSO as a single entity is more biologically relevant and may contribute to a more thorough treatment plan because of the connectedness of the syndrome.

All three conditions of osteoporosis, sarcopenia and obesity have been linked to various elements within an individual cells and hormones, as well as habits. According to research, the largest risks for all three of these illnesses are low oestrogen levels, a lack of vitamin D, and a lack of physical exercise (Clegg, 2012; Messier et al., 2011). Consequently, it is hypothesized that post-menopausal women will have a heightened risk of getting OSO due to their sudden decrease in oestrogen, age-related increase in body fat and lack of physical activity.

Age-related disorders such as osteopenia/osteoporosis and sarcopenia have similar mechanisms of diseases (Ormsbee et al., 2014). It was assumed that if obesity was added to these conditions, metabolic issues would become more severe, resulting in poorer quality of life, an elevated risk of illness and death (Corica et al., 2015). At present, there are numerous theories on what could be the cause of OSO. Cooper et al., (2013) proposed that a higher level of pro-inflammatory cytokines due to an increase in overall and/or abdominal fat, combined with some hormonal imbalances, causes harm to bone and muscle tissue by several different ways, leading to various clinical issues such as higher risks of falls and fractures. It is anticipated that those with all three conditions will experience worse clinical outcomes than those with only one of the conditions, which was evidenced in a Chinese study on elderly women with OSO, who had a poorer quality of blood lipid profile (Mo et al., 2018) compared to those without OSO. Additionally, a Mexican study also found that women with OSO had a significantly lower physical performance and poorer frailty scores compared to those without the syndrome (Szlejf et al., 2017). Moreover, a study by Ilich et al., (2015) determined that elderly women with OSO had poorer handgrip strength, balance and mobility than those of the same age who were obese alone (Ilich et al., 2015). Kalinkovich & Livshits (2017) also uncovered that the simultaneous presence of all three disorders led to even more serious metabolic irregularities, such as dyslipidaemia, and insulin resistance (Kalinkovich & Livshits, 2017).

Importance of Body Composition Measurement

Changes in a person's body composition as they age are inevitable. It is critical to get a precise assessment of body composition in medical settings where there might be perceived or expected irregularities. For example, in an elderly person who is of normal body weight and BMI, dynapenia (low muscle strength) and sarcopenia (low muscle mass) may go unnoticed if no measurements of muscle strength or muscle mass are taken. Individuals may also have undiagnosed osteopenia/osteoporosis, which can only be discovered through bone density screening (Sozen et al., 2017).

Currently, investigations into OSO as a single entity are still in the early stages (Ma et al., 2020; Nasabian et al., 2017b; Ilich et al., 2016a; Ilich et al., 2015). Evidence suggesting that obesity has a positive effect on bone density may have caused researchers to neglect its relationship with osteopenia/osteoporosis and sarcopenia (Hou et al., 2020). It was once thought that obese people had a lower chance of breaking a bone since they usually had stronger bones. Moreover, obese people were also believed to have more fat tissue to cushion any impact from a fall, thus were less likely to get hurt (Hou et al., 2020). The application of mechanical pressure to cortical bone resulting from an individual's excessive body weight was also proposed to be beneficial for bone development despite being a cause of many long-term health problems (Hou et al., 2020).

However, despite a variety of research revealing connections between body mass and bone mineral density (Qiao et al., 2020; Lins Vieira et al., 2021), there is data from epidemiological and animal studies that show otherwise (Palermo et al., 2016; Greco et al., 2010; Hou et al., 2020). Studies have also shown a strong link between fat deposition and adverse outcomes (Gilsanz et al., 2009; Bredella et al., 2011). Investigations conducted by Gilsanz et al., (2009) and Bredella et al., (2011) revealed that visceral fat, which is in the abdominal region, is more damaging to the body, especially the bones, than subcutaneous fat, which was determined to be protective for the bones. Gilsanz et al. (2009) discovered that subcutaneous and visceral fat have powerful, albeit conflicting, correlations with bone structure and strength. They discovered that subcutaneous fat had positive correlations with cross-sectional area (CSA), and cortical bone area (CBA), however visceral fat had negative associations with all bone characteristics.

Diagnostic Criteria for OSO

Since OSO has only recently been identified (less than 10 years ago), there is currently no standard definition, which makes it difficult to diagnose. At present, several tools could be used to screen for OSO in the general population based on two diagnostic principles; 1) through physical measurements of bone and body composition (i.e., QUS and BIA) and/or 2) via functional performance measures as a proxy for bone and body composition data (i.e., Short Physical Performance Battery Test) (Kelley et al., 2019).

Other methods, such as underwater weighing and deuterium oxide (D_2O) dilution, are more accurate but expensive, time-consuming and not patient-friendly, which makes them more suitable for research settings (Peppa et al., 2017). Currently, bone-density scan (DXA), computed tomography (CT) and magnetic resonance imaging (MRI) are considered the most accurate methods for directly assessing body composition and bone density. Despite their accuracy, they can be difficult to access due to the cost, lack of equipment and the potential exposure to radiation with MRI and CT scans.

Ilich et al., (2015) proposed a diagnostic system for OSO in postmenopausal women, which involves both physical and functional evaluations. The physical evaluation criteria are as follows: 1) T-score for BMD $\leq$-1.0 SD at the femoral neck, proximal femur, or lumbar spine; 2) 20th percentile of appendicular lean mass (ALM), with the equation: ALM = -17.4 +18.3 x height (m) + 0.16 x body fat (kg) (Ilich et al., 2015); and, 3) fat mass $\geq$ 32% of body weight for women. All three criteria were required to be assessed using dual energy DXA. The functional assessment includes handgrip strength ($\leq$20 kg for women), and modified components of short physical performance battery test (SPPB): one leg stance: $\leq$16 sec, gait speed: $\leq$0.8 m/sec, sit-to-stand chair test: $\leq$20 times. However, these criteria may not be suitable for all individuals owing to factors such as ethnicity and feasibility in extensive epidemiological research.

Due of the advancing nature of OSO, early diagnosis of the syndrome is essential for effective intervention and management. Recognising OSO as a potential danger to public health can assist in containing the rate of prevalence before it becomes an epidemic. The early diagnosis may also lower the expenses of public health by avoiding the requirement for behaviour, dietary or medicinal interventions in the future. The combined consequences of osteoporosis, obesity, and sarcopenia on general health are now poorly understood. Despite this, a scenario where the unfavourable health consequences connected with these disorders may be avoided in the future if tackled early.

Getting to Know the Trifecta of Trouble

Osteosarcopenic obesity (OSO) is a complex condition with a variety of associated pathways. It is a combination of three health conditions: osteopenia, sarcopenia and obesity. The combination in question has the potential to have a devastating effect on overall health. In the first subtopic, the effects of this triple threat on the body will be examined, as well as any potential health problems that could result.

Osteopenia/osteoporosis is a condition that is characterised by a decrease in bone mineral density (BMD). Normal BMD is defined as a T-score of -1 or above. A T-score between -1 and -2.5 indicates osteopenia, while a T-score below -2.5 indicates osteoporosis. Osteopenia and osteoporosis can lead to weakened bones and an increased risk of fractures, especially in the spine, wrist, and hip (Barnsley et al., 2021). Sarcopenia is a condition characterised by the age-related loss of skeletal muscle mass and strength. It is a common occurrence in older adults and can lead to a decline in physical function and mobility. The combination of osteopenia and sarcopenia can lead to an increased risk of falls and fractures, as well as a decline in overall quality of life (Kalinkovich & Livshits, 2017).

Obesity is associated with several health issues, including an increased risk of heart disease, Type-2 diabetes, and certain types of cancer. It is also associated with metabolic syndrome, which is a cluster of conditions that increase the risk of developing cardiovascular disease. According to one theory, obesity is the condition that most frequently triggers osteoporosis and sarcopenia (Ezzat-Zadeh et al., 2017a). Obesity is the primary factor contributing to the development of OSO, as it causes chronic inflammation and the release of harmful cytokines that damage bone and muscle tissue. This inflammation also leads to the infiltration of fat in muscle tissue, which weakens and reduces the efficiency of muscles. Additionally, the release of specific muscle cytokines, such as myostatin, during sarcopenia has been observed to inhibit the differentiation and mineralisation of osteogenic and osteoblast cells (Qin et al., 2017) (He et al., 2020).

The combination of osteopenia, sarcopenia and obesity can have a variety of adverse effects on health, particularly, on the immune system. Obese individuals tend to have a weakened immune system, which puts them at an increased risk of infection (de Frel et al., 2020). The combination of osteopenia and sarcopenia can also lead to decreased physical activity, which can add to the risk of infection. Overall, the combination of osteopenia, sarcopenia and obesity can lead to a number of serious health issues. The risks associated with having OSO include higher chances of fractures, difficulty with everyday tasks, physical disability, insulin resistance, greater risk of infections, longer hospital stays, and lower chances of survival (Ormsbee et al., 2014). It is important to be aware of this triple threat and to take steps to manage it, such as maintaining a healthy diet, exercising regularly, and managing obesity.

The Pathophysiology of Osteosarcopenic Obesity: How Do Osteopenia, Sarcopenia and Obesity Interact?

Age-related disorders such as osteopenia/osteoporosis and sarcopenia have been seen to have a similar pathophysiology as demonstrated by Ormsbee et al., (2014). Both muscles and bones come from the same mesenchymal cells in the bone marrow and show similar development patterns (Hamrick et al., 2016). Obesity, when added to the combined presence of osteopenia/osteoporosis and sarcopenia, was expected to make any existing abnormalities worse, causing a decreased quality of life, and increasing the likelihood of illness and even death (Corica et al., 2015; Ormsbee et al., 2014).

Ilich et al., (2014) outlined the connection among muscle, fat, and bone. As one ages, alterations in body composition take place due to interplay between various processes, resulting in a decline in bone and muscle mass, and an increase in fatty tissue. OSO is theorised to be caused by the age-related redistribution of fat which infiltrates bone and muscle (Ormsbee et al., 2014). Generally, the cells that form bone, muscle, and fat differentiate at the same time, making it possible for the normal growth of tissue. However, in OSO, the differentiation patterns are impaired, fat production becomes more prominent, resulting in fat entering the bone and muscle (Ilich et al., 2014). This fat infiltration is a characteristic of sarcopenia and osteoporosis (al Saedi et al., 2019; Hardouin et al., 2016). Studies have found that there is a connection between having an abundance of fat in the bone marrow and having reduced bone strength and susceptibility to osteoporosis (Hardouin et al., 2016). Adipocytes in marrow adipose tissue produce adipocytokines and fatty acids that are detrimental to nearby cells, decreasing bone formation and increasing bone resorption (Singh et al., 2018). Cell malfunction can also be caused by fatty deposits within the muscle fibres (Schaap et al., 2013). In 2013, Cooper et al., proposed that heightened levels of pro-inflammatory cytokines, potentially originating from an increase in abdominal fat tissue, may be involved in the formation of OSO. Hamrick et al., (2016) proposed a potential connection between osteoporosis, sarcopenia and obesity, which involves age-associated fat accumulation in bone and muscle. For example, in the bones, fat build-up happens in the marrow spaces of long bones, and this is directly associated with low estrogen levels and drugs that incorporate glucocorticoids. The cause of the build-up of fat in and around muscle cells is still not understood, however, there are indications that myosteatosis may be linked to an inactive lifestyle, a disruption in leptin communication, and the use of glucocorticoid drugs (Correa-de-Araujo et al., 2020). Studies have also discovered a direct relationship between fat in bones and skeletal muscle and low muscle strength, decreased insulin sensitivity and higher mortality in elderly people (Hamrick et al., 2016).

It is safe to say that individuals who concurrently have all three of the disorders can anticipate worse clinical outcomes than people with just one of the conditions. For example, sarcopenia is linked with dyslipidaemia and insulin resistance (IR), and the condition can be exacerbated if obesity and osteoporosis are also present (Kalinkovich & Livshits, 2017). It has been suggested that a primary cause of IR may be caused by the build-up of lipid metabolic by-products such as diacylglycerol and ceramides in myocytes (Consitt et al., 2009). Furthermore, research revealed that IR is associated with a decrease in the breakdown of fatty acids in the mitochondria in cases of obesity (Hafizi Abu Bakar et al., 2015; Dela & Helge, 2013) and in aging (Hepple, 2016; Romanello & Sandri, 2016; Carter et al., 2015; Leduc-Gaudet et al., 2015). In addition, IR can be caused by high amounts of oxidative stress which are a result of lipotoxicity and dysfunctional mitochondria.

Despite the absence of a study on a large scale, 32 of 258 postmenopausal women, or 12%, were identified with OSO in the research conducted by Ilich, Inglis, Kelly, and McGee (2015). The study found that there is a strong correlation between OSO and functional disability; including weakened handgrip, slow regular and rapid walking pace, and reduced balance capacity (Ilich et al., 2015). Hong et al., (2015) discovered that Chinese men with vertebral fractures, hip fractures and ankle fractures had a much higher prevalence of OSO than the non-fractured group and women with ankle fracture exhibited a similar pattern, suggesting a strong link between osteoporosis, sarcopenia, and obesity (Hong et al., 2015). In a study that included more than 500 overweight and obese women of various ages, Inglis, et al., (2013) revealed 25% of them were diagnosed with OSO in a subsequent analysis (Inglis, Panton, Ormsbee, Kelly, & Ilich, 2013). It was also interesting to discover that OSO is not only found in elderly people. Research that involved more than 2,500 young adults aged 18 to 21 found overweight/obese individuals had poorer body composition consisting of less muscle and bone and higher pro-inflammatory markers when compared with those that have a normal body weight, indicating the presence of OSO (Stefanaki et al., 2016). Perhaps, taking action sooner rather than later is necessary to stop the condition from appearing later in life.

So far, it has been suggested that the cause of OSO could be a lack of proper nutrition and/or not enough exercise (Kelly et al., 2019a). It's a Catch-22 with regards to physical inactivity: as bone and muscle deteriorate, it's harder to remain active, thus creating a cycle of degeneration, weight gain, and further inactivity (Ormsbee et al., 2014). Consequently, being overweight causes a build-up of pro-inflammatory cytokines which affects the body's musculoskeletal abilities (Issa & Griffin, 2012; Meyer et al., 2011). A lack of physical activity could be a factor in the decrease in bone and muscle mass. It appears that both an inadequate diet (Ormsbee et al., 2014) and a lack of exercise (Li & Heber, 2012) could be contributing to osteoporosis-related issues, which can lead to reduced mobility and a lower quality of life.

Research has also indicated that vitamin D could be a contributing factor to OSO in addition to an unhealthy diet and lack of physical activity (Bruyère et al., 2017). People who are overweight usually have low levels of 25(OH)D, which causes an increase in parathyroid hormones, which can lead to the breakdown of bones (Earthman et al., 2012). A lack of vitamin D has also been linked to an inability to absorb calcium, alterations in bone structure and a decrease in bone density (Sadat-Ali et al., 2011). Research conducted by Roth et al., (2004) has demonstrated a strong relationship between particular vitamin D receptor variations and diminished muscular mass and performance in older people, indicating that vitamin D is associated with sarcopenia (Roth et al., 2004). Research conducted on human subjects also found that vitamin D deficiency correlates with weak muscles and poor performance (Visser et al., 2003) as well as a heightened chance of falling (Snijder et al., 2006). Figure 1 shows the pathogenic hypothesis of OSO, which described a possible interrelationship between bone, muscle, and adipose tissue.

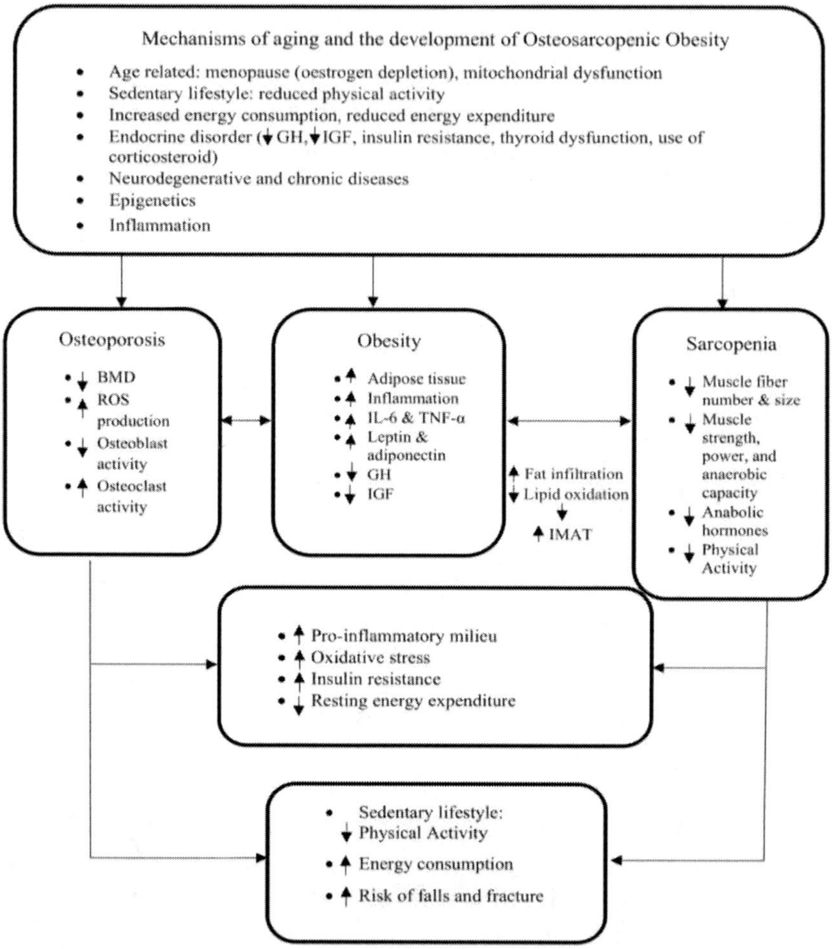

Figure 1. The pathogenic hypothesis of OSO. Hypothesised inter-relationship between bone, muscle and adipose tissue. IMAT = intramuscular adipose tissue; GH = growth hormone; IGF = insulin-like growth factor I; ROS = reactive oxygen species, BMD = bone mineral density. Adapted and modified from (Kelly et al., 2019b; Zamboni et al., 2008, Ezzat-Zadeh et al., 2017, Roubenoff & Hughes, 2000).

The Impact of Nutrition on the Development and Progression of Osteosarcopenic Obesity

Osteosarcopenic obesity (OSO) is a rapidly emerging public health challenge, with an estimated prevalence of up to 20 % among adults aged 50 and above

(Ilich et al., 2020, Kelly et al., 2019) Although the pathogenesis of OSO is not fully understood, there is a growing body of evidence suggesting that nutrition plays an important role in its development and progression (Ilich et al., 2020). This part of the Subtopic 3 discusses the impact of nutrition on the development and progression of OSO, and how different dietary patterns, macronutrient composition and micronutrient deficiencies may affect the development and progression of OSO.

Dietary Patterns

An effective technique to gauge how well people follow dietary advice and comprehend the influence of diet on health outcomes is to examine general dietary patterns. Instead of only focusing on the individual nutrients in a single meal, this method allows for the evaluation of the interaction and cumulative impacts of the complete diet. Recent studies have shown that dietary habits have a significant impact on the onset and progression of OSO (Ilich et al., 2020; Kelly et al., 2019a). There is evidence that suggests an increased risk of OSO is linked to a diet heavy in processed and calorie-dense foods. Saturated fat, trans fats, and refined carbohydrates are frequently found in processed and energy-dense meals, which can hasten the onset of obesity (Kim et al., 2017, Kelly et al., 2019a). Conversely, a diet rich in plant foods, such as fruits, vegetables, and legumes, has been associated with a reduced risk of OSO (Kim et al., 2017). Moreover, a Mediterranean-style diet, which is high in monounsaturated fats, whole grains, and low-fat dairy products, has been shown to be associated with a lower risk of OSO (Ramadas et al., 2022). Therefore, incorporating a Mediterranean-style diet into daily eating habits may help to reduce the risk of OSO and improve overall health and well-being.

Macronutrient Composition

Studies have also found that macronutrient composition plays a role in the development and progression of OSO. Diets high in saturated fat, trans fats and refined carbohydrates have been associated with an increased risk of OSO (Kim et al., 2017). In contrast, diets higher in monounsaturated fats, such as those found in nuts, seeds and fish, have been associated with a reduced risk of OSO (Ilich et al., 2020). Switching to complex carbohydrates such as fruits, vegetables, and whole grains can provide more dietary fibre, regulate blood sugar better, and prevent severe rises in serum insulin levels that could be detrimental to health (Kelly et al., 2017). There is no specific recommendation for total fat intake, but it is suggested that increasing the intake of EPA, DHA (n-3 polyunsaturated fatty acids) and alpha-linolenic acid to more than 1 g per day may be beneficial (Nasabian et al., 2017). Additionally, higher intakes of protein, particularly from animal sources, have been linked to a reduced risk of OSO (Ilich et al., 2020).

Dietary protein is anabolic in muscle tissue. However, it is important to be cautious because higher protein intakes may be detrimental to bone by increasing excretion of Ca (Barzel & Massey, 1998). Barzel and Massey (1998) found that because of their high acidogenic composition, diets high in acid-ash proteins produce excessive calcium loss. However, a high protein diet that also contains exogenous alkali buffers, such as chemical salts or fruits and vegetables, leads to less acid urine, decreased net acid excretion, decreased ammonium and titratable acid excretion, and decreased calciuria, halted bone resorption. Therefore, it is best to consume protein-rich foods with alkali-rich foods or supplements.

Micronutrients

Finally, micronutrient deficiencies have been found to be linked to an increased risk of OSO (Kelly et al., 2016). Low intakes of calcium, vitamin D and potassium have been associated with an increased risk of OSO, while higher intakes of these micronutrients have been associated with a reduced risk (Ilich, 2021). The minerals and vitamins most closely linked to OSO and its components are calcium (Ca), Magnesium (Mg), Phosphorus (P), Potassium (K), Sodium (Na), vitamin D, and vitamin K (Ilich, 2021). Research has found that the intake of all these minerals (except P and Na) and vitamins is lower or marginal when compared to the official recommendations, worldwide (O'Connor et al., 2020). This is especially true for vitamin D, due to its scarcity in food. To overcome this, some improvements could be achieved with the use of supplements (although uncontrolled supplementation is not recommended) or with the use of home-delivered or congregate meals in community-dwelling older adults.

In conclusion, nutrition plays an important role in the development and progression of OSO. Adherence to a healthy dietary pattern, such as a Mediterranean-style diet, and adequate intake of macronutrients and micronutrients, are important for reducing the risk of OSO (Kim et al., 2017). Therefore, it is important for clinicians to educate patients about the importance of a balanced and nutritious diet to reduce the risk of OSO, and its associated health complications.

The Role of Physical Activity in the Management of Osteosarcopenic Obesity

There are currently no clinical studies that have specifically examined treatment approaches for individuals with osteosarcopenic obesity (OSO) (Bauer et al., 2019). It is believed that the components of OSO, such as low muscle mass and low bone density, may be related to a sedentary lifestyle and a lack of regular physical activity, among other factors (dos Santos & Gobbo, 2020). Physical activity plays a crucial role in the management of OSO, as it can help to improve body composition, muscle strength, and bone density, as well as overall health and wellbeing (Yang et al., 2022).

Different types of physical activity can have different effects on the body. Aerobic exercise, such as walking, running, cycling, or swimming, can help to improve cardiovascular fitness and burn calories, which can lead to weight loss and a reduction in body fat (Ormsbee et al., 2014). Resistance exercise, such as weightlifting or bodyweight exercises, can help to build and maintain muscle mass and strength, as well as improve bone density (Yang et al., 2022, Cunha et al., 2018). Flexibility exercises, such as yoga or stretching, can help to improve mobility and reduce the risk of injury (Yang et al., 2022, Kelly et al., 2019b).

The specific effects of physical activity on body composition, muscle strength, and bone density will depend on the intensity, duration, and frequency of the activity, as well as the individual's age, gender, and overall health. In general, engaging in a combination of aerobic, resistance, and flexibility exercises is recommended for the management of OSO (Kelly et al., 2019a).

It is important to consult with a healthcare provider or a certified exercise professional before starting a new physical activity programme, particularly if a person has any underlying health conditions or has been inactive for an extended period. The right physical activity programme can help to improve body composition, muscle strength, and bone density, as well as overall health and wellbeing in persons with OSO (Kelly et al., 2019a). Expert guidelines recommend a varied exercise programme for individuals with OSO, as it is a complex condition. In certain cases, whole body vibration or electrical muscle stimulation may be used as alternatives to traditional resistance training or other exercises. The overall goal of these exercise interventions is to preserve bone density, increase muscle strength, reduce body fat, particularly abdominal fat, improve balance and prevent falls, and enhance quality of life.

The Impact of Psychosocial Factors on the Development, Progression and Management of Osteosarcopenic Obesity

Osteosarcopenic obesity (OSO) can develop and grow as a result of psychological variables such as stress, depression, anxiety, and a negative body image that can influence a person's eating and exercise habits (Brennan-Olsen et al., 2022; Sarwer & Polonsky, 2016). Social elements that might affect behaviour and contribute to the onset and course of the illness include social support, social norms, and resource availability (Sarwer & Polonsky, 2016). Environmental elements can also influence a person's behaviours and contribute to the onset and progression of OSO. These elements include the availability and accessibility of good dietary selections and chances for physical activity (Sallis & Glanz, 2009). Psychosocial elements may also have an impact on a person's capacity to follow a treatment plan and maintain a healthy lifestyle in terms of management and therapy. For instance, stress, depression, and anxiety can make it more challenging for someone to adopt and sustain healthy behaviour changes, but access to resources and social support can help with these adjustments (Sarwer & Polonsky, 2016; Yuenyongchaiwat & Boonsinsukh, 2020). Therefore, managing and treating OSO may need addressing and resolving these psychological variables.

It is important to consult with a healthcare provider or a mental health professional if experiencing any psychological or social difficulties that may be affecting the ability to manage and treat OSO. Healthcare providers or a mental health professional can provide support and guidance to help overcome these challenges and adopt healthy behaviours to manage and treat the condition.

Genetic Predisposition of Osteosarcopenic Obesity

Recent study indicates that genetic predisposition may potentially play a role in the development of OSO, in addition to a few environmental and lifestyle variables (Kirk et al., 2019, Yoshimura et al., 2017). The term "genetic predisposition" refers to inherited genetic differences that raise a person's risk of inheriting a certain characteristics or ailments. Genetic factors may have a role in the development of OSO through their impact on bone density, muscular mass, and control of body weight (Kirk et al., 2019). The existence of specific genetic variations, or alleles, in a person's genome can be one of the main genetic variables that might affect their risk of having OSO. According to studies, sarcopenia and osteoporosis share a substantial amount of the hereditary variables that lead to the development of both diseases. It is believed that 60 to70% of the risk for these disorders are hereditary (Urano & Inoue, 2015) (Karasik & Kiel, 2008). Both muscle and bone tissue are impacted in a variety of ways by these common genetic variables. The same type of cell known as a mesenchymal precursor gives rise to osteogenic and myogenic cells, which are responsible for generating bone and muscle tissue, respectively. This might help to explain why young monozygotic twins have a high genetic link between their bone and muscle mass (Bogl et al., 2011). According to research, this genetic association is between 30 and 45 percent for both proximal and distal regions in the body.

Numerous genetic variations in people have been shown to be linked to a higher risk of osteoporosis. Variants in genes like type I collagen alpha 1 chain (*COL1A1)*, which codes for collagen, a protein necessary for maintaining the strength and shape of bones, are among these variations (Ralston & Uitterlinden, 2010). There are also other genetic variations in the genes low-density lipoprotein receptor-related protein 5 *(LRP5)* and estrogen receptor 1 (*ESR1)* that have been associated with an increased risk of osteoporosis (Ralston & Uitterlinden, 2010). Moreover, there are genetic variations connected to an increased risk of obesity and sarcopenia in addition to those that are directly linked to osteoporosis. Such as, it has been demonstrated that changes in the FTO alpha-ketoglutarate dependent dioxygenase (*FTO)* gene are linked to a higher risk of obesity (Heffernan et al., 2017), while variants in the alpha-actinin 3 *(ACTN3)* gene have been linked to a higher risk of sarcopenia and osteoporosis (Cho et al., 2017).

Interestingly, the sterol regulatory element binding transcription factor 1 (*SREBF1*), which functions in fat metabolism and is expressed in cells that form both muscle and bone tissue, has a substantial effect on both lean mass and bone mineral density, according to a recent study that analysed genetic data from over 10,000 people. This implies that *SREBF1* may be an important regulator of bone and muscle homeostasis (Medina-Gomez et al., 2017). There are also several other genetic variations that have been identified as being associated with osteosarcopenia, which is the simultaneous loss of bone and muscle mass. These include variations in the genes glycine-N-acyltransferase (*GLYAT*), methyltransferase like 21C (*METTL21C*), myostatin, *ACTN3*, peroxisome proliferator-activated receptor-gamma coactivator 1 alpha (*PGC-1alpha*), and myocyte enhancer factor 2C (*MEF-2C*) (Hirschfeld et al., 2017). These genetic variations may influence the balance and stability of muscle and bone tissue in the body.

Another factor that can contribute to the genetic predisposition of OSO is the presence of certain inherited genetic syndromes. These syndromes are caused by mutations in specific genes, and they can lead to a variety of health problems, including osteoporosis, obesity, and sarcopenia. For example, individuals with Prader-Willi syndrome, which is caused by a mutation in the gene that codes for the hormone leptin, are at an increased risk of developing obesity and osteoporosis (Irizarry et al., 2016). Similarly, individuals with Down syndrome, which is caused by a mutation in the chromosome that carries the gene for amyloid precursor protein, are at an increased risk of developing osteoporosis (Carfì et al., 2017) and sarcopenia (Coelho-Junior et al., 2019). Researchers have been able to discover how several epigenetic alterations, such the loss of heterochromatin and core histone proteins, genomic instability, DNA methylation and altered RNA expression, contribute to cellular senescence through the study of model organisms (Pal & Tyler, 2016). The biology of muscle and bone tissue is also influenced by these epigenetic variables, which show the impact of both heredity and environment on cells (Picca et al., 2018).

In addition to genetic variations and inherited genetic disorders, hormonal variables can also affect the chance of developing OSO. For example, low testosterone levels have been connected to a higher risk of sarcopenia, whilst high cortisol levels have been linked to a higher risk of obesity (Diago-Galmés et al., 2021).

It is challenging to predict with confidence who would develop OSO due to the intricate and multidimensional character of the genetic predisposition. Understanding the numerous genetic and environmental variables that might affect a person's risk, however, can assist to identify individuals who may be at a higher risk and enable the successful implementation of early intervention and preventive programmes. It is crucial to understand that these genetic variations do not always increase a person's chance of having OSO. Most of the recent research on the function of epigenetic processes in the development of muscle, bone, and fat has concentrated on examining these tissues independently. It is not yet clear whether epigenetic mechanisms play a role in the development of OSO, or whether they could be used as reliable biomarkers for this syndrome. However, this is an area of active investigation. Genetic factors are just one piece of the puzzle, and other factors such as diet, physical activity, and lifestyle habits can also contribute to the development of these conditions.

In conclusion, genetic predisposition may play a role in the development of OSO. Understanding the genetic basis of this condition may help to identify individuals at a higher risk and may allow for targeted interventions to prevent or delay the onset of OSO.

The Effectiveness of Interventions for Managing and Treating Osteosarcopenic Obesity

There are several evidence-based strategies that can be effective for managing and treating osteosarcopenic obesity (OSO) (JafariNasabian, 2018). These include:

- *Diet and nutrition*: Muscle mass, bone density, and general health may all be enhanced by a nutritious diet high in nutrients like protein, calcium, and vitamin D. A balanced diet is essential, consisting of a range of fruits, vegetables, whole grains, lean meats, and healthy fats. (JafariNasabian, 2018).
- *Physical activity*: Regular physical activity can assist to enhance body composition, muscular strength, bone density, and general health and wellness. This includes aerobic exercise, resistance training, and flexibility exercises. Before beginning a new physical activity programme, it is crucial to speak with a healthcare physician or a qualified exercise specialist (JafariNasabian, 2018).
- *Medications*: Some medications, such as bisphosphonates, can help to improve bone density and reduce the risk of fractures in individuals with osteoporosis (Tu et al., 2018). Other medications, such as testosterone or estrogen, may be recommended for individuals with low hormone levels that may be contributing to muscle loss and

osteoporosis (Tu et al., 2018). Pharmacological osteoporosis treatments can also be used to reduce bone marrow fat (Paccou et al., 2019). In a small study of 16 subjects, the impact of hormone replacement therapy (HRT) on body composition in postmenopausal women was compared to a placebo. During the 12-week intervention, HRT not only prevented the loss of lean body mass that occurred with the placebo, but also increased it. Additionally, HRT has also been found to be able to reduce abdominal fat mass while total body weight remained unchanged. This finding is in addition to the already well-known positive effect of HRT on bone density (Sørensen et al., 2001). Nevertheless, it is important to discuss the potential risks and benefits of these medications with a healthcare provider.

- *Lifestyle changes*: Making healthy lifestyle adjustments, such as giving up smoking, drinking less alcohol, and getting enough sleep, can help to enhance general health and lower the risk of OSO-related problems (Petroni et al., 2019).

To find the best management and treatment options for OSO, it is crucial to speak with a healthcare professional. They can help you develop healthy behaviours and adhere to a treatment plan that is catered to your requirements and objectives by offering advice and assistance.

Knowledge Gaps in Osteosarcopenic Obesity

Researchers are actively attempting to bridge a number of knowledge gaps in the area of osteosarcopenic obesity (OSO). A few of these are:

1. Understanding the underlying mechanisms of OSO and how it affects general health.
2. Determining efficient methods for treating and managing OSO.
3. Investigating the long-term effects of OSO on metabolic, cardiovascular, and musculoskeletal health
4. Investigating how hormones, diet, and lifestyle affect the onset and development of OSO.
5. Investigating the genetic and environmental components that contribute to OSO.

6. Understanding the association between OSO and other chronic diseases.
7. How OSO is affected by concomitant conditions like diabetes and hypertension.
8. The effect of age, gender, and other demographic factors on the development of OSO.
9. The correlation of the gut microbiome to OSO and how it interacts with the immune system.
10. The effect of long-term exposure to environmental toxins on the development of OSO.
11. The effects of psychosocial factors on the development of OSO.
12. The effects of lifestyle modifications and medications on the prevention and treatment of OSO.
13. The economic impact of OSO on health systems and society.
14. Determining the most effective interventions for reducing the prevalence and/or severity of OSO.

Conclusion

The aetiology of osteosarcopenic obesity (OSO) syndrome and the technical and diagnostic challenges that hinder an accurate assessment of its prevalence were explored in this chapter. Additionally, published studies, particularly those with a nutritional focus, were reviewed and updated. It has been determined that a range of factors, including aging, chronic inflammation, stress, immobility, poor nutrition, and certain chronic diseases, contribute to the development of OSO, leading to functional impairment, an increased risk of falls and fractures, metabolic dysfunction, decreased quality of life, increased morbidity, and potentially even mortality. The health concerns associated with OSO are more than the sum of its parts. The prevention and treatment of OSO depends heavily on nutrition, and healthy lifestyle. The roles of calcium, magnesium, potassium, phosphorus, salt, and vitamins D and K in each of the three aspects of OSO have also been discussed. It is important to highlight that it is not advised to supplement any of these nutrients without proper monitoring and control. OSO tends to get worse with time, and there aren't any well-established ways to stop it right now. However, OSO can be managed using the therapeutic methods and philosophies discussed in this chapter.

References

al Saedi, A., Hassan, E. B., & Duque, G. (2019). The diagnostic role of fat in osteosarcopenia. *Journal of Laboratory and Precision Medicine*, *4*, 7–7. https://doi.org/10.21037/jlpm.2019.02.01.

Barnsley, J., Buckland, G., Chan, P. E., Ong, A., Ramos, A. S., Baxter, M., Laskou, F., Dennison, E. M., Cooper, C., & Patel, H. P. (2021). Pathophysiology and treatment of osteoporosis: challenges for clinical practice in older people. *Aging Clinical and Experimental Research*, *33*(4), 759–773. https://doi.org/10.1007/s40520-021-01817-y.

Barzel, U. S., & Massey, L. K. (1998). Excess Dietary Protein Can Adversely Affect Bone. *The Journal of Nutrition*, *128*(6), 1051–1053. https://doi.org/10.1093/jn/128.6.1051.

Bauer, J. M., Cruz-Jentoft, A. J., Fielding, R. A., Kanis, J. A., Reginster, J.-Y., Bruyère, O., Cesari, M., Chapurlat, R., Al-Daghri, N., Dennison, E., Kaufman, J.-M., Landi, F., Laslop, A., Locquet, M., Maggi, S., McCloskey, E., Perna, S., Rizzoli, R., Rolland, Y., Rondanelli, M., Szulc, P., Vellas, B., Vlaskovska, M. & Cooper, C. (2019). Is There Enough Evidence for Osteosarcopenic Obesity as a Distinct Entity? A Critical Literature Review. *Calcified Tissue International*, *105*(2), 109–124. https://doi.org/10.1007/s00223-019-00561-w.

Bogl, L. H., Latvala, A., Kaprio, J., Sovijärvi, O., Rissanen, A., & Pietiläinen, K. H. (2011). An investigation into the relationship between soft tissue body composition and bone mineral density in a young adult twin sample. *Journal of Bone and Mineral Research*, *26*(1), 79–87. https://doi.org/10.1002/jbmr.192.

Bredella, M. A., Torriani, M., Ghomi, R. H., Thomas, B. J., Brick, D. J., Gerweck, A. v., Harrington, L. M., Breggia, A., Rosen, C. J., & Miller, K. K. (2011). Determinants of bone mineral density in obese premenopausal women. *Bone*, *48*(4), 748–754. https://doi.org/10.1016/j.bone.2010.12.011.

Bruyère, O., Cavalier, E., & Reginster, J.-Y. (2017). Vitamin D and osteosarcopenia. *Current Opinion in Clinical Nutrition & Metabolic Care*, *20*(6), 498–503. https://doi.org/10.1097/MCO.0000000000000411.

Carfì, A., Liperoti, R., Fusco, D., Giovannini, S., Brandi, V., Vetrano, D. L., Meloni, E., Mascia, D., Villani, E. R., Manes Gravina, E., Bernabei, R., & Onder, G. (2017). Bone mineral density in adults with Down syndrome. *Osteoporosis International*, *28*(10), 2929–2934. https://doi.org/10.1007/s00198-017-4133-x.

Carter, H. N., Chen, C. C. W., & Hood, D. A. (2015). Mitochondria, Muscle Health, and Exercise with Advancing Age. *Physiology*, *30*(3), 208–223. https://doi.org/10.1152/physiol.00039.2014.

Cho, J., Lee, I., & Kang, H. (2017). ACTN3 Gene and Susceptibility to Sarcopenia and Osteoporotic Status in Older Korean Adults. *BioMed Research International*, *2017*, 1–8. https://doi.org/10.1155/2017/4239648.

Clegg, D. J. (2012). Minireview: The Year in Review of Estrogen Regulation of Metabolism. *Molecular Endocrinology*, *26*(12), 1957–1960. https://doi.org/10.1210/me.2012-1284.

Coelho-Junior, H. J., Villani, E. R., Calvani, R., Carfì, A., Picca, A., Landi, F., Bernabei, R., Onder, G., & Marzetti, E. (2019). Sarcopenia-related parameters in adults with

Down syndrome: A cross-sectional exploratory study. *Experimental Gerontology, 119*, 93–99. https://doi.org/10.1016/j.exger.2019.01.028.

Consitt, L. A., Bell, J. A., & Houmard, J. A. (2009). Intramuscular lipid metabolism, insulin action, and obesity. *IUBMB Life, 61*(1), 47–55. https://doi.org/10.1002/iub.142.

Cooper, C., Fielding, R., Visser, M., van Loon, L. J., Rolland, Y., Orwoll, E., Reid, K., Boonen, S., Dere, W., Epstein, S., Mitlak, B., Tsouderos, Y., Sayer, A. A., Rizzoli, R., Reginster, J. Y., & Kanis, J. A. (2013). Tools in the Assessment of Sarcopenia. *Calcified Tissue International, 93*(3), 201–210. https://doi.org/10.1007/s00223-013-9757-z.

Corica, F., Bianchi, G., Corsonello, A., Mazzella, N., Lattanzio, F., & Marchesini, G. (2015). Obesity in the Context of Aging: Quality of Life Considerations. *PharmacoEconomics, 33*(7), 655–672. https://doi.org/10.1007/s40273-014-0237-8.

Correa-de-Araujo, R., Addison, O., Miljkovic, I., Goodpaster, B. H., Bergman, B. C., Clark, R. v., Elena, J. W., Esser, K. A., Ferrucci, L., Harris-Love, M. O., Kritchevsky, S. B., Lorbergs, A., Shepherd, J. A., Shulman, G. I., & Rosen, C. J. (2020). Myosteatosis in the Context of Skeletal Muscle Function Deficit: An Interdisciplinary Workshop at the National Institute on Aging. *Frontiers in Physiology, 11*. https://doi.org/10.3389/fphys.2020.00963.

Cunha, P. M., Ribeiro, A. S., Tomeleri, C. M., Schoenfeld, B. J., Silva, A. M., Souza, M. F., Nascimento, M. A., Sardinha, L. B., & Cyrino, E. S. (2018). The effects of resistance training volume on osteosarcopenic obesity in older women. *Journal of Sports Sciences, 36*(14), 1564–1571. https://doi.org/10.1080/02640414.2017.1403413.

de Frel, D. L., Atsma, D. E., Pijl, H., Seidell, J. C., Leenen, P. J. M., Dik, W. A., & van Rossum, E. F. C. (2020). The Impact of Obesity and Lifestyle on the Immune System and Susceptibility to Infections Such as COVID-19. *Frontiers in Nutrition, 7*. https://doi.org/10.3389/fnut.2020.597600.

Dela, F., & Helge, J. W. (2013). Insulin resistance and mitochondrial function in skeletal muscle. *The International Journal of Biochemistry & Cell Biology, 45*(1), 11–15. https://doi.org/10.1016/j.biocel.2012.09.019.

Diago-Galmés, A., Guillamón-Escudero, C., Tenías-Burillo, J. M., Soriano, J. M., & Fernández-Garrido, J. (2021). Salivary Testosterone and Cortisol as Biomarkers for the Diagnosis of Sarcopenia and Sarcopenic Obesity in Community-Dwelling Older Adults. *Biology, 10*(2), 93. https://doi.org/10.3390/biology10020093.

dos Santos, V. R., & Gobbo, L. A. (2020). Physical activity is associated with functional capacity of older women with osteosarcopenic obesity: 24-month prospective study. *European Journal of Clinical Nutrition, 74*(6), 912–919. https://doi.org/10.1038/s41430-019-0505-y.

Earthman, C. P., Beckman, L. M., Masodkar, K., & Sibley, S. D. (2012). The link between obesity and low circulating 25-hydroxyvitamin D concentrations: considerations and implications. *International Journal of Obesity, 36*(3), 387–396. https://doi.org/10.1038/ijo.2011.119.

Ezzat-Zadeh, Z., Kim, J.-S., Chase, P. B., & Arjmandi, B. H. (2017a). The Cooccurrence of Obesity, Osteoporosis, and Sarcopenia in the Ovariectomized Rat: A Study for

Modeling Osteosarcopenic Obesity in Rodents. *Journal of Aging Research*, *2017*, 1–11. https://doi.org/10.1155/2017/1454103.

Ezzat-Zadeh, Z., Kim, J.-S., Chase, P. B., & Arjmandi, B. H. (2017b). The Cooccurrence of Obesity, Osteoporosis, and Sarcopenia in the Ovariectomized Rat: A Study for Modeling Osteosarcopenic Obesity in Rodents. *Journal of Aging Research*, *2017*, 1–11. https://doi.org/10.1155/2017/1454103.

Gilsanz, V., Chalfant, J., Mo, A. O., Lee, D. C., Dorey, F. J., & Mittelman, S. D. (2009). Reciprocal Relations of Subcutaneous and Visceral Fat to Bone Structure and Strength. *The Journal of Clinical Endocrinology & Metabolism*, *94*(9), 3387–3393. https://doi.org/10.1210/jc.2008-2422.

Greco, E. A., Fornari, R., Rossi, F., Santiemma, V., Prossomariti, G., Annoscia, C., Aversa, A., Brama, M., Marini, M., Donini, L. M., Spera, G., Lenzi, A., Lubrano, C., & Migliaccio, S. (2010). Is obesity protective for osteoporosis? Evaluation of bone mineral density in individuals with high body mass index. *International Journal of Clinical Practice*, *64*(6), 817–820. https://doi.org/10.1111/j.1742-1241.2009.02301.x.

Hafizi Abu Bakar, M., Kian Kai, C., Wan Hassan, W. N., Sarmidi, M. R., Yaakob, H., & Zaman Huri, H. (2015). Mitochondrial dysfunction as a central event for mechanisms underlying insulin resistance: the roles of long chain fatty acids. *Diabetes/Metabolism Research and Reviews*, *31*(5), 453–475. https://doi.org/10.1002/dmrr.2601.

Hamrick, M. W., McGee-Lawrence, M. E., & Frechette, D. M. (2016). Fatty Infiltration of Skeletal Muscle: Mechanisms and Comparisons with Bone Marrow Adiposity. *Frontiers in Endocrinology*, *7*. https://doi.org/10.3389/fendo.2016.00069.

Hardouin, P., Rharass, T., & Lucas, S. (2016). Bone Marrow Adipose Tissue: To Be or Not To Be a Typical Adipose Tissue? *Frontiers in Endocrinology*, *7*. https://doi.org/10.3389/fendo.2016.00085.

He, C., He, W., Hou, J., Chen, K., Huang, M., Yang, M., Luo, X., & Li, C. (2020). Bone and Muscle Crosstalk in Aging. *Frontiers in Cell and Developmental Biology*, *8*. https://doi.org/10.3389/fcell.2020.585644.

Heffernan, S. M., Stebbings, G. K., Kilduff, L. P., Erskine, R. M., Day, S. H., Morse, C. I., McPhee, J. S., Cook, C. J., Vance, B., Ribbans, W. J., Raleigh, S. M., Roberts, C., Bennett, M. A., Wang, G., Collins, M., Pitsiladis, Y. P., & Williams, A. G. (2017). Fat mass and obesity associated (FTO) gene influences skeletal muscle phenotypes in non-resistance trained males and elite rugby playing position. *BMC Genetics*, *18*(1), 4. https://doi.org/10.1186/s12863-017-0470-1.

Hepple, R. T. (2016). Impact of aging on mitochondrial function in cardiac and skeletal muscle. *Free Radical Biology and Medicine*, *98*, 177–186. https://doi.org/10.1016/j.freeradbiomed.2016.03.017.

Hirschfeld, H. P., Kinsella, R., & Duque, G. (2017). Osteosarcopenia: where bone, muscle, and fat collide. *Osteoporosis International*, *28*(10), 2781–2790. https://doi.org/10.1007/s00198-017-4151-8.

Hong, W., Cheng, Q., Zhu, X., Zhu, H., Li, H., Zhang, X., Zheng, S., Du, Y., Tang, W., Xue, S., & Ye, Z. (2015). Prevalence of Sarcopenia and Its Relationship with Sites of Fragility Fractures in Elderly Chinese Men and Women. *PLOS ONE*, *10*(9), e0138102. https://doi.org/10.1371/journal.pone.0138102.

Hou, J., He, C., He, W., Yang, M., Luo, X., & Li, C. (2020). Obesity and Bone Health: A Complex Link. *Frontiers in Cell and Developmental Biology*, *8*. https://doi.org/10.3389/fcell.2020.600181.

Ilich, J. Z. (2021). Osteosarcopenic adiposity syndrome update and the role of associated minerals and vitamins. *Proceedings of the Nutrition Society*, *80*(3), 344–355. https://doi.org/10.1017/S0029665121000586.

Ilich, J. Z., Gilman, J. C., Cvijetic, S., & Boschiero, D. (2020). Chronic Stress Contributes to Osteosarcopenic Adiposity via Inflammation and Immune Modulation: The Case for More Precise Nutritional Investigation. *Nutrients*, *12*(4), 989. https://doi.org/10.3390/nu12040989.

Ilich, J. Z., Inglis, J. E., Kelly, O. J., & McGee, D. L. (2015). Osteosarcopenic obesity is associated with reduced handgrip strength, walking abilities, and balance in postmenopausal women. *Osteoporosis International*, *26*(11), 2587–2595. https://doi.org/10.1007/s00198-015-3186-y.

Ilich, J. Z., Kelly, O. J., & Inglis, J. E. (2016). Osteosarcopenic Obesity Syndrome: What Is It and How Can It Be Identified and Diagnosed? *Current Gerontology and Geriatrics Research*, *2016*, 1–7. https://doi.org/10.1155/2016/7325973.

Irizarry, K. A., Miller, M., Freemark, M., & Haqq, A. M. (2016). Prader Willi Syndrome. *Advances in Pediatrics*, *63*(1), 47–77. https://doi.org/10.1016/j.yapd.2016.04.005.

Issa, RitaI., & Griffin, TimothyM. (2012). Pathobiology of obesity and osteoarthritis: integrating biomechanics and inflammation. *Pathobiology of Aging & Age-Related Diseases*, *2*(1), 17470. https://doi.org/10.3402/pba.v2i0.17470.

J. Kelly, O., C. Gilman, J., Kim, Y., & Z. Ilich, J. (2016). Micronutrient Intake in the Etiology, Prevention and Treatment of Osteosarcopenic Obesity. *Current Aging Science*, *9*(4), 260–278. https://doi.org/10.2174/1874609809666160509122001.

Jafari Nasabian, P., Inglis, J., Kelly, O., & Ilich, J. (2017a). Osteosarcopenic obesity in women: impact, prevalence, and management challenges. *International Journal of Women's Health*, *Volume 9*, 33–42. https://doi.org/10.2147/IJWH.S106107.

Jafari Nasabian, P., Inglis, J., Kelly, O., & Ilich, J. (2017b). Osteosarcopenic obesity in women: impact, prevalence, and management challenges. *International Journal of Women's Health*, *Volume 9*, 33–42. https://doi.org/10.2147/IJWH.S106107.

Jafari Nasabian, P. (2018). How Exercise and Dietary Intervention Affect the Outcome of Osteosarcopenic Obesity Syndrome? *Journal of Functional Morphology and Kinesiology*, *3*(2), 31. https://doi.org/10.3390/jfmk3020031.

Kalinkovich, A., & Livshits, G. (2017). Sarcopenic obesity or obese sarcopenia: A cross talk between age-associated adipose tissue and skeletal muscle inflammation as a main mechanism of the pathogenesis. *Ageing Research Reviews*, *35*, 200–221. https://doi.org/10.1016/j.arr.2016.09.008.

Karasik, D., & Kiel, D. P. (2008). Genetics of the Musculoskeletal System: A Pleiotropic Approach. *Journal of Bone and Mineral Research*, *23*(6), 788–802. https://doi.org/10.1359/jbmr.080218.

Kelly, O., Gilman, J., Boschiero, D., & Ilich, J. (2019a). Osteosarcopenic Obesity: Current Knowledge, Revised Identification Criteria and Treatment Principles. *Nutrients*, *11*(4), 747. https://doi.org/10.3390/nu11040747.

Kelly, O., Gilman, J., Boschiero, D., & Ilich, J. (2019b). Osteosarcopenic Obesity: Current Knowledge, Revised Identification Criteria and Treatment Principles. *Nutrients*, *11*(4), 747. https://doi.org/10.3390/nu11040747.

Kim, J., Lee, Y., Kye, S., Chung, Y. S., Kim, J. H., Chon, D., & Lee, K. E. (2017). Diet quality and osteosarcopenic obesity in community-dwelling adults 50 years and older. *Maturitas*, *104*, 73–79. https://doi.org/10.1016/J.MATURITAS.2017.08.007.

Kim, J., Wei, Y., & Sowers, J. R. (2008). Role of Mitochondrial Dysfunction in Insulin Resistance. *Circulation Research*, *102*(4), 401–414. https://doi.org/10.1161/CIRCRESAHA.107.165472.

Kirk, B., al Saedi, A., & Duque, G. (2019). Osteosarcopenia: A case of geroscience. *AGING MEDICINE*, *2*(3), 147–156. https://doi.org/10.1002/agm2.12080.

Leduc-Gaudet, J.-P., Picard, M., Pelletier, F. S.-J., Sgarioto, N., Auger, M.-J., Vallée, J., Robitaille, R., St-Pierre, D. H., & Gouspillou, G. (2015). Mitochondrial morphology is altered in atrophied skeletal muscle of aged mice. *Oncotarget*, *6*(20), 17923–17937. https://doi.org/10.18632/oncotarget.4235.

Li, Z., & Heber, D. (2012). Sarcopenic obesity in the elderly and strategies for weight management. *Nutrition Reviews*, *70*(1), 57–64. https://doi.org/10.1111/j.1753-4887.2011.00453.x.

Lins Vieira, N. F., da Silva Nascimento, J., do Nascimento, C. Q., Barros Neto, J. A., & Oliveira Dos Santos, A. C. (2021). Association Between Bone Mineral Density and Nutritional Status, Body Composition and Bone Metabolism in Older Adults. *The Journal of Nutrition, Health & Aging*, *25*(1), 71–76. https://doi.org/10.1007/s12603-020-1452-y.

Ma, Y., Zhang, W., Han, P., Kohzuki, M., & Guo, Q. (2020). Osteosarcopenic Obesity Associated with Poor Physical Performance in the Elderly Chinese Community. *Clinical Interventions in Aging*, *Volume 15*, 1343–1352. https://doi.org/10.2147/CIA.S257739.

Medina-Gomez, C., Kemp, J. P., Dimou, N. L., Kreiner, E., Chesi, A., Zemel, B. S., Bønnelykke, K., Boer, C. G., Ahluwalia, T. S., Bisgaard, H., Evangelou, E., Heppe, D. H. M., Bonewald, L. F., Gorski, J. P., Ghanbari, M., Demissie, S., Duque, G., Maurano, M. T., Kiel, D. P., Hsu, Y. H., van der Eerden, B. C. J., Ackert-Bicknell, C., Reppe, S., Gautvik, K. M., Raastad, T., Karasik, D., van de Peppel, J., Jaddoe, V. W. V., Uitterlinden, A. G., Tobias, J. H., Grant, S. F. A., Bagos, P. G., Evans, D. M., & Rivadeneira, F. (2017). Bivariate genome-wide association meta-analysis of pediatric musculoskeletal traits reveals pleiotropic effects at the SREBF1/TOM1L2 locus. *Nature Communications*, *8*(1), 121. https://doi.org/10.1038/s41467-017-00108-3.

Messier, V., Rabasa-Lhoret, R., Barbat-Artigas, S., Elisha, B., Karelis, A. D., & Aubertin-Leheudre, M. (2011). Menopause and sarcopenia: A potential role for sex hormones. *Maturitas*, *68*(4), 331–336. https://doi.org/10.1016/j.maturitas.2011.01.014.

Meyer, M. R., Clegg, D. J., Prossnitz, E. R., & Barton, M. (2011). Obesity, insulin resistance and diabetes: sex differences and role of oestrogen receptors. *Acta Physiologica*, *203*(1), 259–269. https://doi.org/10.1111/j.1748-1716.2010.02237.x.

Migliaccio, S., Greco, E. A., Aversa, A., & Lenzi, A. (2014). Age-associated (cardio)metabolic diseases and cross-talk between adipose tissue and skeleton:

endocrine aspects. *Hormone Molecular Biology and Clinical Investigation*, *20*(1). https://doi.org/10.1515/hmbci-2014-0030.

Mo, D., Hsieh, P., Yu, H., Zhou, L., Gong, J., Xu, L., Liu, P., Chen, G., Chen, Z., & Deng, Q. (2018). Osteosarcopenic obesity and its relationship with dyslipidemia in women from different ethnic groups of China. *Archives of Osteoporosis*, *13*(1), 65. https://doi.org/10.1007/s11657-018-0481-1.

O'Connor, J.-L. P., Milledge, K. L., O'Leary, F., Cumming, R., Eberhard, J., & Hirani, V. (2020). Poor dietary intake of nutrients and food groups are associated with increased risk of periodontal disease among community-dwelling older adults: a systematic literature review. *Nutrition Reviews*, *78*(2), 175–188. https://doi.org/10.1093/nutrit/nuz035.

Ormsbee, M. J., Prado, C. M., Ilich, J. Z., Purcell, S., Siervo, M., Folsom, A., & Panton, L. (2014). Osteosarcopenic obesity: the role of bone, muscle, and fat on health. *Journal of Cachexia, Sarcopenia and Muscle*, *5*(3), 183–192. https://doi.org/10.1007/s13539-014-0146-x.

Paccou, J., Penel, G., Chauveau, C., Cortet, B., & Hardouin, P. (2019). Marrow adiposity and bone: Review of clinical implications. *Bone*, *118*, 8–15. https://doi.org/10.1016/j.bone.2018.02.008.

Pal, S., & Tyler, J. K. (2016). Epigenetics and aging. *Science Advances*, *2*(7). https://doi.org/10.1126/sciadv.1600584.

Palermo, A., Tuccinardi, D., Defeudis, G., Watanabe, M., D'Onofrio, L., Lauria Pantano, A., Napoli, N., Pozzilli, P., & Manfrini, S. (2016). BMI and BMD: The Potential Interplay between Obesity and Bone Fragility. *International Journal of Environmental Research and Public Health*, *13*(6), 544. https://doi.org/10.3390/ijerph13060544.

Pang, B. W. J., Wee, S.-L., Chen, K. K., Lau, L. K., Jabbar, K. A., Seah, W. T., Ng, D. H. M., Tan, Q. L. L., Jagadish, M. U., & Ng, T. P. (2021). Coexistence of osteoporosis, sarcopenia and obesity in community-dwelling adults – The Yishun Study. *Osteoporosis and Sarcopenia*, *7*(1), 17–23. https://doi.org/10.1016/j.afos.2020.12.002.

Qiao, D., Li, Y., Liu, X., Zhang, X., Qian, X., Zhang, H., Zhang, G., & Wang, C. (2020). Association of obesity with bone mineral density and osteoporosis in adults: a systematic review and meta-analysis. *Public Health*, *180*, 22–28. https://doi.org/10.1016/j.puhe.2019.11.001.

Qin, Y., Peng, Y., Zhao, W., Pan, J., Ksiezak-Reding, H., Cardozo, C., Wu, Y., Divieti Pajevic, P., Bonewald, L. F., Bauman, W. A., & Qin, W. (2017). Myostatin inhibits osteoblastic differentiation by suppressing osteocyte-derived exosomal microRNA-218: A novel mechanism in muscle-bone communication. *Journal of Biological Chemistry*, *292*(26), 11021–11033. https://doi.org/10.1074/jbc.M116.770941.

Ralston, S. H., & Uitterlinden, A. G. (2010). Genetics of Osteoporosis. *Endocrine Reviews*, *31*(5), 629–662. https://doi.org/10.1210/er.2009-0044.

Ramadas, A., Law, H. H., Krishnamoorthy, R., Ku, J. W. S., Mohanty, P., Lim, M. Z. C., & Shyam, S. (2022). Diet Quality and Measures of Sarcopenia in Developing Economies: A Systematic Review. *Nutrients*, *14*(4), 868. https://doi.org/10.3390/nu14040868.

Romanello, V., & Sandri, M. (2016). Mitochondrial Quality Control and Muscle Mass Maintenance. *Frontiers in Physiology*, *6*. https://doi.org/10.3389/fphys.2015.00422.

Roth, S. M., Zmuda, J. M., Cauley, J. A., Shea, P. R., & Ferrell, R. E. (2004). Vitamin D Receptor Genotype Is Associated with Fat-Free Mass and Sarcopenia in Elderly Men. *The Journals of Gerontology Series A: Biological Sciences and Medical Sciences*, *59*(1), B10–B15. https://doi.org/10.1093/gerona/59.1.B10.

Roubenoff, R., & Hughes, V. A. (2000). Sarcopenia: Current Concepts. *The Journals of Gerontology Series A: Biological Sciences and Medical Sciences*, *55*(12), M716–M724. https://doi.org/10.1093/gerona/55.12.M716.

Sadat-Ali, M., al Elq, A. H., Al-Turki, H. A., Al-Mulhim, F. A., & Al-Ali, A. K. (2011). Influence of vitamin D levels on bone mineral density and osteoporosis. *Annals of Saudi Medicine*, *31*(6), 602–608. https://doi.org/10.4103/0256-4947.87097.

Schaap, L. A., Koster, A., & Visser, M. (2013). Adiposity, Muscle Mass, and Muscle Strength in Relation to Functional Decline in Older Persons. *Epidemiologic Reviews*, *35*(1), 51–65. https://doi.org/10.1093/epirev/mxs006.

Singh, L., Tyagi, S., Myers, D., & Duque, G. (2018). Good, Bad, or Ugly: The Biological Roles of Bone Marrow Fat. *Current Osteoporosis Reports*, *16*(2), 130–137. https://doi.org/10.1007/s11914-018-0427-y.

Snijder, M. B., van Schoor, N. M., Pluijm, S. M. F., van Dam, R. M., Visser, M., & Lips, P. (2006). Vitamin D Status in Relation to One-Year Risk of Recurrent Falling in Older Men and Women. *The Journal of Clinical Endocrinology & Metabolism*, *91*(8), 2980–2985. https://doi.org/10.1210/jc.2006-0510.

Sørensen, M. B., Rosenfalck, A. M., Højgaard, L., & Ottesen, B. (2001). Obesity and Sarcopenia after Menopause Are Reversed by Sex Hormone Replacement Therapy. *Obesity Research*, *9*(10), 622–626. https://doi.org/10.1038/oby.2001.81.

Sozen, T., Ozisik, L., & Calik Basaran, N. (2017). An overview and management of osteoporosis. *European Journal of Rheumatology*, *4*(1), 46–56. https://doi.org/10.5152/eurjrheum.2016.048.

Stefanaki, C., Peppa, M., Boschiero, D., & Chrousos, G. P. (2016). Healthy overweight/obese youth: early osteosarcopenic obesity features. *European Journal of Clinical Investigation*, *46*(9), 767–778. https://doi.org/10.1111/eci.12659.

Szlejf, C., Parra-Rodríguez, L., & Rosas-Carrasco, O. (2017). Osteosarcopenic Obesity: Prevalence and Relation With Frailty and Physical Performance in Middle-Aged and Older Women. *Journal of the American Medical Directors Association*, *18*(8), 733.e1-733.e5. https://doi.org/10.1016/j.jamda.2017.02.023.

Tu, K. N., Lie, J. D., Wan, C. K. V., Cameron, M., Austel, A. G., Nguyen, J. K., Van, K., & Hyun, D. (2018). Osteoporosis: A Review of Treatment Options. *P & T : A Peer-Reviewed Journal for Formulary Management*, *43*(2), 92–104.

Urano, T., & Inoue, S. (2015). Recent genetic discoveries in osteoporosis, sarcopenia and obesity [Review]. *Endocrine Journal*, *62*(6), 475–484. https://doi.org/10.1507/endocrj.EJ15-0154.

Vaidya, R. (2014). Obesity, sarcopenia and postmenopausal osteoporosis: An interlinked triad! *Journal of Mid-Life Health*, *5*(1), 1. https://doi.org/10.4103/0976-7800.127778.

Visser, M., Deeg, D. J. H., & Lips, P. (2003). Low Vitamin D and High Parathyroid Hormone Levels as Determinants of Loss of Muscle Strength and Muscle Mass

(Sarcopenia): The Longitudinal Aging Study Amsterdam. *The Journal of Clinical Endocrinology & Metabolism*, *88*(12), 5766–5772. https://doi.org/10.1210/jc.2003-030604.

Yang, J., Ye, H., Zhu, Q., Zhang, J., Liu, Q., Xie, H., Long, Y., Huang, H., Niu, Y., Luo, Y., & Wang, M. (2022). Effects of resistance training on body composition and physical function in elderly patients with osteosarcopenic obesity: a systematic review and meta-analysis. *Archives of Osteoporosis*, *17*(1), 82. https://doi.org/10.1007/s11657-022-01120-x

Yoshimura, N., Muraki, S., Oka, H., Iidaka, T., Kodama, R., Kawaguchi, H., Nakamura, K., Tanaka, S., & Akune, T. (2017). Is osteoporosis a predictor for future sarcopenia or vice versa? Four-year observations between the second and third ROAD study surveys. *Osteoporosis International*, *28*(1), 189–199. https://doi.org/10.1007/s00198-016-3823-0.

Zamboni, M., Mazzali, G., Fantin, F., Rossi, A., & di Francesco, V. (2008). Sarcopenic obesity: A new category of obesity in the elderly. *Nutrition, Metabolism and Cardiovascular Diseases*, *18*(5), 388–395. https://doi.org/10.1016/j.numecd.2007.10.002.

Chapter 2

Fragile X Syndrome

Marjanu Hikmah Elias*

Faculty of Medicine & Health Sciences, Universiti Sains Islam Malaysia, Nilai, Negeri Sembilan, Malaysia

Abstract

Fragile X syndrome is a genetic disease that manifests as a neurodevelopmental disorder. The patients have a high number of repeated CGG codons at the 5' untranslated flanking region the Fragile X Messenger Ribonucleoprotein 1 (*FMR1*) gene, located at the extended arm of the X chromosome, which causes it to undergo a high rate of localized methylation. This leads to a high level of transcription, but the translation process is disrupted. The *FMR1* protein, known as FMRP, is a vital regulator that interacts with around 180 other proteins in various pathways. Hence, disruption in protein production will lead to developmental defects, particularly those relating to mental capabilities, with patients suffering from cognitive disabilities. Thus, fragile X syndrome is a disease inherited through the X-linked recessive pattern. This chapter discusses its clinical, molecular, and diagnostic aspects. It consists of six subtopics that include: 1) The introduction of fragile X syndrome, which highlights its clinical symptoms and prevalence in Malaysia and southeast Asia; 2) The molecular mechanism of the disease, including mutations in the *FMR1* gene and other related mechanisms that contribute to the phenotype; 3) Disease diagnosis using the gold standard and other latest methods; 4) Therapies and medical treatment; 5) Research updates; and 6) Treatment limitations and future of disease management.

---

* Corresponding Author's Email: marjanuhikmah@usim.edu.my.

In: Genetic Disorders and Rare Diseases
Editors: Shazlin Shaharudin, Hisham Atan Edinur and Nor Fazila Che Mat
ISBN: 979-8-88697-953-4

Keywords: mental retardation, DNA methylation, repeated codon, fragile X messenger ribonucleoprotein1, X-linked, chromosome

Introduction

Fragile X syndrome (FXS) is the most common sex-linked disease that impairs mental development. It occurs due to mutation of a very important gene in the X chromosome that regulates many other gene and protein functions in the human neurological system. It reportedly has a higher preponderance in males, with a ratio of 1:5,000 compared with females, which the ratio is between 1:4,000 and 8,000 (Hagerman et al., 2017). In Indonesia, FXS has been diagnosed in 1.7% to 1.9% of individuals with intellectual disability of unknown aetiology (Sihombing et al., 2021). The disease was first diagnosed in a Malaysian family in 1985 (Ten et al., 1985). However, due to the complexity of the diagnostic process, no other reports, or studies on FXS had been conducted in Malaysia. It was only in 2006 that researchers from Universiti Sains Malaysia started a population survey on FXS nationwide via cytogenetic analysis.

Interestingly, even in a developed country, the reported prevalence is much lower than actual cases, as many individuals with FXS did not receive a proper clinical diagnosis. In the United States, the estimated rate of those underdiagnosed of the disease was between 58% and 61% in men and 72% to 87% in women (Movaghar et al., 2021). Thus, in developing countries like Malaysia, it is estimated that the rate of FXS underdiagnosis is even higher. The high rate may be attributed to a lack of knowledge and awareness of FXS and its genetic screening, as well as the lack of access to molecular genetic testing.

Clinical Symptoms

Individuals affected by FXS typically have normal life span because they are not afflicted by severe growth or health problems and thus, may have the opportunity to lead normal lives. This is unlike other chromosomal disorders such as Down syndrome, where congenital heart anomalies and respiratory conditions are the leading causes of death among patients. Patients with FXS show a wide variability of clinical characteristics that are significantly differed by gender. Males generally present with severe conditions compared with females, who show lesser symptoms (Marlborough et al., 2021).

The clinical symptoms are mostly related to impaired mental development, such as autism spectrum disorder, extreme aggression, intellectual disability, speech and language delay, social anxiety, sensory hyperstimulation, attention deficit hyperactivity disorder (ADHD), sleep disorder, seizures and obsessive-compulsive disorder (Davidson et al., 2022). These cause the individuals to face problems in maintaining short-term memory, performing executive functions (cognitive control, reasoning and problem-solving), and communicating with others. In terms of intellectual development, males who tend to be severely affected will have very low intelligence quotient (IQ), whereas females may have an IQ that is normal or at slight learning difficulty. As the individuals suffer from social anxiety, they are usually withdrawn and are prone to suffer extreme shyness and panic attacks in places with unfamiliar people. The physical characteristics of FXS patients include dysmorphic appearances like long and narrow face, large protruding ears, and prominent jawline and forehead (Lozano et al., 2014). They may also display hyper extensible fingers, flat feet, low muscle tone, soft skin and macroorchidism (large testicles). A Thai study found that ADHD and large ears were the most common clinical and physical characteristics, respectively, in pre-pubertal boys with FXS (Charalsawadi et al., 2017). In the same study, the researchers observed that female patients also presented with similar features but were less severe than males.

Related Health Problems

Like other chromosomal diseases, FXS patients may also be at risk of developing certain health problems, such as otitis media, mitral valve prolapses, gastrointestinal problems, strabismus (misaligned eyes) and joint laxity. Otitis media, which is an infection of the middle ear, is the most frequently observed. Approximately 85% of FXS patients are diagnosed with recurring otitis media in their lifetime that results in conductive hearing loss, thus impairing their behaviour, language, and cognitive development. Thus, FXS patients suffering from otitis media are usually subjected to aggressive treatment of antibiotics (Lozano et al., 2016).

Seizures occur in approximately 14 to 44% of FXS patients, with the major type being complex partial seizures. The seizures mainly occur during childhood and are not severe. Nevertheless, the onset of seizures at a young age may impact brain function and has been associated with development of autism spectrum disorder (Lozano et al., 2016).

As high as 50% of FXS patients may suffer mitral valve prolapse. This heart condition occurs due to dislocation of an irregularly thickened mitral valve leaflet into the left atrium during systole. FXS patients with mitral valve prolapse but do not show symptoms like an irregular heartbeat may require no treatment. However, they are at higher risk of bacterial infection in the heart lining and valve.

The most serious health condition may probably be obstructive sleep apnoea, which affects up to 38% of FXS patients (Curran et al., 2017). This condition can reduce the body's oxygen level due to airflow obstruction in the oral-nasal airway while sleeping, resulting in organ dysfunction, brain damage and even death. FXS patients with obstructive sleep apnoea will exhibit disruptive sleep patterns, such as heavy breathing and loud snoring, in addition to sudden awaking and gasping for air. As the patients are sleep-deprived, they may also suffer from urinary incontinence and daytime lethargy.

Gastrointestinal problems, like diarrhoea and gastro-oesophageal reflux disease (GERD), are the least observed in FXS patients, with a prevalence of approximately 11%. The episodes of patients passing loose stools have been associated with sympathetic hyperarousal and chronic anxiety (Lozano et al., 2016). It is also noted that FXS patients may have the ability to suppress abdominal pain and other gastrointestinal symptoms due to their higher pain threshold. Communication difficulties also made it difficult to determine if they have gastrointestinal problems, hence contributing to the low prevalence.

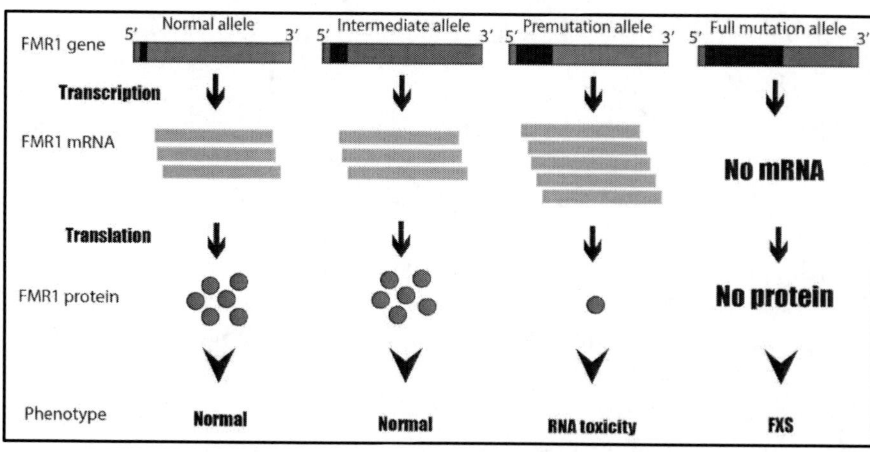

Figure 1. Expression of *FMR1* based on CGG repeats changes at the 5' region that disrupts the production of FMRP, leading to fragile X syndrome (FXS).

Molecular Mechanism

FXS is a unifactorial disease associated with a single gene known as the Fragile X Messenger Ribonucleoprotein 1 (*FMR1*). *FMR1* is located in the X chromosome, specifically near the edge of the q arm (Xq27.3). The gene's size is about 40 kilobases (kb) and it encodes a 3.9kb mRNA. The mRNA consists of approximately a 5' untranslated flanking region (0.2 kb), a 1.9 kb protein-coding region and a 3' untranslated flanking region (1.8 kb) (Tassanakijpanich et al., 2020). The protein-coding region of the *FMR1* is composed of 17 exons. The 5' untranslated region contains trinucleotide repeats (CGG). The number of CGG repetitions varies between individuals.

According to the American College of Medical Genetics guidelines on paediatric testing, a normal allele has a 5' untranslated region that ranges from six to 44 CGG repeats. Individuals in the intermediate or grey zone allele range has between 45 and 54 CGG repeats. A pre-mutation individual has a 5' untranslated region ranging from 55 to 200 repeats. FXS-positive individuals have full mutation with more than 200 repeats.

In the full mutation allele, gene transcription becomes suppressed when the CGG repeats are stretched and methylated, resulting in the reduction or absence of fragile X messenger ribonucleoprotein (FMRP) production. In the premutation allele, the *FMR1* is actively transcripted, resulting in high levels of *FMR1* mRNA, but normal to low levels of FMRP. A high level of *FMR1* mRNA has been associated with clinical complications caused by RNA toxicity (Schneider et al., 2020; Tassanakijpanich et al., 2021) such as Fragile X-associated Tremor/Ataxia Syndrome (FXTAS), psychiatric disorder, endocrine dysfunction and immunologic disorders. The CGG repeats in the pre-mutation allele become progressively unstable as the number increases when the gene is passed down from generation to generation. The expansion of the CGG codon is believed to be a consequence of strand slippage during DNA replication or repair. The higher the number of CGG repeats in a pre-mutation woman, the higher the risk of extension to a full mutation in her next offspring (Sherman et al., 2005). Figure 1 shows the gene expression of *FMR1* based on the expansion of CGG repeats at the 5' untranslated region.

Although FXS is a unifactorial disease caused by mutation of a single gene (*FMR1*), this syndrome is a complex disease as FMRP (the protein encoded by *FMR1*) interacts with approximately 180 other proteins from various pathways (Taha et al., 2021). RNA-binding proteins, such as FXR1P, FXR2P and 82-FIP, are some of its interacting proteins. Thus, the lack of FMRP in FXS patients will result in the downregulation of mRNA translation in non-neuronal cells, which reduces their co-localisation with the translational machinery in neurons (Cook et al., 2014). The absence of FMRP causing protein synthesis in the brain is excessive, which in turn impairs neuronal circuit formation and higher cognitive function (Ritcher & Zhao, 2021). (Richter & Zhao, 2021). The molecular mechanisms of FMRP include:

1. Regulating translation:
   (a) Influencing the initiation of RNA translation.
   (b) Controlling RNA synthesis through regulated translation of critical transcriptional factors or chromatin modulators.
   (c) Reduces or stops ribosome translocation, thus reducing the polypeptide elongation rate.
2. Regulating nuclear activities, including transcription and splicing.
3. Regulating RNA modification and maintaining its stability.

FMRP is mostly found within the brain and testes. It appears to be responsible for selectively binding to around 4% of mRNA in animal brain cells and transporting them out of the nucleus to the synapses of neurons. Most of these mRNA targets have been found to be located in dendrites, and brain tissues of FXS individuals and mouse models have been observed to have abnormal dendritic spines, Dendritic spines are required to increase contact with other neurons, and subsequent abnormalities in their formation will affect the function of synapses and development of neural circuits, which will result in disruptions to the integral part of memory and learning (Malecki et al., 2020).

Many studies have proved that the absence of FMRP leads to FXS via various pathways, one of which is by disrupting the GABAergic system. Gamma amino-butyric acid (GABA) is a neurotransmitter that blocks impulses between nerve cells in the central nervous system, and the GABAergic system regulates the releasing and binding of GABA in neuronal cells. In normal individuals, FMRP binds to the GABA receptor and increases the activity of the single-channel receptor. However, in FXS, the loss of FMRP markedly reduces tonic inhibition in the GABAergic system and suppresses critical aspects of signal processing in the brain (Deng et al., 2022).

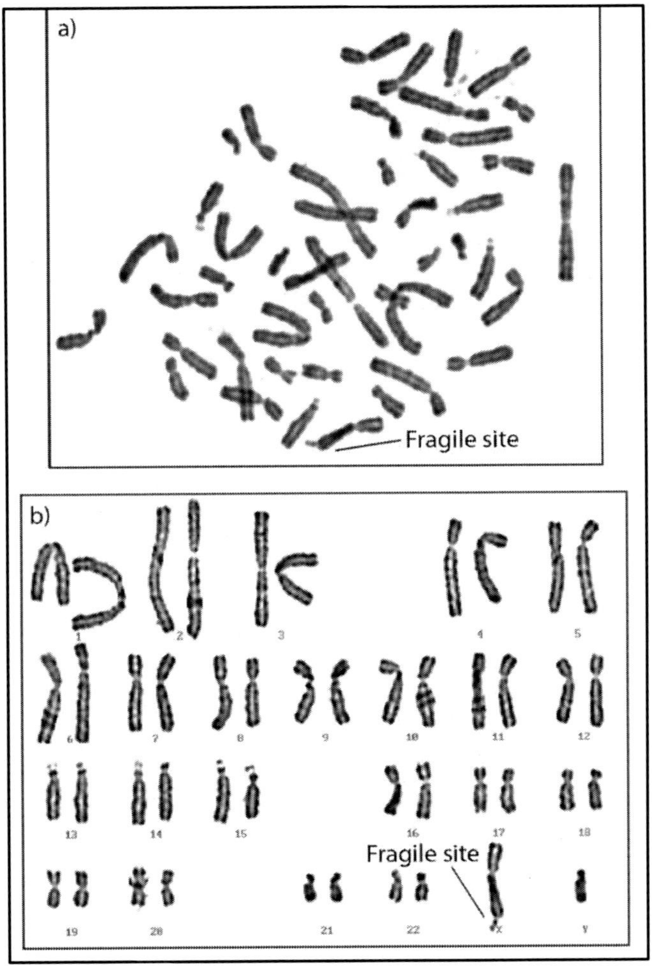

Figure 2. Karyotype showing fragile site at the X chromosome. (a) Chromosomes of white blood cells arrested in metaphase. (b) The 23 pairs of arranged chromosomes, including Y and fragile X at q27.3.

Diagnostic Methods

Cytogenetic Analysis

Cytogenetic analysis is a conventional technique used to confirm the diagnosis of FXS. The fragile site of the X chromosome may be identified through karyotyping with unbanded Giemsa staining. The white blood cells of patients are extracted and cultured with folate-deficient phytohaemagglutinin media for three days to induce mitosis. On the third day, the cells are transferred to a hypotonic solution with colchicine to expand the cells and arrest them in mitotic metaphase. The cell culture will be gently dripped onto a slide, causing the expanded cells to burst and spread their chromosomes. The slide is then subjected to Giemsa staining and the image of each chromosome is captured using a microscope camera and arranged for karyotyping. This chromosomal examination may be done on affected males and female carriers of the disease. The prenatal diagnosis of FXS may also be performed using amniotic fluid cells from a carrier mother, although there is a risk of causing miscarriage when obtaining such cells. Figure 2 shows an example of the cytogenetic karyotyping result of an FXS patient.

Although cytogenetic methods have improved tremendously, the fragile site manifestation at X q27.3 does not occur in all the patients' chromosomes. The fragile site is usually seen in 2% to 60% only of the metaphase cells. Moreover, heterozygous females tend to show a lower frequency of X chromosomes with fragile sites than affected males. Thus, for diagnostic purposes, the minimum frequency of fragile X metaphases is recommended at 4%. Nevertheless, there are diagnostic laboratories that apply even lower cut-off points. However, the cytogenetic test is unable to detect clinically normal carriers. Currently, the diagnosis trend is shifting towards sensitive and specific molecular techniques, which can detect full-mutation and pre-mutation carriers simultaneously.

Molecular Analysis

The gold standard for laboratory confirmation of FXS is the combination of polymerase chain reaction (PCR) and Southern blot analysis (Sachdeva et al., 2019). However, methylation-specific PCR also may also be used in lieu of Southern blot to assess the methylation status of the *FMR1* allele.

Specific primers are used to amplify the CGG repeats, and the size of the CGG repeats can be measured using agarose gel electrophoresis or quantitative PCR. However, the high CG content of the CGG repeat reduces the efficiency of the PCR, making it hard to amplify fully mutated alleles with high CGG repeats.

Table 1. The supportive strategies used in management of FXS

Therapy	**Beneficial group**
Behavioural therapy	Those with autism spectrum disorder who need help in managing anxiety
Functional communication training	Those with self-injurious and aggressive behaviour
Occupational therapy	Those having sensory integration problems that affect cognitive development
Speech therapy	Those experiencing speech difficulties
Toilet training	Those having problems with bowel movement and bladder control

Southern blot can only produce estimated size of large CGG repeat segments, but a precise sizing is impossible. Still, an accurate assessment of the methylation status can be examined simultaneously. Moreover, Southern blot analysis needs high quantity of genomic DNA from sample, and it is also more laborious than PCR (Ramos et al., 2020).

Other than Southern blot, the *FMR1* methylation status of the FXS patients can be identified using methylation-specific PCR. However, this method can only detect the full mutation of *FMR1* allele. Unfortunately, methylation-specific PCR cannot differentiate the pre-mutation allele from the normal allele. However, a new and improved method known as the "Methylation-Specific Triplet-Primed PCR and Melting Curve Analysis" (Rajan-Babu & Chong, 2019) has been introduced, with high sensitivity and specificity, and can concurrently detect the *FMR1* CGG-repeat expansions and their methylation status.

Therapies and Medical Treatment

Supportive Strategies

FXS patients will fully benefit from supportive strategies, such as speech therapy, special educational services, occupational therapy, and behavioural intervention when started from a very young age. However, the supportive strategies need to be individualised according to the patient's specific problems. Thus, treatment management requires coordination between physicians, occupational therapists, physical therapists, psychologists, speech therapists and educators (Lozano et al., 2016). Table 1 shows the type of therapies used in the management of FXS.

Apart from supportive strategies, FXS patients and their family members are recommended to join a support group. In Malaysia, there is the Malaysian Rare Disorders Society (MRDS) in which family members can meet and share experiences in managing patients with rare diseases such as FXS. The members also can get the latest information on FXS and its management through various health professionals. The group also organizes specialized activities that can help improve the social wellbeing of FXS patients.

Medication Strategies

Symptoms of autism, aggressive and self-injurious behaviour, and anxiety-related issues among FXS patients can be controlled through medication. The use of medication enhances the patients' ability to take part in activities with their family and in school. Table 2 shows the common medicines prescribed to control the symptoms in FXS patients.

The medical problems associated with FXS are treated based on the severity of symptoms. Table 3 shows the medication used to treat medical problems that tend to affect FXS patients.

Table 2. Medication to treat clinical symptoms in FXS patients

Medication	Symptoms
Methylphenidate	Hyperactivity, lack of concentration and impulsivity.
Alpha-2-adrenergic agonists Clonidine and Guanfacine	Hyperactivity, hyper-arousal to sensory stimuli Impulsivity, aggressive behaviour and sleep problem
Melatonin	Sleep problem
Selective serotonin re-uptake inhibitors (e.g., Sertraline)	Mood disorders, anxiety, hyper-arousal, communication deficiencies and tantrums related to autism and obsessive-compulsive disorder
Cannabidiol	Anxiety, seizures, and depression
Antipsychotics (e.g., Risperidone)	Aggressive and self-injurious behaviour
Riluzole	Aggressive, self-injurious and repetitive behaviour

Table 3. Medication used to treat diseases that commonly affect FXS patients

Medical problem	Treatment and management
Otitis media	• Antibiotics • Pneumococcal and influenza vaccine • Pressure equalizing tube therapy
Seizures	• Carbamazepine • Valproic acid
Mitral valves prolapse	In rare cases, surgery is performed to repair or replace the mitral valve
Obstructive sleep apnoea	• Steroids to reduce tonsillar hypertrophy • Tonsillectomy

Genetic Counselling

Family members of FXS patients will usually be provided with genetic counselling irrespective whether the patient has pre- or fully mutated *FMR1* genes (Sachdeva et al., 2019). Women with pre-mutation are carriers of the disease, and the higher the frequency of CGG repeats in the mother's genes, the higher the risk of her offspring inheriting the elongated repeats. Thus, there is higher risk of her bearing children with full mutation. Meanwhile, men with pre-mutation genes will pass down the extended alleles to their daughters only.

Genetic counsellors are medical specialists with background knowledge in clinical or medical genetics and psychosocial counselling. They have the expertise to interpret patients' medical information and genetic test results to provide guidance on family planning to those at risk of producing offspring with FXS and other inheritable diseases. They also advise family members on how to cope with emotional and psychosocial problems encountered by FXS patients.

In Malaysia, genetic counselling is conducted by clinical geneticists in the hospital setting, in which family and medical histories are taken into consideration before recommending treatment and advising patients and family members on how to cope with the disease. Generally, the aim of counselling includes:

1. Helping family members to understand the variability of clinical characteristics in FXS.

2. Offering molecular screening to family members and explaining the results.
3. Advising pre-mutation adults on their risk of developing ataxia, anxiety, depression, ovarian insufficiency, or other medical problems.
4. Providing family planning and reproductive advice to affected people to avoid passing down the disease to their children.

Research Updates

The main objective in treating FXS is to reverse the dysregulated functions in brain development due to the disruption in FRMP synthesis. Therefore, early supportive strategies combined with medication are mainly used in managing FXS patients (Protic et al., 2022).

Currently, more researchers are focusing on targeted treatments and drug repurposing. The objective of targeted treatments in FXS is to identify specific proteins that control gene expression, besides maintaining cell growth integrity and signalling, especially in neuron cells. In the case FXS, targeted treatments will naturally focus on proteins that can reverse the neurobiological deformities caused by the lack of FMRP. Although many new and existing drugs have been proposed or repurposed to treat FXS, there is still no medication specifically approved by the United States Food and Drug Agency for its treatment,

Gaboxadol is being studied to alleviate FXS symptoms in preclinical and clinical trials. This drug is an agonist that targets GABA receptors in the synapse of neuron cells, triggering anti-excitation brain signals that relieve mood, thought and cognition. GABA signalling induces a soothing effect; hence the drug was initially developed as an analgesic and anti-anxiety medication in the 1980s. It was further tested as a drug to reduce insomnia in the late 1990s and early 2000s. However, trials were not promising in this aspect and focus had then shifted to using it in FXS patients (Krogsgaard-Larsen et al., 2004). Activation of GABA receptors with Gaboxadol has been potentially shown to treat fundamental problems related to FXS, such as restoration of distorted synapse structure, reduction of hypersensitivity to noises, relieving hyperactivity, and alleviating seizures. However, common side-effects include nausea, vomiting, headache and fatigue (Budimirovic et al., 2021).

Another group of drugs (mavoglurant and basimglurant) is designed to act as antagonists of metabotropic glutamate receptors (mGluRs). The mGluR family comprises G-protein-coupled receptors that are important in regulating synaptic transmission and neuronal excitability throughout the central nervous system. Unfortunately, although these drugs have shown positive neuronal and behavioural effects in preclinical studies, they failed to demonstrate any behavioural benefits in clinical trials (Berry-Kravis et al., 2018).

Drug repurposing has become frequent in FXS treatment. Metformin, an antihyperglycemic medication used to treat type 2 diabetes and promote weight loss, has been observed to reverse dendritic spine dysgenesis and electrophysiological anomalies related to long-term depression in FXS patients. It promotes positive changes by reducing their irritability, social avoidance and aggressive behaviour (Protic et al., 2022). Interestingly, apart from correcting behavioural problems, metformin treatment is also useful in managing the weight of FXS patients. However, bloating, gas, diarrhoea, constipation, and reduced appetite have been reported as side-effects.

The antibiotic minocycline is another example of a drug that is being repurposed for FXS treatment. However, further research is still ongoing. Minocycline has been reported to restore the normal synaptic structure in the neuromuscular junction of FXS patients. Minocycline treatment among FXS patients has reportedly improved their mood-related behaviour and social function. However, the side effects include nausea, vomiting, diarrhoea and dizziness.

Treatment Limitations and Future of Disease Management

Medications, including non-specific demethylating agents, have been studied for FXS treatment for many years. However, these drugs are toxic and produce many sides effect. Recently, research is changing towards the direct elimination of the primary genetic cause of FXS. The advancement of this treatment strategy is made possible with the development of the Clustered Regularly Interspaced Short Palindromic Repeats (CRISPR) genome editing strategy. This technology allows the splicing and rejoining of DNA sequences at certain locations of a gene with the use of the Cas-9 enzyme. For FXS treatment, researchers have used a CRISPR-based epigenetic approach to promote the demethylation of full-mutation CGG repeats in the *FMR1* promoter region by targeting the TET1 gene (Liu et al., 2018). The demethylation of the expended CGG then restores the FMRP level in the stem cells and neurons of the FXS patient. However, there are numerous hurdles in this promising research. One of them is on the best way to deliver the CRISPR tools to the central nervous system of FXS patients although three different strategies have been proposed. 1) Intracranial injection, 2) intranasal administration, 3) Oral drug (Cota-Coronado et al., 2019). Therefore, the procurement of more knowledge regarding the molecular pathogenesis of the FXS, understanding if the symptoms can be reverted after the onset, identifying the minimal number of cells to be corrected and determining the ideal therapeutic window to achieve a significant improvement would help to accelerate the therapeutic translation from preclinical to clinical trial (Ricci & Colasante, 2021).

Conclusion

FXS is a neurodevelopmental disorder caused by the silencing of FMRP production due to the DNA methylation as a result of elongated CGG repeats in the *FMR1* gene. Although FXS is a unifactorial disease, the molecular pathogenesis is very complex, involving various pathways, thus producing various medical problems and mental disabilities. Therefore, comprehensive management strategies are needed to manage FXS, including supportive and medicinal strategies. Due to the complexity of the FXS pathogenesis and treatment, further studies are needed to design the best treatment to cure FXS.

Acknowledgment

The author would like to thank staff members in the Biochemistry Unit, Department of Biomedical 1, Faculty of Medicine and Health Sciences, Universiti Sains Islam Malaysia, for their assistance. The review is produced as part of a study supported by Universiti Sains Islam Malaysia.

References

Berry-Kravis, E. M., Lindemann, L., Jonch, A. E., Apostol, G., Bear, M. F., Carpenter, R. L., Crawley, J. N., Curie, A., Des Portes, V., Hossain, F., Gasparini, F., Gomez-Mancilla, B., Hessl, D., Loth, E., Scharf, S. H., Wang, P. P., Von Raison, F., Hagerman, R., Spooren, W., and Jacquemont, S. (2018). Drug development for neurodevelopmental disorders: lessons learned from fragile X syndrome. *Nat Rev Drug Discov*, 17(4), 280-299. https://doi.org/10.1038/nrd.2017.221.

Budimirovic, D. B., Dominick, K. C., Gabis, L. V., Adams M., Adera, M., Huang, L., Ventola, P., Tartaglia, N. R., and Berry-Kravis, E. (2021) Gaboxadol in Fragile X Syndrome: A 12-Week Randomized, Double-Blind, Parallel-Group, Phase 2a Study. *Front Pharmacol*, 8(12), 757825. doi: 10.3389/fphar.2021.757825.

Charalsawadi, C., Wirojanan, J., Jaruratanasirikul, S., Ruangdaraganon, N., Geater, A., and Limprasert, P. (2017). Common Clinical Characteristics and Rare Medical Problems of Fragile X Syndrome in Thai Patients and Review of the Literature. *Int J Pediatr*, 2017, 9318346. https://doi.org/10.1155/2017/9318346.

Cook, D., Nuro, E., Jones, E. V., Altimimi, H. F., Farmer, W. T., Gandin, V., Hanna, E., Zong, R., Barbon, A., Nelson, D. L., Topisirovic, I., Rochford, J., Stellwagen, D., Beique, J. C., and Murai, K. K. (2014). FXR1P limits long-term memory, long-lasting synaptic potentiation, and de novo GluA2 translation. *Cell Rep*, 9(4), 1402-1416. https://doi.org/10.1016/j.celrep.2014.10.028.

Curran, C., Debbarma, S., and Sedky, K. (2017). Fragile X and Obstructive Sleep Apnea Syndrome: Case Presentation and Management Challenges. *J Clin Sleep Med*, 13(1), 137-138. https://doi.org/10.5664/jcsm.6408.

Davidson, M., Sebastian, S. A., Benitez, Y., Desai, S., Quinonez, J., Ruxmohan, S., Stein, J. D., and Cueva, W. (2022). Behavioral Problems in Fragile X Syndrome: A Review of Clinical Management. *Cureus*, 14(2), e21840. https://doi.org/10.7759/cureus.21840.

Deng, P. Y., Kumar, A., Cavalli, V., and Klyachko, V. A. (2022). FMRP regulates GABAA receptor channel activity to control signal integration in hippocampal granule cells. *Cell Rep*, 39(7), 110820. https://doi.org/10.1016/j.celrep.2022.110820.

Hagerman, R. J., Berry-Kravis, E., Hazlett, H. C., Bailey, D. B., Moine, H., Kooy, R. F., Tassone, F., Gantois, I., Sonenberg, N., Mandel, J. L., and Hagerman, P. J. (2017). Fragile X syndrome. *Nature Reviews Disease Primers*, 3(1), 17065. https://doi.org/10.1038/nrdp.2017.65.

Krogsgaard-Larsen, P., Frølund, B., Liljefors, T., and Ebert, B. (2004) GABAA agonists and partial agonists: THIP (Gaboxadol) as a non-opioid analgesic and a novel type of hypnotic. *Biochem Pharmacol*, 68(8), 1573-1580.

Liu, X. S., Wu, H., Krzisch, M., Wu, X., Graef, J., Muffat, J., Hnisz, D., Li, C. H., Yuan, B., Xu, C., Li, Y., Vershkov, D., Cacace, A., Young, R. A., and Jaenisch, R. (2018). Rescue of Fragile X Syndrome Neurons by DNA Methylation Editing of the FMR1 Gene. *Cell*, 172(5), 979-992. https://doi.org/10.1016/j.cell.2018.01.012.

Lozano, R., Azarang, A., Wilaisakditipakorn, T., and Hagerman, R. J. (2016). Fragile X syndrome: A review of clinical management. *Intractable Rare Dis Res*, 5(3), 145-157. https://doi.org/10.5582/irdr.2016.01048.

Lozano, R., Rosero, C. A., and Hagerman, R. J. (2014). Fragile X spectrum disorders. *Intractable Rare Dis Res*, 3(4), 134-146. https://doi.org/10.5582/irdr.2014.01022.

Malecki, C., Hambly, B. D., Jeremy, R. W., and Robertson, E. N. (2020). The RNA-binding fragile-X mental retardation protein and its role beyond the brain. *Biophys Rev*, 12(4), 903-916. https://doi.org/ 10.1007/s12551-020-00730-4.

Marlborough, M., Welham, A., Jones, C., Reckless, S., and Moss, J. (2021). Autism spectrum disorder in females with fragile X syndrome: a systematic review and meta-analysis of prevalence. *J Neurodev Disord*, 13(1), 28. https://doi.org/10.1186/s11689-021-09362-5.

Movaghar, A., Page, D., Brilliant, M., and Mailick, M. (2021). Prevalence of Underdiagnosed Fragile X Syndrome in 2 Health Systems. *JAMA Netw Open*, 4(12), e2141516. https://doi.org/10.1001/jamanetworkopen.2021.41516.

Protic, D. D., Aishworiya, R., Salcedo-Arellano, M. J., Tang, S. J., Milisavljevic, J., Mitrovic, F., Hagerman, R. J., and Budimirovic, D. B. (2022). Fragile X Syndrome: From Molecular Aspect to Clinical Treatment. *Int J Mol Sci*, 23(4). https://doi.org/10.3390/ijms23041935.

Rajan-Babu, I. S., and Chong, S. S. (2019). Triplet-Repeat Primed PCR and Capillary Electrophoresis for Characterizing the Fragile X Mental Retardation 1 CGG Repeat Hyperexpansions. *Methods Mol Biol*, 1972, 199-210. https://doi.org/10.1007/978-1-4939-9213-3_14.

Ramos, C., Ocampos, M., Barbato, I. T., Graca Bicalho, M. D., and Nisihara, R. (2020). Molecular analysis of FMR1 gene in a population in Southern Brazil: Comparison of four methods. *Pract Lab Med*, 21, e00162. https://doi.org/10.1016/j.plabm.2020.e00162.

Ricci, R., and Colasante, G. (2021). CRISPR/dCas9 as a Therapeutic Approach for Neurodevelopmental Disorders: Innovations and Limitations Compared to Traditional Strategies. *Dev Neurosci*, 43(3-4), 253-261. https://doi.org/10.1159/000515845.

Richter, J. D., and Zhao, X. (2021). The molecular biology of FMRP: new insights into fragile X syndrome. *Nat Rev Neurosci*, 22(4), 209-222. https://doi.org/10.1038/s41583-021-00432-0.

Sachdeva, A., Jain, P., Gunasekaran, V., Mahay, S. B., Mukherjee, S., Hagerman, R., Shankar, S., Kapoor, S., Kedia, S. N., Indian Academy of Pediatrics Consensus in, D., Management of Fragile, X. S. C., Indian Academy of Pediatrics Consensus in, D., and Management of Fragile, X. S. C. (2019). Consensus Statement of the Indian Academy of Pediatrics on Diagnosis and Management of Fragile X Syndrome in India. *Indian Pediatr*, 56(3), 221-228. https://www.ncbi.nlm.nih.gov/pubmed/30954995.

Schneider, A., Winarni, T. I., Cabal-Herrera, A. M., Bacalman, S., Gane, L., Hagerman, P., Tassone, F., and Hagerman, R. (2020). Elevated FMR1-mRNA and lowered FMRP - A double-hit mechanism for psychiatric features in men with FMR1 premutations. *Transl Psychiatry, 10*(1), 205. https://doi.org/10.1038/s41398-020-00863-w.

Sherman, S., Pletcher, B. A., and Driscoll, D. A. (2005). Fragile X syndrome: diagnostic and carrier testing. *Genet Med*, 7(8), 584-587. https://doi.org/10.1097/01.gim.0000182468.22666.dd.

Sihombing, N. R. B., Winarni, T. I., Utari, A., van Bokhoven, H., Hagerman, R. J., and Faradz, S. M. (2021). Surveillance and prevalence of fragile X syndrome in Indonesia. *Intractable Rare Dis Res*, 10(1), 11-16. https://doi.org/10.5582/irdr.2020.03101.

Taha, M. S., Haghighi, F., Stefanski, A., Nakhaei-Rad, S., Kazemein Jasemi, N. S., Al Kabbani, M. A., Gorg, B., Fujii, M., Lang, P. A., Haussinger, D., Piekorz, R. P., Stuhler, K., and Ahmadian, M. R. (2021). Novel FMRP interaction networks linked to cellular stress. *FEBS J*, 288(3), 837-860. https://doi.org/10.1111/febs.15443.

Tassanakijpanich, N., Cohen, J., Cohen, R., Srivatsa, U. N., and Hagerman, R. J. (2020). Cardiovascular Problems in the Fragile X Premutation. *Front Genet*, 11, 586910. https://doi.org/10.3389/fgene.2020.586910.

Tassanakijpanich, N., McKenzie, F. J., McLennan, Y. A., Makhoul, E., Tassone, F., Jasoliya, M. J., Romney, C., Petrasic, I. C., Napalinga, K., Buchanan, C. B., Hagerman, P., Hagerman, R., and Casanova, E. L. (2021). Hypermobile Ehlers-Danlos syndrome (hEDS) phenotype in fragile X premutation carriers: case series. *J Med Genet*, https://doi.org/10.1136/jmedgenet-2020-107609.

Ten, S. K., Chin, Y. M., Jamilatul Noor, M. B., and Hassan, K. (1985). The fragile X syndrome: first family reported in Malaysia. *Singapore Med J*, 26(4-5), 372-378. https://www.ncbi.nlm.nih.gov/pubmed/4071092.

Chapter 3

Apolipoprotein E (APOE) Genetic Mutation in Alzheimer's Disease Amongst Malaysians

Muhammad Syahir Hakimi Mohd Hazli and Azalina Zainuddin*

Chemical Pathology Department, School of Medical Sciences,
Universiti Sains Malaysia, Kota Bharu, Kelantan, Malaysia

Abstract

Alzheimer's disease (AD) is a complex medical condition involving the degeneration of brain cells among ageing people. It is a progressive deterioration of cognition, characterized by memory loss, disturbances in behaviour and psychotic episodes. AD is associated with several neuropathological risk factors, such as production of amyloid beta plaques, accumulation of intracellular neurofibrillary tangles (NFT) containing hyperphosphorylated tau protein, cytosolic TDP-43 and α-synuclein, and carrier of the apolipoprotein E (APOE) ε4 allele. The APOE gene is localised on chromosome 19 and contains three common alleles (ε2, ε3, and ε4). It generally involves producing carrier proteins for cholesterol and lipids in plasma. APOE ε4 has been identified to be the most common genetic risk factor associated with late-onset AD amongst the elderly across the population. In Malaysia, alleles ε3 and ε4 have the highest frequency compared with ε2 in Malays, Chinese and Indians. Specifically, among ethnicity groups, Malays have the highest frequency of heterozygous ε3/ε4 alleles, followed by Indians and Chinese. Prevalence of dementia across the ethnicity in Malaysia is also reflected by the frequency of APOE alleles, where the Malay population has the highest incidence of dementia, followed by Chinese and Indians.

* Corresponding Author's Email: azalina@usm.my.

In: Genetic Disorders and Rare Diseases
Editors: Shazlin Shaharudin, Hisham Atan Edinur and Nor Fazila Che Mat
ISBN: 979-8-88697-953-4

However, the ε2 allele is silenced among Indians. This article reviews the prevalence of the APOE mutation in the Malaysian population that contributes to Alzheimer's disease, the relationship of APOE allele frequencies with the prevalence of dementia, and recent technologies targeting the APOE gene that are useful in the prevention of late onset AD.

Keywords: Alzheimer's disease, apolipoprotein E, genetic mutation, alleles frequency

Introduction

Alzheimer's disease (AD) is a neurological degenerative disease that is common in an ageing population. The disorder is a leading cause of dementia and can be characterised by several hallmarks, including memory loss, progressive cognitive impairment, amyloid-β plaque accumulation, tau hyperphosphorylation, and activity of oxygen reactive species resulting in neuronal cell death (Anand et al., 2014; Rodríguez-Martín et al., 2013). Patients with AD typically project a progressive impairment as it is progressive in nature and affects the ability of the patient to perform daily life routines (World Health Organisation, 2017).

According to World Alzheimer Report (2019), the prevalence of dementia increases from year to year as the global population ages. It is estimated that about 36 million people live with dementia in 2010 and the figure may double by 2030. The report also predicted that by 2050, the prevalence of people with dementia may reach about 152 million, sparking great concern about the burden on healthcare services globally.

Association of Apolipoprotein E (APOE) with the late onset of AD has been determined among 95% of the total AD population (Yamazaki et al., 2019). There are three major allelic variants of APOE (ε2, ε3, and ε4), with the ε4 allele posing the greatest risk of late onset AD compared to ε2 and ε3 (Saunders et al., 1993). Carrying one ε4 allele has been determined to increase the risk of AD 3-4 fold, whilst carrying two alleles may increase the risk by 9-15 fold (Genin et al., 2011; Neu et al., 2017).

Ironically, carrying allele ε2 either homozygous or heterozygous was associated with a decrease of beta-amyloid accumulation, hence decreasing the risk of late-onset AD in the elderly (Grothe et al., 2017). Although the genetic inheritance of the APOE gene contributes to the development of AD, the pathophysiology of how the alleles result in AD development is incomplete. Further study by Foraker et al., (2015) has shown that the presence of a single allele of the APOE gene is neither sufficient nor necessary for the development of AD.

Biological Structure of APOE

APOE consists of three common alleles (ε2, ε3, and ε4) that are defined by two single nucleotide polymorphisms (SNPs). The alleles reside in the exon 4 coding region, and localised with a cytosine-phosphate-guanine (CpG) rich region known as the "CPG island" (CGI) (Foraker et al., 2015). APOE is a glycoprotein approximately 34 kDa in size. It is identified in triglyceride-rich lipoproteins and is composed of 299 amino acids after cleavage of the 18-amino-acid signal peptide (Mahley, 1988). Each allele differs in its frequencies: ε2 about five to 10%, ε3 about 65 to 70%, and ε4 about 15 to 20%. These three isoforms contribute to three homozygous (ε2/ε2, ε3/ε3, ε4/ε4) and three heterozygous (ε2/ε3, ε2/ε4, ε3/ε4) phenotypes (Zannis et al., 1982).

The glycoprotein structure of APOE has two structural domains; the N-terminal and C-terminal, both are separated by a hinge region. The N-terminal consists of four main helices (helix 2, helix 3, helix 4 and helix 5) and a receptor-binding region, with two hinge helices. Meanwhile, the C-terminal domains consist of helices and lipid-binding residues. The APOE isoforms differ from each other at two residues: ε2 at Cys112 and Cys158, ε3 at Cys112 and Arg158, and ε4 at Arg112 and Arg158 (Mahley et al., 2009).

Structural modelling of human APOE protein has been well documented in the Protein Data Bank (PDB) (Berman et al., 2000), which allows the 3D modelling of proteins from multiple structural templates to be built and visualised using advanced Mol* Viewer (Sehnal et al., 2021). The 3D structural model of APOE ε4 (PDB ID: 1B68) and ε3 (PDB ID: 1NFN) retrieved from RCSB PDP website shows difference peptides at locus 112 between Arg and Cys. The major lipid binding region, mainly at C-terminal (residues 244-272), interacts directly with lipid particles like LDL and HDL (Segelke et al., 2000). The binding of the C-terminal of APOE with lipid particles will enhance the affinity of the receptor binding region on N-terminal (residues 130 150), hence increasing the delivery of cholesterol particles (Guttman et al., 2010).

APOE Pathogenesis in AD

APOE is the major known genetic risk factor for AD and has a potential role in other neurological diseases and traumatic brain injury (Mahley et al., 2006). In AD, the ε4 allele has a significant contribution to neuropathology by interacting with the amyloid pathway, mainly to modulate the β-amyloid peptide clearance. APOE ε4 allele can also cause neuropathology directly and establish the next stages to precipitate neuropathology. These next stages could be genetically inherited (α-synuclein, tau aggregation, and presenilin), metabolic (ischemia and oxidative stress), or environmental (aging, inflammation, and central nervous system trauma). The neuropathologic effects of the ε4 allele are mediated by its structural features (e.g., domain interaction) due to the presence of Arg112 and Arg158 residues (Mahley et al., 2009).

APOE in β-Amyloid Clearance and Aggregation

β-amyloid is primarily produced in neurons via cleavage of proteolytic amyloid precursor protein (APP). The protein is cleared from the brain by several pathways such as degradation by enzymes, perivascular drainage via interstitial fluid, glymphatic clearance, and blood-brain barrier (BBB) clearance (O'Brien & Wong, 2011). Receptor binding of APOE includes LDL receptor-related protein 1 (LRP1), LDL receptor (LDLR), and heparan sulphate proteoglycan (HSPG) (Guttman et al., 2010). These receptors allow the APOE to mediate cellular uptake of β-amyloid and clear the β-amyloid into the blood flow.

However, the ε4 allele of APOE increases the seeding and aggregation of β-amyloid and lowers the clearance by increasing the lipidation of β-amyloid inside the brain parenchyma (Foraker et al., 2015). This leads to the accumulation of insoluble β-amyloid plaque in the brain and the vascular wall (Yamazaki et al., 2019).

APOE in Tau Hyperphosphorylation

Emerging evidence suggests that the APOE gene is capable of modulating tau-mediated neurodegeneration, one of the hallmarks of AD. A study reported individuals with primary tauopathies may exhibit tau pathology when carrying homozygous ε4/ε4 allele (Tiraboschi et al., 2004). The study also suggested individuals with two ε4 alleles have more tau aggregates than individuals with one ε4 allele when β-amyloid pathology is present. In the mice model, a strong correlation was demonstrated between neuron-specific overexpression of APOE4 and increased tau phosphorylation (Brecht et al., 2004). In addition, a study using human iPSC-derived APOE*ε4-expressing neurons in animal models also demonstrated higher levels of tau phosphorylation compared to APOE*ε3-expressing neurons (Wang et al., 2018).

Prevalence of APOE Gene in Malaysian Populations

Findings have been determined that the ε4 allele has a clear association with elevated serum cholesterol and increased the risk of late onset of AD. In contrast, allele ε2 can suppress the effect of serum cholesterol elevation, hence potentially lowering the risk of diseases related to dementia and heart disease (Seet et al., 2004). Table 1 shows the comparison between a meta-analysis of all published AD association studies globally and a study conducted by Seet et al., (2004) on the distribution of the different APOE alleles and genotypes amongst Malaysian population. It is interesting that both data project almost similar frequencies between APOE genotypes of patients with AD globally and among races in Malaysia.

Table 1. Comparison of the APOE genotype frequency between patients with AD and races in Malaysia

APOE genotype	**Frequency in patients with AD (%)** [a]	**Frequency amongst races in Malaysia (%)** [b]			
		Malay	**Chinese**	**Indian**	**Total**
ε2/ ε2	0.3	1.04	0.58	0	0.68
ε2/ ε3	4.6	8.33	12.28	0	9.83
ε3/ ε3	34.3	65.63	69.01	71.43	68.13
ε2/ ε4	2.6	0	0.58	0	0.33
ε3/ ε4	43.4	22.92	16.37	28.57	19.66
ε4/ ε4	14.8	2.08	1.17	0	1.37

a. Meta-analysis of all published AD association studies (n = 38) (AlzGene, 2010).

b. A study on the distribution of the different APOE alleles and genotypes amongst the Malaysian population (n = 295) (Seet et al., 2004).

According to Table 1, alleles ε3 and ε4 of APOE have higher frequency compared with ε2 in Malays, Chinese and Indians. Malays have the highest frequency of heterozygous ε3/ε4 alleles, followed by Indians and Chinese. Prevalence of dementia across ethnicities in Malaysia is also reflected by the frequency of APOE alleles. According to a study by Hamid et al., (2011), Malay and Bumiputera populations have the highest prevalence of dementia, at 14.8% and 32% respectively, followed by the Chinese (6.3%) and the Indians (5.8%). A similar figure was also reported by Krishnaswamy et al., (1997), in which the Malay population who were urban settlers in Kuala Lumpur and better educated has a higher prevalence of dementia (6%).

An earlier report by Kua (1993) on the prevalence of dementia in Singapore also stated similar results in the three main races. The study used the Geriatric Mental Scale (GMS-AGECAT) by Copeland et al., (1976), a diagnostic instrument to assess cognitive functions, namely memory and orientation-information. It reported that higher dementia prevalence was observed among Malays (9.4%), followed by Indians (8.8%) and Chinese (4.2%). Although these reports only showed the prevalence of dementia and are not specific to AD, the observations are important to understand the correlation between the APOE gene and its contribution to AD across populations in Malaysia. Hence, further research is required to collect greater data regarding AD among races in Malaysia, with special attention to Malay and Bumiputera patients.

Recent Technologies for Targeting Apoe

Observations from previous reports and findings have determined the most firmly established genetic risk factor contributing to late-onset AD is the ε4 allele, which notorious for its hyperfunction of protein stability and increased overall APOE expression. Current technologies are focused on therapeutic strategies to mitigate the hyperfunction of the ε4 and ε3 allele, which also involves in increase protein production and β-amyloid pathogenesis (Yang et al., 2021). Several technologies that have recently become the focus of precision medicine include antisense oligonucleotide therapy, monoclonal antibody therapy, and the most advance, is gene editing using CRISPR-Cas9.

Antisense Oligonucleotide (ASO) Therapy

ASO therapy uses short, single-stranded deoxyribonucleotides (~25 nucleotides) that are complementary and capable of hybridizing to specific mRNA sequences (Rinaldi & Wood, 2018). The therapy aims to down-regulate protein production that contributes to a disease by targeting specific RNA molecules from which the protein is translated (Yang et al., 2021). These ASO-based drugs have been used to treat several diseases, such as Etepliersen and Golodirsen for Duchene Muscular Dystrophy (DMD) (Frank et al., 2020); Nusinersen for spinal muscular atrophy (SMA), which was approved by FDA in 2016 and European Medicines Agency in 2017 (Mercuri et al., 2018); and, superoxide dismutase 1 (SOD1) RNA inhibitors, which has shown promising results to treat amyotrophic lateral sclerosis (ALS) in animal models (McCampbell et al., 2018). There are two mechanisms of ASO therapy: splicing modulation and target degradation (knockdown). These approaches are recently used to target the APOE ε4 and ε3 alleles to decrease the β-amyloid pathology in a mouse model (Huynh et al., 2017).

Monoclonal Antibody (mAb) Therapy

The development of mAb therapy is mainly to target specific epitopes of a protein, resulting in its deactivation. This is achieved by blocking the protein binding site and activating the protein degradation by recruiting the immune system (Yang et al., 2021). The therapy usually uses direct protein delivery, however, it also can be paired with virus-mediated gene transfer, such as adeno-associated vector (AAV) or lentiviral (LV) vectors (Bakker et al., 2004). This therapy has been used to treat immune-related diseases such as inflammatory diseases, autoimmune, cancer, and osteoporosis (Drewe & Powell, 2002).

In targeting the APOE gene, anti-APOE immunotherapy has been developed to inhibit the pathology of late-onset AD. A study by Kim et al., (2012) reported that passive immunisation using HJ6.3 APOE mAb has resulted 60% to 80% reduction in β-amyloid accumulation in a mouse model. The study also reported that anti-APOE antibody HJ6.3 could prevent the formation of new plaques, significantly inhibit the production of β-amyloid and improve cognitive function. Another study also reported that delivery of the anti-human APOE4 antibody (HAE-4) is consistently capable of reducing the β-amyloid pathology in an animal model by targeting the non-lipid aggregated APOE before the onset of the plaque (Liao et al., 2018).

Gene Therapy Using CRISPR-Cas9

CRISPR-Cas9 offers gene editing by removing, revising, or replacing particular gene mutations that cause disease with healthy copies of genes. This therapy is approved in precision medicine for its accuracy, and efficiency, and is highly safe for clinical purposes (Li et al., 2020). The therapy is suggested for targeting the APOE gene, especially the ε4 allele at locus 112, which edits the locus to become a "natural" allele of ε3 (Yang et al., 2021). Another study explored the use of human-induced pluripotent stem cell (hiPSC)-derived neurons characterised with ε4/ε4 genotype. It demonstrated an increase of β-amyloid production and high tau phosphorylation. Converting the genotype to a natural ε3/ε3 isoform has been found to decrease plaque production and reduce the phosphorylation of tau protein in the model (Wang et al., 2018).

Conclusion

APOE gene has strong evidence of contributing to the pathology of Alzheimer's disease with late onset symptoms. The allele ε4 of the APOE gene has strong evidence to become a major risk factor for the accumulation of β-amyloid, tau hyperphosphorylation, and other AD hallmarks. Although allele ε2 may become a preventive allele for late-onset AD, the single presence of ε4 in heterozygous genotype may disrupt the preventive functionality. In Malaysia, the presence of the ε4 allele is abundantly observed in the Malays and Bumiputeras compared with Chinese and Indians. Malay and Bumiputera populations make up the majority of the Malaysian population; hence, the high incidence of AD in these communities may become a great burden for the country's healthcare system in future. Recent technologies mentioned in this article, such as ASO therapy, mAb therapy and gene therapy using CRISPR-Cas9 can become leading preventive strategies in targeting the APOE gene to mitigate the hyperfunction of its alleles that contributes to the late onset of AD. Although statistics on Alzheimer's patients in Malaysia is still lacking, the World Alzheimer Report has predicted the number to expand by 2050. Therefore, more effort should be devoted to raising awareness on AD among the elderly and their caregivers, besides adopting a healthy lifestyle to prevent the disease.

Acknowledgments

Mohd Hazli MSH is supported by Universiti Sains Malaysia Graduate Fellowship Scheme (GFUSM) and the research for Alzheimer's disease is supported by Fundamental Research Grant Scheme (FRGS/1/2019/ SKK06/USM/02/2) from the Ministry of Higher Education Malaysia.

References

AlzGene. (2010). *Meta-analysis of all published AD association studies (case-control only) APOE_E2/3/4*. AlzGene. http://www.alzgene.org/Meta.asp?GeneID=83.

Alzheimer's Disease International. (2019). World Alzheimer Report 2019: Attitudes to dementia. In *Alzheimer's Disease International: London*.

Anand, R., Gill, K. D., & Mahdi, A. A. (2014). Therapeutics of Alzheimer's disease: Past, present and future. *Neuropharmacology*, *76*, 27–50. https://doi.org/10.1016/j.neuropharm.2013.07.004.

Bakker, J. M., Bleeker, W. K., & Parren, P. W. H. I. (2004). Therapeutic antibody gene transfer: An active approach to passive immunity. *Molecular Therapy*, *10*(3), 411–416. https://doi.org/10.1016/j.ymthe.2004.06.865.

Berman, H. M., Westbrook, J., Feng, Z., Gilliland, G., Bhat, T. N., Weissig, H., Shindyalov, I. N., & Bourne, P. E. (2000). The Protein Data Bank. *Nucleic Acids Research*, *28*, 235–242. https://doi.org/10.1093/nar/28.1.235.

Brecht, W. J., Harris, F. M., Chang, S., Tesseur, I., Yu, G. Q., Xu, Q., Fish, J. D., Wyss-Coray, T., Buttini, M., Mucke, L., Mahley, R. W., & Huang, Y. (2004). Neuron-Specific Apolipoprotein E4 Proteolysis Is Associated with Increased Tau Phosphorylation in Brains of Transgenic Mice. *Journal of Neuroscience*, *24*(10), 2527–2534. https://doi.org/10.1523/JNEUROSCI.4315-03.2004.

Copeland, J. R. M., Kelleher, M. J., Kellett, J. M., Gourlay, A. J., Gurland, B. J., Fleiss, J. L., & Sharpe, L. (1976). A semi-structured clinical interview for the assessment of diagnosis and mental state in the elderly: The geriatric mental state schedule. *Psychological Medicine*, *6*(3), 439–449. https://doi.org/10.1017/S0033291700015889.

Dong, J., Peters-Libeu, C. A., Weisgraber, K. H., Segelke, B. W., Rupp, B., Capila, I., Hernáiz, M. J., LeBrun, L. A., & Linhardt, R. J. (2001). Interaction of the N-terminal domain of apolipoprotein E4 with heparin. *Biochemistry*, *40*, 2826–2834. https://doi.org/10.1021/bi002417n.

Dong, L. M., Parkin, S., Trakhanov, S. D., Rupp, B., Simmons, T., Arnold, K. S., Newhouse, Y. M., Innerarity, T. L., & Weisgraber, K. H. (1996). Novel mechanism for defective receptor binding of apolipoprotein E2 in type III hyperlipoproteinemia. *Nature Structural Biology*, *3*(718–722). https://doi.org/10.1038/nsb0896-718.

Drewe, E., & Powell, R. J. (2002). Clinically useful monoclonal antibodies in treatment. *Journal of Clinical Pathology*, *55*(2), 81–85. https://doi.org/10.1136/jcp.55.2.81.

Foraker, J., Millard, S. P., Leong, L., Thomson, Z., Chen, S., Keene, C. D., Bekris, L. M., Yu, C. E., & Fischer, A. (2015). The APOE Gene is Differentially Methylated in Alzheimer's Disease. *Journal of Alzheimer's Disease*, *48*(3), 745–755. https://doi.org/10.3233/JAD-143060.

Frank, D. E., Schnell, F. J., Akana, C., El-Husayni, S. H., Desjardins, C. A., Morgan, J., Charleston, J. S., Sardone, V., Domingos, J., Dickson, G., Straub, V., Guglieri, M., Mercuri, E., Servais, L., & Muntoni, F. (2020). Increased dystrophin production with golodirsen in patients with Duchenne muscular dystrophy. *Neurology*, *94*(21), e2270–e2282. https://doi.org/10.1212/WNL.0000000000009233.

Genin, E., Hannequin, D., Wallon, D., Sleegers, K., Hiltunen, M., Combarros, O., Bullido, M. J., Engelborghs, S., De Deyn, P., Berr, C., Pasquier, F., Dubois, B., Tognoni, G., Fiévet, N., Brouwers, N., Bettens, K., Arosio, B., Coto, E., Del Zompo, M., Mateo, I., Epelbaum, J., Frank-Garcia, A., Helisalmi, S., Porcellini, E., Pilotto, A., Forti, P., Ferri, R., Scarpini, E., Siciliano, G., Solfrizzi, V., Sorbi, S., Spalletta, G., Valdivieso, F., Vepsäläinen, S., Alvarez, V., Bosco, P., Mancuso, M., Panza, F., Nacmias, B., Bossù, P., Hanon, O., Piccardi, P., Annoni, G., Seripa, D., Galimberti, D., Licastro, F., Soininen, H., Dartigues, J. F., Kamboh, M. I., Van Broeckhoven, C., Lambert, J. C., Amouyel, P., & Campion, D. (2011). APOE and Alzheimer disease: A major gene with semi-dominant inheritance. *Molecular Psychiatry*, *16*(9), 903–907. https://doi.org/10.1038/mp.2011.52.

Grothe, M. J., Villeneuve, S., Dyrba, M., Bartrés-Faz, D., & Wirth, M. (2017). Multimodal characterization of older APOE2 carriers reveals selective reduction of amyloid load. *Neurology*, *88*(6), 569–576. https://doi.org/10.1212/WNL.0000000000003585.

Guttman, M., Prieto, J. H., Handel, T. M., Domaille, P. J., & Komives, E. A. (2010). Structure of the minimal interface between ApoE and LRP. *Journal of Molecular Biology*, *398*(2), 306–319. https://doi.org/10.1016/j.jmb.2010.03.022.

Hamid, T. A., Krishnaswamy, S., Abdullah, S. S., & Momtaz, Y. A. (2011). Sociodemographic risk factors and correlates of dementia in older Malaysians. *Dementia and Geriatric Cognitive Disorders*, *30*(6), 533–539. https://doi.org/10.1159/000321672.

Huynh, T. P. V., Liao, F., Francis, C. M., Robinson, G. O., Serrano, J. R., Jiang, H., Roh, J., Finn, M. B., Sullivan, P. M., Esparza, T. J., Stewart, F. R., Mahan, T. E., Ulrich, J. D., Cole, T., & Holtzman, D. M. (2017). Age-Dependent Effects of apoE Reduction Using Antisense Oligonucleotides in a Model of β-amyloidosis. *Neuron*, *95*(5), 1013–1023. https://doi.org/10.1016/j.neuron.2017.11.014.

Kim, J., Eltorai, A. E. M., Jiang, H., Liao, F., Verghese, P. B., Kim, J., Stewart, F. R., Basak, J. M., & Holtzman, D. M. (2012). Anti-apoE immunotherapy inhibits amyloid accumulation in a transgenic mouse model of Aβ amyloidosis. *Journal of Experimental Medicine*, *209*(12), 2149–2156. https://doi.org/10.1084/jem.20121274.

Krishnaswamy, S., Kadir, K., Ali, R., Sidi, H., & Mathew, S. (1997). Prevalence of dementia among Malaysia in an urban settlement in Malaysia. *Neurology Journal Southeast Asia*, *2*, 154–162.

Kua, E. H. (1993). Dementia in elderly Malays--preliminary findings of a community survey. *Singapore Medical Journal*, *34*, 26–26.

Li, H., Yang, Y., Hong, W., Huang, M., Wu, M., & Zhao, X. (2020). Applications of genome editing technology in the targeted therapy of human diseases: mechanisms, advances and prospects. *Signal Transduction and Targeted Therapy*, *5*(1), 1. https://doi.org/10.1038/s41392-019-0089-y.

Liao, F., Li, A., Xiong, M., Bien-Ly, N., Jiang, H., Zhang, Y., Finn, M. B., Hoyle, R., Keyser, J., Lefton, K. B., Robinson, G. O., Serrano, J. R., Silverman, A. P., Guo, J. L., Getz, J., Henne, K., Leyns, C. E. G., Gallardo, G., Ulrich, J. D., Sullivan, P. M., Lerner, E. P., Hudry, E., Sweeney, Z. K., Dennis, M. S., Hyman, B. T., Watts, R. J., & Holtzman, D. M. (2018). Targeting of nonlipidated, aggregated apoE with antibodies inhibits amyloid accumulation. *Journal of Clinical Investigation*, *128*(5), 2144–2155. https://doi.org/10.1172/JCI96429.

Mahley, R. W. (1988). Apolipoprotein E: Cholesterol transport protein with expanding role in cell biology. *Science*, *240*(4852), 622–630. https://doi.org/10.1126/science.3283935.

Mahley, R. W., Weisgraber, K. H., & Huang, Y. (2006). Apolipoprotein E4: A causative factor and therapeutic target in neuropathology, including Alzheimer's disease. *Proceedings of the National Academy of Sciences of the United States of America*, *103*(15), 5644–5651. https://doi.org/10.1073/pnas.0600549103.

Mahley, R. W., Weisgraber, K. H., & Huang, Y. (2009). Apolipoprotein E: Structure determines function, from atherosclerosis to Alzheimer's disease to AIDS. *Journal of Lipid Research*, *50*, S183–S188. https://doi.org/10.1194/jlr.R800069-JLR200.

McCampbell, A., Cole, T., Wegener, A. J., Tomassy, G. S., Setnicka, A., Farley, B. J., Schoch, K. M., Hoye, M. L., Shabsovich, M., Sun, L., Luo, Y., Zhang, M., Thankamony, S., Salzman, D. W., Cudkowicz, M., Graham, D. L., Bennett, C. F., Kordasiewicz, H. B., Swayze, E. E., & Miller, T. M. (2018). Antisense oligonucleotides extend survival and reverse decrement in muscle response in ALS models. *Journal of Clinical Investigation*, *128*(8), 3558–3567. https://doi.org/10.1172/JCI99081.

Mercuri, E., Darras, B. T., Chiriboga, C. A., Day, J. W., Campbell, C., Connolly, A. M., Iannaccone, S. T., Kirschner, J., Kuntz, N. L., Saito, K., Shieh, P. B., Tulinius, M., Mazzone, E. S., Montes, J., Bishop, K. M., Yang, Q., Foster, R., Gheuens, S., Bennett, C. F., Farwell, W., Schneider, E., De Vivo, D. C., Finkel RS; CHERISH Study Group. (2018). Nusinersen versus Sham Control in Later-Onset Spinal Muscular Atrophy. *New England Journal of Medicine*, *378*(7), 625–635. https://doi.org/10.1056/nejmoa1710504.

Neu, S. C., Pa, J., Kukull, W., Beekly, D., Kuzma, A., Gangadharan, P., Wang, L. S., Romero, K., Arneric, S. P., Redolfi, A., Orlandi, D., Frisoni, G. B., Au, R., Devine, S., Auerbach, S., Espinosa, A., Boada, M., Ruiz, A., Johnson, S. C., Koscik, R., Wang, J. J., Hsu, W. C., Chen, Y. L., & Toga, A. W. (2017). Apolipoprotein E genotype and sex risk factors for Alzheimer disease: A meta-analysis. *JAMA Neurology*, *74*(10), 1178–1189. https://doi.org/10.1001/jamaneurol.2017.2188.

O'Brien, R. J., & Wong, P. C. (2011). Amyloid precursor protein processing and Alzheimer's disease. *Annual Review of Neuroscience*, *34*, 185–204. https://doi.org/10.1146/annurev-neuro-061010-113613.

Rinaldi, C., & Wood, M. J. A. (2018). Antisense oligonucleotides: The next frontier for treatment of neurological disorders. *Nature Reviews Neurology*, *14*(1), 9–21. https://doi.org/10.1038/nrneurol.2017.148.

Rodríguez-Martín, T., Cuchillo-Ibáñez, I., Noble, W., Nyenya, F., Anderton, B. H., & Hanger, D. P. (2013). Tau phosphorylation affects its axonal transport and degradation. *Neurobiology of Aging*, *34*(9), 2146–2157. https://doi.org/10.1016/j.neurobiolaging.2013.03.015.

Saunders, A. M., Strittmatter, W. J., Schmechel, D., George-Hyslop, P. H., Pericak-Vance, M. A., Joo, S. H., Rosi, B. L., Gusella, J. F., Crapper-MacLachlan, D. R., & Alberts, M. J. (1993). Association of apolipoprotein E allele epsilon 4 with late-onset familial and sporadic Alzheimer's disease. *Neurology*, *43*(8), 1467–1467.

Seet, W. T., Ai Mary Anne, T. J., & Yen, T. S. (2004). Apolipoprotein e genotyping in the Malay, Chinese and Indian ethnic groups in Malaysia - A study on the distribution of the different apoE alleles and genotypes. *Clinica Chimica Acta*, *340*(1–2), 201–205. https://doi.org/10.1016/j.cccn.2003.11.001.

Segelke, B. W., Forstner, M., Knapp, M., Trakhanov, S. D., Parkin, S., Newhouse, Y. M., Bellamy, H. D., Weisgraber, K. H., & Rupp, B. (2000). Conformational flexibility in the apolipoprotein E amino-terminal domain structure determined from three new crystal forms: Implications for lipid binding. *Protein Science*, *9*(5), 886–897. https://doi.org/10.1110/ps.9.5.886.

Sehnal, D., Bittrich, S., Deshpande, M., Svobodová, R., Berka, K., Bazgier, V., Velankar, S., Burley, S. K., Koča, J., & Rose, A. S. (2021). Mol*Viewer: Modern web app for 3D visualization and analysis of large biomolecular structures. *Nucleic Acids Research*, *49*(W1), W431–W437. https://doi.org/10.1093/nar/gkab314.

Tiraboschi, P., Hansen, L. A., Masliah, E., Alford, M., Thal, L. J., & Corey-Bloom, J. (2004). Impact of APOE genotype on neuropathologic and neurochemical markers of Alzheimer disease. *Neurology*, *62*(11), 1977–1983. https://doi.org/10.1212/01.WNL.0000128091.92139.0F.

Wang, C., Najm, R., Xu, Q., Jeong, D. E., Walker, D., Balestra, M. E., Yoon, S. Y., Yuan, H., Li, G., Miller, Z. A., Miller, B. L., Malloy, M. J., & Huang, Y. (2018). Gain of toxic apolipoprotein E4 effects in human iPSC-derived neurons is ameliorated by a small-molecule structure corrector article. *Nature Medicine*, *24*(5), 647–657. https://doi.org/10.1038/s41591-018-0004-z.

World Health Organisation. (2017). Global action plan on the public health response to dementia 2017 - 2025. *Geneva: World Health Organization.*

Yamazaki, Y., Zhao, N., Caulfield, T. R., Liu, C. C., & Bu, G. (2019). Apolipoprotein E and Alzheimer disease: pathobiology and targeting strategies. *Nature Reviews Neurology*, *15*(9), 501–518. https://doi.org/10.1038/s41582-019-0228-7.

Yang, A., Kantor, B., & Chiba-Falek, O. (2021). APOE: The new frontier in the development of a therapeutic target towards precision medicine in late-onset alzheimer's. *International Journal of Molecular Sciences*, *22*(3), 1244. https://doi.org/10.3390/ijms22031244.

Zannis, V. I., Breslow, J. L., Utermann, G., Mahley, R. W., Weisgraber, K. H., Havel, R. J., Goldstein, J. L., Brown, M. S., Schonfeld, G., Hazzard, W. R., & Blum, C. (1982). Proposed nomenclature of apoE isoproteins, apoE genotypes, and phenotypes. *Journal of Lipid Research*, *23*(6), 911–914. https://doi.org/10.1016/s0022-2275(20)38094-9.

Chapter 4

Brain-Derived Neurotrophic Factor (BDNF) *VAL66MET* Gene Polymorphism in Alzheimer's and Parkinson's Diseases

Noor Azila Ismail
Rohayu Hami
Mohammad Farris Iman Leong Abdullah
and Hazwani Ahmad Yusof Hanafi*
Department of Community Health, Advanced Medical and Dental Institute, Universiti Sains Malaysia, Kepala Batas, Pulau Pinang, Malaysia

Abstract

The percentage of elderly people in Malaysia is expected to increase almost three-fold in 2040 to about 14.5% of the total population. With an ageing population, dementia becomes an important health issue to address in Malaysia and across the world. Mild cognitive impairment (MCI) is the prodromic stage of dementia, whereby about 10 to 54% of patients will progress into advanced stages of the condition, and about 10 to15% will further develop Alzheimer's disease (AD) annually. Currently, no curative treatments are available for this neurodegenerative condition, hence strategies to prevent and delay the progression of MCI to dementia, AD or Parkinson's disease (PD) need to be examined and implemented. Exercise is a non-pharmacological therapy considered helpful in the prevention of MCI and to decelerate its progression to AD. Potential neurobiological mechanisms include exercise-induced exerkines, such as brain-derived neurotrophic factor (BDNF), which

* Corresponding Author's Email: hazwanihanafi@usm.my.

In: Genetic Disorders and Rare Diseases
Editors: Shazlin Shaharudin, Hisham Atan Edinur and Nor Fazila Che Mat
ISBN: 979-8-88697-953-4

plays a role in maintaining cerebral plasticity, neurogenesis, and angiogenesis, besides making the brain more resistant to structural and functional degeneration. The functional BNDF is believed to be affected by gene polymorphisms, such as *BDNF Val66Met* that causes a substitution of valine to methionine in the pro-region part related to the probability and prevalence of various neurological disorders. This chapter discusses the present state of understanding on the impact of the *BDNF Val66Met* gene polymorphism in neurological disorders, with emphasis on AD and PD.

Keywords: ageing, cognitive, neurodegenerative, dementia

Introduction

Neurological disorders have become a major and increasing concern, affecting approximately 450 million individuals worldwide (Ventriglia et al., 2013). It is characterised by a slow and steady decline in neuronal functions, which may eventually lead to complete neuronal death. This condition frequently leads to progressive functional, and behavioural changes, which manifest as dysfunctional motor and cognitive deficits. Neurological disorders are a global socioeconomic burden. The likelihood of developing a disease rises exponentially over time (Hou et al., 2019). Consequently, the number of affected individuals is expected to rise as the population ages, forcing the establishment of effective treatments capable of preventing or halting the deterioration process. Neurological disorders have complex and diverse disorders with numerous risk factors, treatments, causes and consequences. As a result of the extensive study undertaken by professionals from a number of clinical disciplines, numerous correlations and overlaps have been uncovered with the genetic components of the disease mechanisms, such as vulnerability and variables that contribute to the expression of phenotypic, and genetic inheritance, becoming an increasing interest to the researchers (Balaratnasingam & Janca, 2012).

Recently, there is burgeoning evidence that alterations in signalling and expression of brain-derived neurotrophic factor (BDNF) may contribute to neurodegeneration (Giacobbo et al., 2019). BDNF is a member of the protein family known as neurotrophins and is coded by the *BDNF Val66Met* gene that is crucial for maintaining synaptic plasticity and neuronal survival in the adult brain, in addition to appropriate functioning of the central and peripheral nervous systems (Giacobbo et al., 2019). Altered BDNF functioning has been linked to several neurological diseases, such as dementia (Giacobbo et al., 2019). This chapter intends to highlight the significance of BDNF protein and *BDNF Val66Met* gene polymorphism that expresses different variants of this protein in relation to the development and clinical manifestations dementia, especially Alzheimer's (AD) and Parkinson's disease (PD).

Brain-Derived Neurotrophic Factor (BDNF) Gene and Protein

BDNF is a neurotrophin (NT) that was originally identified in 1982 by Barde et al. (1982). It is a member of the NT family of growth factors, which are crucial for regulating the survival, maintenance, and development of neurons (Urbina-Varela et al., 2020). The gene that encodes for BDNF protein is found on the short arm of chromosome 11 (p14.1) (Figure 1) (Urbina-Varela et al., 2020). BDNF is synthesised in the endoplasmic reticulum in the form of a 32-35 kDa precursor protein (pro-BDNF) and transported through the Golgi and trans-Golgi networks (Bathina & Das, 2015). It is then cleaved either intracellularly or extracellularly, and a mature BDNF (mBDNF) protein is formed (Brigadski & Leßmann, 2020; Colucci-D'amato et al., 2020). In human brain, these two variants of BDNF (pro-BDNF and mBDNF) have been shown to exist (Miranda et al., 2019). Dysregulation of BDNF has been associated with greater susceptibility to neurodegenerative diseases (Shen et al., 2018).

A common variant known as single-nucleotide polymorphism (SNP) has been discovered in the human BDNF gene. This variant causes a change in the gene's protein-coding sequence from G to A at nucleotide position 196, which in turn, causes a change in the amino acid sequence from valine to methionine at location 66 (e.g., *Val66Met*) as in the BDNF protein's pro-domain (Faris et al., 2020). This *Met* variant of BDNF carriers, namely BDNF *Val/Met* and *Met/Met*, have an altered pro-domain structure of the gene. This polymorphism can cause BDNF proteins to fold abnormally and make it harder for mBDNF to bind to its receptor tyrosine receptor kinase B (TrkB), which is observed to impair the function of the hippocampus (Egan et al., 2003). This polymorphism may result to deficiencies in hippocampus function even though it does not impact the mBDNF protein's intrinsic biological functioning (Egan et al., 2003). Furthermore, neuronal activity-dependent of BDNF secretion is inhibited by the changes in Met for Val substitution (Egan et al., 2003). Numerous genetic investigations on the effects of this *BDNF Val66Met* gene polymorphism on brain activity and behaviour, notably in neurological illnesses, have been undertaken over the past 15 years due to the significance of BDNF in neuron control (De Meo et al., 2021; Giordano et al., 2022; Miyajima et al., 2008). Figure 1 illustrates the conceptual framework on how *BDNF Val66Met* gene polymorphism affects neuro-cognitive function.

The *BDNF* gene is found on chromosome 11 at position 14.1. The *Val* allele codes to produce the normal pro-BDNF protein, and the *Met* allele will encode an altered form that binds to the p75 neurotrophin receptor ($p75^{NTR}$), which has a low affinity for BDNF and is not converted to mBDNF, causing the production of proteins linked to apoptosis and cell death. As mature mBDNF interacts with TrkB, this will promote synaptic plasticity, neuronal survival and cognitive level maintenance.

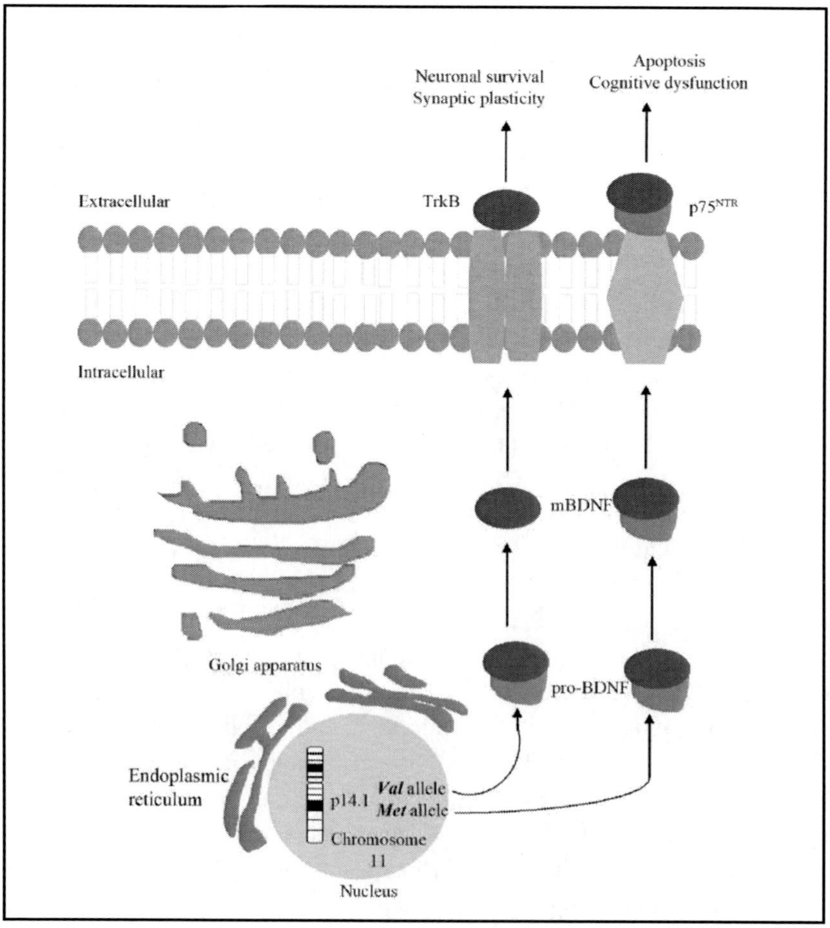

Figure 1. *BDNF Val66Met* gene polymorphism affecting neuro-cognitive function.

The Role of *BDNF VAL66MET* Gene Polymorphism in Neurological Disorders

As neurotrophins are crucial for survival, growth, function and regeneration of neurons, gene variations that encode these proteins may lead to certain l vulnerabilities in neurological conditions (Colardo et al., 2021). mBNDF produced by the gene with a *Met* allele has been predicted to hinder synaptic localisation and intracellular trafficking, as well as substantially lowering the activity-dependent secretion of the protein up to 30%, yet having no effect on its constitutive secretion (Egan et al., 2003). However, genetic association studies showed conflicting outcomes in the concentration of BDNF serum levels in *Met* carriers, which are either greater (Caldieraro et al., 2017; Elzinga et al., 2011), lower (Zhen et al., 2017) or equal (Duncan et al., 2009; Maria De Araujo et al., 2019) than non-carriers. Possible explanations for the conflicting findings include differences in psychopathology, gender and ethnicity (Bus et al., 2012).

In healthy human subjects, BDNF *Val66Met* gene polymorphism has been observed to have deleterious effects on the morphology of both the prefrontal cortex and hippocampus as determined using magnetic resonance imaging (MRI). *Met* carriers had a significant bilateral reduction in hippocampal grey matter sizes in contrast with *Val* homozygotes (*Val/Val*), indicating that functional diversity in multiple brain regions associated with memory and learning may have a moderating impact (Jasińska et al., 2017). Intriguingly, the *Val/Val* carriers, who initially outscored the *Met* carriers on cognitive function tests, showed a significant decline in performance a decade later, as determined by a longitudinal research (Erickson et al., 2008). Such result is in line to some extent with a recent research showing how *Met* homozygotes (*Met/Met*) perform better with age, suggesting that the impact of BDNF upon cognitive performance may vary across the lifespan of an individual, as well as the *Met* allele conferring neuronal protection in old age (Harris et al., 2006). Hence, *BDNF Val66Met* polymorphism may have an impact in human development, as a previous research revealed beneficial effects of *Met/Met* on grey matter volume in healthy Japanese adolescents and children (Hashimoto et al., 2016). The effect of *BDNF Val66Met* polymorphism in modifying cognition and memory in AD and PD are discussed in the next section to provide a better understanding of the effects of this variant on neuron deterioration related to ageing.

BDNF VAL66MET Gene Polymorphism and Alzheimer's Disease

AD is a progressive form of dementia caused by irreversible neurodegeneration accompanied by a set of unique pathological abnormalities. The condition is characterised by the accumulation of beta amyloid (Aβ) as well as hyperphosphorylated Tau protein plaques in the brain and neurofibrillary tangles, which are responsible for behavioural dysfunction, loss of memory and cognitive decline (Abeysinghe et al., 2020). Up to 2006, 26.6 million people around the world have been reported to have AD and by 2050, the estimated number of people living with the disease is expected to triple up to 106 million (Thakur et al., 2018). However, apart from extensive drug developments and studies to reverse the condition, no viable treatment or medication to slow or stop the progression of AD have been found (Gong et al., 2022).

Genetic screening is currently used to diagnose and identify patients at an early stage, especially for those who are at a greater risk of AD, and a risk profile would permit future individualised treatments. Several missense gene variants that significantly increase the susceptibility to AD have been identified. Examples include those encoding for the amyloid precursor protein presenilin 1 and presenilin 2, where mutations are found in early-onset familial AD (Dai et al., 2018). Being more common than very rare mutations in the amyloid precursor protein gene, mutations in the presenilin genes may result in familial AD (Lanoiselée et al., 2017). Meanwhile, a study by Di Battista et al. (2016) reported that the greatest genetic risk of AD is associated with allele variation of the apolipoprotein E (*APOE*) gene. Nevertheless, AD is a genetically complicated condition, and the genes described above cannot entirely explain why some people are more susceptible to developing the disease than others. This suggests that the various AD subtypes may be affected by multiple gene alterations and interactions.

The pathophysiology of AD may involve alterations of the *BDNF* gene. The *BDNF Val66Met* variant has a different impact on males and females when it comes to the onset of AD, as shown in a large-sample meta-analysis using 4,711 patients and 4,537 controls (Fukumoto et al., 2010). The study reported that male carriers of the *Met* allele had a lower risk than female carriers in developing AD. Besides, female carriers of *BDNF Val* were also associated with a lower risk of developing AD and a slower disease progression in a Chinese population-based study (Bian et al., 2005). This suggests that the *BDNF Met* allele might have an influence in the progression of the disorder, as it was also found to be common in AD individuals than in cognitively normal controls in case-control research of a Japanese community (Vepsäläinen et al., 2005). In addition, prodromal AD patients who have elevated initial Aβ levels may benefit from *BDNF Val66Met* gene polymorphism since it slows the progression of hippocampus atrophy and memory loss (Lim et al., 2014). When comparing *Val/Val* genotype to *Met* carriers with amnestic mild cognitive impairment (aMCI) and high Aβ density, the latter showed considerably greater rates of hippocampus shrinkage and faster episodic memory deterioration (Lim et al., 2014). In spite of these findings, this variant did not affect the pace of Aβ deposition, suggesting that it may expedite neurodegeneration and memory impairment through impacting signalling pathways like tau aggregation (Lim et al., 2014). Similarly, healthy *BDNF Met* carriers with increased Aβ levels also showed a marked decrease in hippocampus volume and memory (Lim et al., 2013).

Preclinical autosomal dominant Alzheimer's disease (ADAD) mutation carriers carrying *Met* alleles were also reported to be more vulnerable to the negative impacts of Aβ on hippocampal function, tau and episodic memory (Lim et al., 2016). In addition, according to preliminary research by Ventrigalia et al. (2002), individuals with two copies of the *Val* allele are at a higher likelihood of developing AD. This is because the homozygous *Val* allele frequency was higher in AD patients than in controls. On the other hand, in Chinese (Tsai et al., 2004), Japanese (Nishimura et al., 2005), Spanish (Combarros et al., 2004), Finnish (Vepsäläinen et al., 2005), American (Bodner et al., 2005) and Italian (Bagnoli et al., 2004) populations, such polymorphism was not observed to be related to the risk of late-onset AD. Nevertheless, there was no association between the *BDNF Val66Met* variation and the lower levels of BDNF protein in the temporal neocortex of AD patients' brain (Lee et al., 2005). These contradicting data show that the *BDNF Val66Met* polymorphism may only affect AD with an early onset instead of a late onset. However, it must be validated in larger population studies as the mentioned studies had sample sizes ranging from 163 to 256 patients only, indicating a lack of statistical power that may have contributed to the ambiguous results.

BDNF VAL66MET Polymorphism and Parkinson's Disease

Parkinson's Disease (PD) is regarded as the second most severe form of neurological disorder after AD. This neurological disorder is a result of the death of dopaminergic neurons located in the substantia nigra of the brain, as well as the development of Lewy bodies (Kouli et al., 2018). However, multiple investigations have pointed to a complicated interaction between environmental and genetic variables as a possible cause and other neurological diseases with non-mendelian inheritance (Warner et al., 2003). In an early post-mortem human trial, BDNF mRNA expression was found to be significantly lower among PD substantia nigra pars compacta (SNpc) neurons versus control. However, this difference might be attributable in partiality towards the reduction of SNpc dopaminergic neurons that secrete BDNF. Besides, patients with PD had low BDNF expression in their SNpc surviving dopaminergic neurons compared with healthy controls, suggesting that BDNF deficit may lead to the reduction of nigral dopaminergic neurons and promote the progression of PD (Palasz et al., 2020). It was also discovered that people with PD had reduced levels of BDNF in their serum. The lower BDNF levels in the initial stages of the disease could be useful for early diagnosis of the disease, and increasing BDNF concentrations in blood was a potential therapy (He et al., 2018).

Recent finding reveals that the *BDNF Val66Met* variant may influence the incidence of PD or its clinical progression. Observational studies of 20 target gene SNPs for PD found that the frequency of the *Met/Met* genotype was greater in PD patients than healthy controls (Momose et al., 2002). Furthermore, there was a 5.3-year difference in onset between *Met/Met* and B *Val/Val* in a United Kingdom study (Karamohamed et al., 2005). According to Altmann et al. (2016) presence of the *Met* allele was related to greater likelihood of cognitive deficits in PD patients, suggesting that polymorphism could serve as a significant predictor for cognitive impairment in PD. Foltynie and colleagues (2009) reported that patients with PD who had one or two *Met* alleles were more likely to experience levodopa-induced dyskinesia following therapy with a dopaminergic medication. Furthermore, there was indication that *BDNF* genotypes could significantly affect the planning overall performance outcomes of the Tower of London test in PD patients, even after controlling several probable potential variables. However, the significant improvement in *Met* carriers was observed substantially in female participants only (Thomas Foltynie et al., 2005).

Met carriers with PD have considerably lower loss in set switching, which is a cognitive flexibility that involves the ability to shift concentration throughout tasks across a two-year follow-up examination, showing a potential favourable impact of the *Met* allele on mental ability (van der Kolk et al., 2015). Conversely, previous studies have revealed no relationship involving *Val66Met* with neither the probability nor clinical progression of PD (Białecka et al., 2014; Gao et al., 2010; Karakasis et al., 2011). PD is a complicated neurodegenerative disorder with multiple pathophysiology. Hence, small to substantial involvement of *BDNF Val66Met* polymorphism in conjunction with other genetic or environmental variables cannot be ruled out in specific patients. The relationship between *BDNF Val66Met* polymorphism with PD remains uncertain though, necessitating more data from population-based studies.

Conclusion

Neurological disorders impose a significant socioeconomic burden on individuals and society. Understanding the underlying molecular and cellular pathogenic processes is crucial, since there are currently no promising treatments available to prevent and reverse this deteriorating state. In this chapter, we discuss the potential role of *BDNF Val66Met* polymorphism in neurological disorders, with particularly emphasis on AD and PD. There are inconsistent and limited data to support the association of this variant with the discussed diseases that warrants larger and concrete future study. The main rationale of investigating *BDNF Val66Met* polymorphism is the beneficial focus in gaining information on disease pathophysiology and therapies. The results so far suggest that it has a homeostatic function in the regulation of appetite, as well as memory, emotion, perceptions, sensory and motor systems. This is because BDNF has substantial influence on both neuronal and non-neuronal cell proliferation, differentiation, survival, and death, making it critical to the nervous system's health and well-being. Besides, the interaction between environmental stress and gene expression also seems to be mediated by the gene.

It is also crucial to investigate whether *BDNF Val66Met* polymorphism may impact the phenotypes and neurons in people who are otherwise healthy, as well as the possible consequences that come with advancing age. Given that there is evidence associating this variant to late onset of AD (Egan et al., 2003), decline in executive and reasoning ability with ageing (Erickson et al.,

2008; Harris et al., 2006), and also impaired cognitive ability in the elderly (Miyajima et al., 2008), ageing then becomes a factor that increases the risk of neurological illnesses and can intensify the consequences of the gene's polymorphism. *Met* allele carriers have been shown to be at higher risk for AD in early adulthood, whereas *Val* homozygotes were prone to AD later in life (Voineskos et al., 2011).

Therefore, it is essential to investigate whether the *BDNF Val66Met* polymorphism controls long-term neurodegeneration in an age-dependent manner, since this could lead the way for the establishment of new treatment strategies for the vulnerable groups. Hence, the presence of *BDNF Val66Met* polymorphism may serve as potential prognostic or diagnostic markers, contribute to treatment planning and facilitate early diagnosis evaluation of treatment efficacy using novel medications.

Acknowledgment

The study is supported by the Malaysian Higher Education Ministry through the Fundamental Research Grant Scheme (Project Code: FRGS/1/2019/SKK05/USM/03/2).

References

Abeysinghe, A. A. D. T., Deshapriya, R. D. U. S., & Udawatte, C. (2020). Alzheimer's disease; a review of the pathophysiological basis and therapeutic interventions. *Life Sciences*, *256*, 117996. https://doi.org/10.1016/J.LFS.2020.117996.

Altmann, V., Schumacher-Schuh, A. F., Rieck, M., Callegari-Jacques, S. M., Rieder, C. R. M., & Hutz, M. H. (2016). Val66Met BDNF polymorphism is associated with Parkinson's disease cognitive impairment. *Neuroscience Letters*, *615*, 88–91. https://doi.org/10.1016/J.NEULET.2016.01.030.

Bagnoli, S., Nacmias, B., Tedde, A., Guarnieri, B. M., Cellini, E., Petruzzi, C., Bartoli, A., Ortenzi, L., & Sorbi, S. (2004). Brain-derived neurotrophic factor genetic variants are not susceptibility factors to Alzheimer's disease in Italy. *Annals of Neurology*, *55*(3), 447–448. https://doi.org/10.1002/ANA.10842.

Balaratnasingam, S., & Janca, A. (2012). Brain Derived Neurotrophic Factor: A novel neurotrophin involved in psychiatric and neurological disorders. In *Pharmacology and Therapeutics* (Vol. 134, Issue 1, pp. 116–124). Elsevier B.V. https://doi.org/10.1016/j.pharmthera.2012.01.006.

Barde, Y. A., Edgar, D., & Thoenen, H. (1982). Purification of a new neurotrophic factor from mammalian brain. *The EMBO Journal*, *1*(5), 549. https://doi.org/10.1002/J.1460-2075.1982.TB01207.X.

Bathina, S., & Das, U. N. (2015). Brain-derived neurotrophic factor and its clinical Implications. *Archives of Medical Science*, *11*(6), 1164–1178. https://doi.org/10.5114/aoms.2015.56342.

Bhang, S., Ahn, J. H., & Choi, S. W. (2011). Brain-derived neurotrophic factor and serotonin transporter gene-linked promoter region genes alter serum levels of brain-derived neurotrophic factor in humans. *Journal of Affective Disorders*, *128*(3), 299–304. https://doi.org/10.1016/J.JAD.2010.07.008.

Białecka, M., Kurzawski, M., Roszmann, A., Robowski, P., Sitek, E. J., Honczarenko, K., Mak, M., Deptuła-Jarosz, M., Gołab-Janowska, M., Droździk, M., & Sławek, J. (2014). BDNF G196A (Val66Met) polymorphism associated with cognitive impairment in Parkinson's disease. *Neuroscience Letters*, *561*, 86–90. https://doi.org/10.1016/J.NEULET.2013.12.051.

Bian, J. T., Zhang, J. W., Zhang, Z. X., & Zhao, H. L. (2005). Association analysis of brain-derived neurotrophic factor (BDNF) gene 196 A/G polymorphism with Alzheimer's disease (AD) in mainland Chinese. *Neuroscience Letters*, *387*(1), 11–16. https://doi.org/10.1016/J.NEULET.2005.07.009.

Bodner, S. M., Berrettini, W., Van Deerlin, V., Bennett, D. A., Wilson, R. S., Trojanowski, J. Q., & Arnold, S. E. (2005). Genetic variation in the brain derived neurotrophic factor gene in Alzheimer's disease. *American Journal of Medical Genetics. Part B, Neuropsychiatric Genetics: The Official Publication of the International Society of Psychiatric Genetics*, *134B*(1), 1–5. https://doi.org/10.1002/AJMG.B.30154.

Brigadski, T., & Leßmann, V. (2020). The physiology of regulated BDNF release. *Cell and Tissue Research 2020 382:1*, *382*(1), 15–45. https://doi.org/10.1007/S00441-020-03253-2.

Bus, B. A. A., Arias-Vasquez, A., Franke, B., Prickaerts, J., De Graaf, J., & Voshaar, R. C. O. (2012). Increase in serum brain-derived neurotrophic factor in met allele carriers of the BDNF Val66Met polymorphism is specific to males. *Neuropsychobiology*, *65*(4), 183–187. https://doi.org/10.1159/000336997.

Caldieraro, M. A., McKee, M., Leistner-Segal, S., Vares, E. A., Kubaski, F., Spanemberg, L., Brusius-Facchin, A. C., Fleck, M. P., & Mischoulon, D. (2017). Val66Met polymorphism association with serum BDNF and inflammatory biomarkers in major depression. *World J Biol Psychiatry,* *19*(5), 402–409. https://doi.org/10.1080/15622975.2017.1347713.

Colardo, M., Martella, N., Pensabene, D., Siteni, S., Di Bartolomeo, S., Pallottini, V., & Segatto, M. (2021). Neurotrophins as key regulators of cell metabolism: implications for cholesterol homeostasis. *International Journal of Molecular Sciences*, *22*(11). https://doi.org/10.3390/IJMS22115692.

Colucci-D'amato, L., Speranza, L., & Volpicelli, F. (2020). Neurotrophic factor BDNF, physiological functions and therapeutic potential in depression, neurodegeneration and brain cancer. *International Journal of Molecular Sciences, 21*(20), 7777. https://doi.org/10.3390/IJMS21207777.

Combarros, O., Infante, J., Llorca, J., & Berciano, J. (2004). Polymorphism at codon 66 of the brain-derived neurotrophic factor gene is not associated with sporadic Alzheimer's disease. *Dementia and Geriatric Cognitive Disorders*, *18*(1), 55–58. https://doi.org/10.1159/000077736.

Dai, M. H., Zheng, H., Zeng, L. D., & Zhang, Y. (2018). The genes associated with early-onset Alzheimer's disease. *Oncotarget*, *9*(19), 15132. https://doi.org/10.18632/ONCOTARGET.23738.

De Meo, E., Portaccio, E., Prestipino, E., Nacmias, B., Bagnoli, S., Razzolini, L., Pastò, L., Niccolai, C., Goretti, B., Bellinvia, A., Fonderico, M., Giorgio, A., Stromillo, M. L., Filippi, M., Sorbi, S., De Stefano, N., & Amato, M. P. (2021). Effect of BDNF Val66Met polymorphism on hippocampal subfields in multiple sclerosis patients. *Molecular Psychiatry*, *27*(2), 1010–1019. https://doi.org/10.1038/s41380-021-01345-1.

de Araujo, C. M., Swardfager, W., Zugman, A., Cogo-Moreira, H., Belangero, S. I., Ota, V. K., Spindola, L. M., Hakonarson, H., Pellegrino, R., Gadelha, A., Salum, G. A., Pan, P. M., Mansur, R. B., Hoexter, M., Picon, F., Sato, J. R., Brietzke, E., Grassi-Oliveira, R., Rohde, L. A. P., Miguel, E. C., Bressan, R. A., & Jackowski, A. P. (2020). Are serum brain-derived neurotrophic factor concentrations related to brain structure and psychopathology in late childhood and early adolescence? *CNS Spectr,* 25(6),790-796. https://doi.10.1017/S1092852919001688.

Di Battista, A. M., Heinsinger, N. M., & Rebeck, G. W. (2016). Alzheimer's Disease genetic risk factor APOE-ε4 also affects normal brain function. *Curr Alzheimer Res,* 13(11),1200-1207. https://doi.10.2174/1567205013666160401115127.

Duncan, L. E., Hutchison, K. E., Carey, G., & Craighead, W. E. (2009). Variation in Brain-Derived Neurotrophic Factor (BDNF) Gene is associated with symptoms of depression. *Journal of Affective Disorders*, *115*(1–2), 215. https://doi.org/10.1016/J.JAD.2008.08.016.

Egan, M. F., Kojima, M., Callicott, J. H., Goldberg, T. E., Kolachana, B. S., Bertolino, A., Zaitsev, E., Gold, B., Goldman, D., Dean, M., Lu, B., & Weinberger, D. R. (2003). The BDNF val66met polymorphism affects activity-dependent secretion of BDNF and human memory and hippocampal function. *Cell*, *112*(2), 257–269. https://doi.org/10.1016/S0092-8674(03)00035-7.

Elzinga, B. M., Molendijk, M. L., Oude Voshaar, R. C., Bus, B. A. A., Prickaerts, J., Spinhoven, P., & Penninx, B. J. W. H. (2011). The impact of childhood abuse and recent stress on serum brain-derived neurotrophic factor and the moderating role of BDNF Val66Met. *Psychopharmacology*, *214*(1), 319. https://doi.org/10.1007/S00213-010-1961-1.

Erickson, K. I., Kim, J. S., Suever, B. L., Voss, M. W., Francis, B. M., & Kramer, A. F. (2008). Genetic contributions to age-related decline in executive function: a 10-year longitudinal study of COMT and BDNF polymorphisms. *Frontiers in Human Neuroscience*, *2*(SEP). https://doi.org/10.3389/NEURO.09.011.2008.

Faris, A., Cheah, P., & Ling, K. (2020). Single nucleotide polymorphism of BDNF Val66Met (rs6265) and its association to neuropsychiatric disorders. *Neuroscience Research Notes*, *3*(3), 23. https://doi.org/10.31117/neuroscirn.v3i3.50.

Foltynie, T., Cheeran, B., Williams-Gray, C. H., Edwards, M. J., Schneider, S. A., Weinberger, D., Rothwell, J. C., Barker, R. A., & Bhatia, K. P. (2009). BDNF val66met influences time to onset of levodopa induced dyskinesia in Parkinson's disease. *Journal of Neurology, Neurosurgery, and Psychiatry*, *80*(2), 141–144. https://doi.org/10.1136/JNNP.2008.154294.

Foltynie, Thomas, Lewis, S. G. J., Goldberg, T. E., Blackwell, A. S., Kolachana, B. S., Weinberger, D. R., Robbins, T. W., & Barker, R. A. (2005). The BDNF Val66Met polymorphism has a gender specific influence on planning ability in Parkinson's disease. *Journal of Neurology*, *252*(7), 833–838. https://doi.org/10.1007/S00415-005-0756-5.

Fukumoto, N., Fujii, T., Combarros, O., Kamboh, M. I., Tsai, S. J., Matsushita, S., Nacmias, B., Comings, D. E., Arboleda, H., Ingelsson, M., Hyman, B. T., Akatsu, H., Grupe, A., Nishimura, A. L., Zatz, M., Mattila, K. M., Rinne, J., Goto, Y. I., Asada, T., Nakamura, S., & Kunugi, H. (2010). Sexually dimorphic effect of the Val66Met polymorphism of BDNF on susceptibility to Alzheimer's disease: New data and meta-analysis. *American Journal of Medical Genetics. Part B, Neuropsychiatric Genetics*, *153B*(1), 235–242. https://doi.org/10.1002/AJMG.B.30986.

Gao, L., Díaz-Corrales, F. J., Carrillo, F., Díaz-Martín, J., Caceres-Redondo, M. T., Carballo, M., Palomino, A., López-Barneo, J., & Mir, P. (2010). Brain-derived neurotrophic factor G196A polymorphism and clinical features in Parkinson's disease. *Acta Neurologica Scandinavica*, *122*(1), 41–45. https://doi.org/10.1111/J.1600-0404.2009.01253.X.

Giordano, A., Clarelli, F., Cannizzaro, M., Mascia, E., Santoro, S., Sorosina, M., Ferrè, L., Leocani, L., & Esposito, F. (2022). BDNF Val66Met polymorphism is associated with motor recovery after rehabilitation in progressive multiple sclerosis patients. *Frontiers in Neurology*, *13*, 790360. https://doi.org/10.3389/FNEUR.2022.790360/FULL.

Gong, C. X., Dai, C. L., Liu, F., & Iqbal, K. (2022). Multi-targets: an unconventional drug development strategy for Alzheimer's Disease. *Frontiers in Aging Neuroscience*, *14*, 86. https://doi.org/10.3389/FNAGI.2022.837649/BIBTEX.

Harris, S. E., Fox, H., Wright, A. F., Hayward, C., Starr, J. M., Whalley, L. J., & Deary, I. J. (2006). The brain-derived neurotrophic factor Val66Met polymorphism is associated with age-related change in reasoning skills. *Molecular Psychiatry*, *11*(5), 505–513. https://doi.org/10.1038/SJ.MP.4001799.

Hashimoto, T., Fukui, K., Takeuchi, H., Yokota, S., Kikuchi, Y., Tomita, H., Taki, Y., & Kawashima, R. (2016). Effects of the BDNF Val66Met polymorphism on gray matter volume in typically developing children and adolescents. *Cerebral Cortex (New York, NY)*, *26*(4), 1795. https://doi.org/10.1093/CERCOR/BHW020.

He, R., Yan, X., Guo, J., Xu, Q., Tang, B., & Sun, Q. (2018). Recent advances in biomarkers for Parkinson's disease. *Frontiers in Aging Neuroscience*, *10*(OCT), 305. https://doi.org/10.3389/FNAGI.2018.00305/BIBTEX.

Hou, Y., Dan, X., Babbar, M., Wei, Y., Hasselbalch, S. G., Croteau, D. L., & Bohr, V. A. (2019). Ageing as a risk factor for neurodegenerative disease. *Nature Reviews Neurology 2019 15:10*, *15*(10), 565–581. https://doi.org/10.1038/s41582-019-0244-7.

Jasińska, K. K., Molfese, P. J., Kornilov, S. A., Mencl, W. E., Frost, S. J., Lee, M., Pugh, K. R., Grigorenko, E. L., & Landi, N. (2017). The BDNF Val66Met polymorphism is associated with structural neuroanatomical differences in young children. *Behavioural Brain Research*, *328*, 48–56. https://doi.org/10.1016/J.BBR.2017.03.014.

Karakasis, C., Kalinderi, K., Katsarou, Z., Fidani, L., & Bostantjopoulou, S. (2011). Association of brain-derived neurotrophic factor (BDNF) Val66Met polymorphism with Parkinson's disease in a Greek population. *Journal of Clinical Neuroscience*, *18*(12), 1744–1745. https://doi.org/10.1016/J.JOCN.2011.03.015.

Karamohamed, S., Latourelle, J. C., Racette, B. A., Perlmutter, J. S., Wooten, G. F., Lew, M., Klein, C., Shill, H., Golbe, L. I., Mark, M. H., Guttman, M., Nicholson, G., Wilk, J. B., Saint-Hilaire, M., DeStefano, A. L., Prakash, R., Tobin, S., Williamson, J., Suchowersky, O., Labell, N., Growdon, B. N. J., Singer, C., Watts, R., Goldwurm, S., Pezzoli, G., Baker, K. B., Giroux, M. L., Pramstaller, P. P., Burm, D. J., Chinnery, P., Sherman, S., Vieregge, P., Litvan, I., Gusella, J. F., Myers, R. H. & Parsian, A. (2005). BDNF genetic variants are associated with onset age of familial Parkinson disease: GenePD Study. *Neurology*, *65*(11), 1823–1825. https://doi.org/10.1212/01.WNL.0000187075.81589.FD.

Kouli, A., Torsney, K. M., & Kuan, W.-L. (2018). Parkinson's Disease: etiology, neuropathology, and pathogenesis. *Parkinson's Disease: Pathogenesis and Clinical Aspects*, 3–26. https://doi.org/10.15586/CODONPUBLICATIONS.PARKINSONSDISEASE.2018.CH1.

Kumar Thakur, A., Kamboj, P., Goswami, K., & Ahuja, K. (2018). Pathophysiology and management of Alzheimer's Disease: an overview. *Journal of Analytical & Pharmaceutical Research*, *Volume 7*(Issue 2). https://doi.org/10.15406/JAPLR.2018.07.00230.

Lanoiselée, H. M., Nicolas, G., Wallon, D., Rovelet-Lecrux, A., Lacour, M., Rousseau, S., Richard, A. C., Pasquier, F., Rollin-Sillaire, A., Martinaud, O., Quillard-Muraine, M., de la Sayette, V., Boutoleau-Bretonniere, C., Etcharry-Bouyx, F., Chauviré, V., Sarazin, M., le Ber, I., Epelbaum, S., Jonveaux, T., Rouaud, O., Ceccaldi, M., Félician, O., Godefroy, O., Formaglio, M., Croisile, B., Auriacombe, S., Chamard, L., Vincent, J. L., Sauvée, M., Marelli-Tosi, C., Gabelle, A., Ozsancak, C., Pariente, J., Paquet, C., Hannequin, D., Campion, D; collaborators of the CNR-MAJ project. (2017). APP, PSEN1, and PSEN2 mutations in early-onset Alzheimer disease: A genetic screening study of familial and sporadic cases. *PLOS Medicine*, *14*(3), e1002270. https://doi.org/10.1371/JOURNAL.PMED.1002270.

Lee, J., Fukumoto, H., Orne, J., Klucken, J., Raju, S., Vanderburg, C. R., Irizarry, M. C., Hyman, B. T., & Ingelsson, M. (2005). Decreased levels of BDNF protein in Alzheimer temporal cortex are independent of BDNF polymorphisms. *Experimental Neurology*, *194*(1), 91–96. https://doi.org/10.1016/J.EXPNEUROL.2005.01.026.

Lim, Y. Y., Hassenstab, J., Cruchaga, C., Goate, A., Fagan, A. M., Benzinger, T. L. S., Maruff, P., Snyder, P. J., Masters, C. L., Allegri, R., Chhatwal, J., Farlow, M. R., Graff-Radford, N. R., Laske, C., Levin, J., McDade, E., Ringman, J. M., Rossor, M., Salloway, S., Schofield, P. R., Holtzman, D. M., Morris, J. C., & Bateman, R. J. (2016). BDNF Val66Met moderates memory impairment, hippocampal function and tau in preclinical autosomal dominant Alzheimer's disease. *Brain : A Journal of Neurology*, *139*(Pt 10), 2766–2777. https://doi.org/10.1093/BRAIN/AWW200.

Lim, Y. Y., Villemagne, V. L., Laws, S. M., Ames, D., Pietrzak, R. H., Ellis, K. A., Harrington, K., Bourgeat, P., Bush, A. I., Martins, R. N., Masters, C. L., Rowe, C. C., & Maruff, P. (2014). Effect of BDNF Val66Met on memory decline and hippocampal atrophy in prodromal Alzheimer's Disease: a preliminary study. *PLOS ONE*, *9*(1), e86498. https://doi.org/10.1371/JOURNAL.PONE.0086498.

Lim, Y. Y., Villemagne, V. L., Laws, S. M., Ames, D., Pietrzak, R. H., Ellis, K. A., Harrington, K. D., Bourgeat, P., Salvado, O., Darby, D., Snyder, P. J., Bush, A. I., Martins, R. N., Masters, C. L., Rowe, C. C., Nathan, P. J., & Maruff, P. (2013). BDNF Val66Met, Aβ amyloid, and cognitive decline in preclinical Alzheimer's disease. *Neurobiology of Aging*, *34*(11), 2457–2464. https://doi.org/10.1016/J.NEUROBIOLAGING.2013.05.006.

Lima Giacobbo, B., Doorduin, J., Klein, H. C., Dierckx, R. A. J. O., Bromberg, E., & de Vries, E. F. J. (2019). Brain-Derived Neurotrophic Factor in brain disorders: focus on neuroinflammation. In *Molecular Neurobiology* (Vol. 56, Issue 5, pp. 3295–3312). Humana Press Inc. https://doi.org/10.1007/s12035-018-1283-6.

Miranda, M., Morici, J. F., Zanoni, M. B., & Bekinschtein, P. (2019). Brain-Derived Neurotrophic Factor: a key molecule for memory in the healthy and the pathological brain. *Frontiers in Cellular Neuroscience*, *13*(August), 1–25. https://doi.org/10.3389/fncel.2019.00363.

Miyajima, F., Ollier, W., Mayes, A., Jackson, A., Thacker, N., Rabbitt, P., Pendleton, N., Horan, M., & Payton, A. (2008). Brain-derived neurotrophic factor polymorphism Val66Met influences cognitive abilities in the elderly. *Genes, Brain, and Behavior*, *7*(4), 411–417. https://doi.org/10.1111/J.1601-183X.2007.00363.X.

Momose, Y., Murata, M., Kobayashi, K., Tachikawa, M., Nakabayashi, Y., Kanazawa, I., & Toda, T. (2002). Association studies of multiple candidate genes for Parkinson's disease using single nucleotide polymorphisms. *Annals of Neurology*, *51*(1), 133–136. https://doi.org/10.1002/ANA.10079.

Nishimura, M., Kuno, S., Kaji, R., & Kawakami, H. (2005). Brain-derived neurotrophic factor gene polymorphisms in Japanese patients with sporadic Alzheimer's disease, Parkinson's disease, and multiple system atrophy. *Movement Disorders*, *20*(8), 1031–1033. https://doi.org/10.1002/MDS.20491.

Palasz, E., Wysocka, A., Gasiorowska, A., Chalimoniuk, M., Niewiadomski, W., & Niewiadomska, G. (2020). BDNF as a promising therapeutic agent in Parkinson's Disease. *International Journal of Molecular Sciences 2020, Vol. 21, Page 1170*, *21*(3), 1170. https://doi.org/10.3390/IJMS21031170.

Shen, T., You, Y., Joseph, C., Mirzaei, M., Klistorner, A., Graham, S. L., & Gupta, V. (2018). BDNF polymorphism: a review of its diagnostic and clinical relevance in neurodegenerative disorders. *Aging and Disease*, *9*(3), 523. https://doi.org/10.14336/AD.2017.0717.

Swardfager, W., Herrmann, N., Marzolini, S., Saleem, M., Shammi, P., Oh, P. I., Albert, P. R., Daigle, M., Kiss, A., & Lanctôt, K. L. (2011). Brain derived neurotrophic factor, cardiopulmonary fitness and cognition in patients with coronary artery disease. *Brain, Behavior, and Immunity*, *25*(6), 1264. https://doi.org/10.1016/J.BBI.2011.04.017.

Tsai, S. J., Hong, C. J., Liu, H. C., Liu, T. Y., Hsu, L. E., & Lin, C. H. (2004). Association analysis of brain-derived neurotrophic factor Val66Met polymorphisms with

Alzheimer's disease and age of onset. *Neuropsychobiology*, *49*(1), 10–12. https://doi.org/10.1159/000075332.

Urbina-Varela, R., Soto-Espinoza, M. I., Vargas, R., Quiñones, L., & del Campo, A. (2020). Influence of BDNF Genetic Polymorphisms in the Pathophysiology of Aging-related Diseases. *Aging and Disease*, *11*(6), 1513. https://doi.org/10.14336/AD.2020.0310.

van der Kolk, N. M., Speelman, A. D., van Nimwegen, M., Kessels, R. P. C., IntHout, J., Hakobjan, M., Munneke, M., Bloem, B. R., & van de Warrenburg, B. P. (2015). BDNF polymorphism associates with decline in set shifting in Parkinson's disease. *Neurobiology of Aging*, *36*(3), 1605.e1-1605.e6. https://doi.org/10.1016/J.NEUROBIOLAGING.2014.08.023.

Ventriglia, M., Chiavetto, L. B., Benussi, L., Binetti, G., Zanetti, O., Riva, M. A., & Gennarelli, M. (2002). Association between the BDNF 196 A/G polymorphism and sporadic Alzheimer's disease. *Molecular Psychiatry 2002 7:2*, *7*(2), 136–137. https://doi.org/10.1038/sj.mp.4000952.

Ventriglia, Mariacarla, Zanardini, R., Bonomini, C., Zanetti, O., Volpe, D., Pasqualetti, P., Gennarelli, M., & Bocchio-Chiavetto, L. (2013). Serum brain-derived neurotrophic factor levels in different neurological diseases. *BioMed Research International*, *2013*, 1–7. https://doi.org/10.1155/2013/901082.

Vepsäläinen, S., Castren, E., Helisalmi, S., Iivonen, S., Mannermaa, A., Lehtovirta, M., Hänninen, T., Soininen, H., & Hiltunen, M. (2005). Genetic analysis of BDNF and TrkB gene polymorphisms in Alzheimer's disease. *Journal of Neurology*, *252*(4), 423–428. https://doi.org/10.1007/S00415-005-0667-5.

Voineskos, A. N., Lerch, J. P., Felsky, D., Shaikh, S., Rajji, T. K., Miranda, D., Lobaugh, N. J., Mulsant, B. H., Pollock, B. G., & Kennedy, J. L. (2011). The brain-derived neurotrophic factor Val66Met polymorphism and prediction of neural risk for Alzheimer disease. *Archives of General Psychiatry*, *68*(2), 198–206. https://doi.org/10.1001/ARCHGENPSYCHIATRY.2010.194.

Warner, T. T., Schapira, A. H. V., Tatton, Rascol, Kordower, Olanow, Beal, Marek, Stocchi, & Isacson. (2003). Genetic and environmental factors in the cause of Parkinson's disease. *Annals of Neurology*, *53 Suppl 3*(SUPPL. 3). https://doi.org/10.1002/ANA.10487.

Yu, H., Zhang, Z., Shi, Y., Bai, F., Xie, C., Qian, Y., Yuan, Y., & Deng, L. (2008). Association study of the decreased serum BDNF concentrations in amnestic mild cognitive impairment and the Val66Met polymorphism in Chinese Han. *The Journal of Clinical Psychiatry*, *69*(7), 1104–1111. https://doi.org/10.4088/JCP.V69N0710.

Zhen, Y.-F., Liu, X.-Y., Zhou, D.-H., Du, X., Yin, G., Zhang, Y., Fang, H., Xu, G., Soares, J. C., & Zhang, X. Y. (2018). Cognition, serum BDNF levels, and BDNF Val66Met polymorphism in type 2 diabetes patients and healthy controls. *Oncotarget*, *9*(3), 3653–3662. https://doi.org/10.18632/ONCOTARGET.23342.

Chapter 5

Hereditary Colorectal Cancer in Malaysia

Mohd Nizam Zahary*
Faculty of Health Sciences, Universiti Sultan Zainal Abidin, Kuala Nerus, Terengganu, Malaysia

Abstract

Colorectal cancer (CRC) occurs in the inner epithelium of the colon and rectum, and it is usually a progression of adenomatous polyps towards malignancy. Majority of the tumours develop sporadically, accounting for 70 to 85% of all cases worldwide. CRC is the second-most common cancer among Malaysians. Chinese males have a lifetime risk of 1 in 43 in developing the disease, whereas Malays and Indians have a lower risk at 1 in 65 and 1 in 70, respectively. The lifetime risk for Chinese females is far lower than males at 1 in 57, but still high compared with Malay (1 in 89) and Indian (1 in 95) females. The prevalence of hereditary CRC, however, is low, which is similar to those reported overseas. Lynch syndrome (accounting for 1 to 5% of cases worldwide) seems to be the most common, followed by familial adenomatous polyposis (1 to 2%). Cases of hamartomatous polyposis syndromes, including Peutz-Jeghers syndrome, juvenile polyposis syndrome and Cowden syndrome, have been negligible for the past 30 years. As the disease's five-year survival rate is 40.8 % only, implementation of the latest screening strategies is important to diagnose cases at early stage and ensure better prognosis.

Keywords: Cowden syndrome, familial adenomatous polyposis, juvenile polyposis syndrome, Lynch syndrome, Peutz-Jeghers syndrome

---

* Corresponding Author's Email: nizamzahary@unisza.edu.my.

In: Genetic Disorders and Rare Diseases
Editors: Shazlin Shaharudin, Hisham Atan Edinur and Nor Fazila Che Mat
ISBN: 979-8-88697-953-4

Introduction: Overview of Colorectal Cancer

Colorectal cancer (CRC) occurs in the inner part of the colonic or rectal epithelium, and has a tendency to develop from adenomatous polyps. Its development is linked to a multi-step process known as the adenoma-carcinoma sequence, which explains how normal epithelial cells experience abnormal growth to form polyps that later become malignant (Armaghany et al., 2012). The process involves genetic and epigenetic changes (Armaghany et al., 2012), and this genomic instability provides a desirable environment for the activation of oncogenes, silencing of tumour suppressor genes and allelic imbalance at chromosomal regions that accelerate the transformation to adenocarcinoma (Abbas et al., 2013).

CRC tends to occur sporadically compared with a hereditary trait. Sporadic cancer is defined as a cancer that occurs irrespective of family history. Although such cancer may afflict people from all walks of life, they may exhibit trends that are influenced by demography (age, gender, ethnicity, location), environment (pollution) and lifestyle (smoking, alcohol consumption and physical activity). Genetic variants such as polymorphisms may also contribute towards the risk of developing sporadic cancer, and they are considered a predisposing factor. Sporadic cancer is associated with somatic mutations of the DNA in specific tissues due to pollution, diet, smoking and alcohol consumption (Testa et al., 2018).

Other possible risk factors include abdominal obesity, which may be explained by possible mechanisms, such as insulin resistance, chronic inflammation and hyperinsulinemia (Jochem & Leitzmann, 2016). A lack of physical activity is also observed to be associated with an increased risk of developing CRC (An & Park, 2022). Finally, patients with inflammatory bowel disease also have an increased risk due to chronic inflammation, which may trigger the development of dysplastic precursor lesions in the colon (Shah & Itzkowitz, 2022).

Genetic Predispositions in Hereditary Colorectal Cancer

Sporadic CRC accounts for 70 to 85% of all reported cases of CRC, and the remaining 10 to 15% may be hereditary (Maharaj et al., 2014; Yamagishi et al., 2016). Hereditary CRC is characterised by an early onset, which is usually manifested before age 50. Examples of hereditary CRC include hereditary non-polyposis colorectal cancer (HNPCC) or Lynch syndrome, familial adenomatous polyposis (FAP) and hamartomatous polyposis syndromes. Lynch syndrome represents 1-5% of all hereditary colon cancers, whereas FAP comprises 1-2% of the cases (Duraturo et al., 2019).

Table 1. The number of Lynch syndrome patients with defective MMR genes (Adapted from International Mismatch Repair Consortium (2021) and other studies)

Country	*MLH1*	*MSH2*	*MSH6*	*PMS2*	Total	Reference
United Kingdom	159	206	64	20	449	International Mismatch Repair Consortium (2021)
France	244	254	32	0	530	
Germany	421	517	89	44	1071	
Spain	118	73	49	16	256	
Denmark	66	135	86	17	304	
Finland	12	1	0	0	13	
Italy	3	11	3	0	17	
Norway	15	44	31	11	101	
Poland	6	1	0	0	7	
Switzerland	5	3	2	0	10	
The Netherlands	0	0	36	46	82	
USA	457	560	226	188	1431	
Canada	69	77	16	11	173	
Australia	244	289	159	94	786	
New Zealand	10	8	5	2	25	
Thailand	42	11	5	0	58	Manchana et al., (2021)
Malaysia	0	4	0	0	4	Zahary et al., (2012)
	0	0	5	4	9	Zahary et al., (2014)
	2	4	0	0	6	Wan Juhari et al., (2018)
Singapore	16	7	0	0	23	Liu et al., (2014)
Japan	15	10	4	0	29	Saita et al., (2018)

The development of Lynch syndrome has been associated with the inheritance of defective DNA mismatch repair (MMR) genes. Besides CRC, individuals with MMR gene defects are also at higher risk of developing cancers of the ovary, endometrium, liver, bladder, small intestine, stomach and skin (Chen et al., 2018). Mutations in MMR genes, namely *MLH1*, *MSH2*, *MSH6* and *PMS2,* have been identified as the main culprit that results in the development of Lynch syndrome (Zahary et al., 2012). These genes encode the MMR protein complexes involved in repairing errors after DNA replication. Defects in these genes may result in the accumulation of genomic errors, which may disrupt normal cell function that leads to abnormal growth and cancer. *EPCAM*, a gene located upstream to *MSH2*, is also associated with Lynch syndrome as its variants may lead to the inactivation of *MSH2* (Tutlewska et al., 2013).

Microsatellite instability (MSI) is the hallmark of tumours associated with Lynch syndrome. MSI, however, is not exclusively related to the syndrome, since mostly MSI/MMR deficient tumours are sporadic (Leclerc et al., 2021). Lynch syndrome patients tend to harbour tumours in the ascending colon and rectum as observed by Mas-Moya et al. (2015), where germline mutations in MMR genes were detected in 96 % of their patients who had a "right-sided" colon or rectal carcinoma. The other histopathological characteristics associated with MSI/MMR deficient tumours are poor differentiation, existence of mucinous components and signet ring cells, presence of a large number of tumour-infiltrating lymphocytes and medullary growth pattern (Aysal et al., 2012). The number of Lynch syndrome patients with defective MMR genes reported in several countries are shown in Table 1.

FAP also occurs in the colon and rectum, which may initially develop as multiple non-cancerous growths known as polyps. The reported prevalence of FAP is between 1 in 7000 to 1 in 22,000 (James et al., 2012). There is a variant of this disease with delay in the development of polyps into a malignant tumour, known as attenuated FAP (Ibrahim et al., 2014). The number of polyps will increase with age among FAP patients. The polyps or malignant tumours may also develop in other organs, such as the stomach, skin and duodenum (upper part of the small intestine) (James et al., 2012). Autosomal recessive inheritance of FAP is a milder form of the disease. Affected individuals have fewer polyps compared with classical FAP. Mutations in the adenomatous polyposis coli (*APC*) gene are the causative variants for FAP and attenuated FAP (Leoz et al., 2015). *APC* codes for a tumour suppressor protein involved in the Wnt signalling pathway (Leoz et al., 2015). Abnormalities in Wnt signalling have been associated with many types of cancer, resulting first in cell overgrowth and later, the formation of colon polyps in FAP. Mutation in MutY homolog gene (*MUTYH)* causes a milder type of FAP, which is autosomal recessive FAP (Leoz et al., 2015). *MUTYH* codes for DNA glycosylase that plays a role in apoptosis by inducing single-strand breaks in genomic DNA following oxidative damage (Markkanen et al., 2013). Mutations in this gene will result in the inability of mutant cells to undergo apoptosis, which may eventually end up proliferating as cancer. In FAP cases, the colonic mucosa is covered by hundreds of sessile polyps. Adenomas in FAP demonstrate tubular architecture and these tumours are identical to sporadic CRC (Moriichi et al., 2020). In contrast, fewer colorectal polyps were present in autosomal recessive FAP.

The other rare syndromes related to hereditary CRC include juvenile polyposis syndrome, Peutz-Jeghers syndrome and Cowden syndrome. Juvenile polyposis syndrome is characterised by the development of multiple benign growths (juvenile polyps) (Jelsig et al., 2014). It is believed to occur in approximately 1 in 100,000 individuals worldwide (Gao et al., 2020). Although affected individuals usually develop polyps in their colon before the age of 20, but the word "juvenile" actually refers to the characteristics of the polyp tissues, and not the patients' age of onset. The polyps usually grow in the colon and the numbers may vary from few to hundreds. The polyps may later cause complications, such as gastrointestinal bleeding, diarrhoea and abdominal pain. Genetic mutations of *BMPR1A* and *SMAD4* are found to be associated with juvenile polyposis syndrome (Liu et al., 2020). Protein encoded by *BMPR1A* is a receptor that belongs to the family of transmembrane serine/threonine kinases involved in the cell signalling pathway. *SMAD4* encodes a signal transduction protein belonging to the SMAD family, which is also related to transmembrane serine/threonine receptor kinases that activate cell signalling pathways (McCarthy & Chetty, 2018). Mutations in these genes may interrupt the regulation of cell signalling and promote proliferation. The *STK11* gene codes for a serine/threonine kinase that regulates cell polarity, and it is also a tumour suppressor protein (Zhang et al., 2021). Any abnormalities in this protein may result in its inability to control cell division.

The hamartomas present in juvenile polyposis do not include muscularis mucosae, which is a common feature of Peutz-Jeghers syndrome. It is also characterised by the presence of multiple hamartomatous polyps with or without the adenomatous component. Adenomatous dysplasia may also develop in juvenile polyps (Gao et al., 2020). Peutz-Jeghers syndrome is characterised by the existence of multiple hamartomatous polyps in the gastrointestinal tract. Patients have an increased risk of developing other types of cancers, such as ovarian, cervical and breast cancer (Jelsig et al., 2014). The prevalence of Peutz-Jeghers syndrome is estimated to be 1 in 25,000 to 300,000 individuals. The polyps in Peutz-Jeghers syndrome consist of smooth muscles covered by glandular epithelium (Oliveira & Rodrigues, 2021). They are predominantly located in the small intestine, in clusters and lobulated surfaces that are often seen in larger lesions. Features of pseudoinvasion that cause displacement of epithelial components have also been observed (Okada et al., 2013).

Cowden syndrome is rare and associated with the growth of multiple non-cancerous hamartomas. Affected individuals also face an increased risk of developing kidney, endometrial, thyroid, breast and CRC. The prevalence of Cowden syndrome is unknown, but it is believed to be 1 in 200,000 individuals (Dragoo et al., 2021). Twenty-five per cent of cases may be attributed to mutations in the tumour suppressor *phosphatase* and *tensin homolog* (*PTEN*) gene, and the remaining are due to alterations in the Killin, P53 Regulated DNA Replication Inhibitor (*KLLN)* and WW Domain-Containing E3 Ubiquitin Protein Ligase 1 (*WWP1*) genes (Lee et al., 2020). *PTEN* is found to be commonly mutated in the majority of cancers (Tan et al., 2012). The enzyme encoded by the gene has been negatively implicated in the regulation of AKT/PKB signalling pathway and prevents the cell from rapidly dividing. Polyps found in Cowden syndrome are sessile polyps without surface erosion, and with the appearance of inflamed fibrotic lamina propria with smooth muscle proliferation and lymphoid follicles (Shaco-Levy et al., 2016).

Colorectal Cancer in Malaysia

To date, CRC is the second most common cancer diagnosed among Malaysians (Azizah et al., 2019). According to the National Cancer Registry published in 2019, CRC is the most frequently reported cancer among males (16.9%) and the second-most frequent among females (10.7%) from 2012 until 2016. A total of 15,515 (13.5%) CRC cases were reported in the country from 2012 to 2016, of which 8,701 cases were males and 6,814 were females. The age-standardised rates of this cancer among males and females are 14.8 and 11.1 per 100,000 populations, respectively. The incidence increases with age, especially those 70 years old and above for both genders. However, the Malaysian age-standardised rates for males and females are quite low compared with Europe and the United States, which is 40 per 100,000 populations (Arnold et al., 2017).

The lifetime risk of developing CRC is 1 in 55 among Malaysian males and 1 in 76 among females. However, Chinese males seem to have a strong predisposition towards the disease. The lifetime risk for Chinese males is 1 in 43, whereas Malays and Indians have a lower value at 1 in 65 and 1 in 70, respectively. The lifetime risk for Chinese females is far lower than males at 1 in 57, but still very high compared with Malay (1 in 89) and Indian (1 in 95) women. Unfortunately, majority of cases in Malaysia are detected at advanced stages (stage III and IV), with 72.4% of cases in males and 73.1% of cases in females (Azizah et al., 2019). This scenario results in poor outcome and increases the burden on the country's healthcare system as complex treatments have to be provided to the patients. CRC is a disease with very poor prognosis because patients have been observed to have a five-year survival rate of 40.8% only (Malaysian Study on Cancer Survival, 2018). Therefore, it should be of great concern to health authorities and policymakers because the incidence of this cancer is rising worldwide, and Malaysia is no exception, owing to its huge socioeconomic development and adaptation to urban diets and lifestyle.

Hereditary Colorectal Cancer in Malaysia

Unlike sporadic CRC, the prevalence of hereditary ones is extremely low in Malaysia. A local study reported 34 individuals only who were diagnosed with Lynch syndrome based on revised Bethesda guidelines (Zahary et al., 2012). Four of the cases harboured mutations in two MMR genes, *MLH1* and *MSH2*. A later study by the same researchers reported that nine (18 %) out of 50 Malaysian Lynch syndrome patients had *MSH6* and *PMS2* mutations (Zahary et al., 2014). In screening for Lynch syndrome patients, a study concluded that the use of the revised Bethesda guidelines and immunohistochemical analysis were the most convenient approach in a Malay cohort, with the detection of 17 patients from several collaborating hospitals nationwide (Wan Juhari et al., 2015). A more recent study enrolled 12 patients from six Malay Lynch syndrome families, with the patients found to harbour multiple mutations in *MLH1* and *MSH2* (Wan Juhari et al., 2018).

The reported cases of FAP in Malaysia is lower compared with Lynch syndrome. There was a study reported on one Chinese family with nine affected members in three generations (Mohamed et al., 2003). A rare case of papillary thyroid cancer associated with FAP was also reported in five Malaysian patients (Rohaizak et al., 2003, Suhaimi et al., 2015). The reported cases for rare syndromes, such as juvenile polyposis syndrome, Peutz-Jeghers syndrome and Cowden syndrome, are almost negligible. Over the last 30 years, two patients from one family only were reported to have Peutz-Jeghers syndrome, with the presence of multiple polyps in their gastrointestinal tract (Vishvanathan et al., 1992).

Conclusion

The prevalence of hereditary CRC in Malaysia is low. The precise strategy for hereditary CRC screening, however, is still important to discriminate between sporadic MSI/dMMR tumours and those arising from hereditary gene defects. The high cost and burden of treating CRC is undeniable. Therefore, it is imperative for the government and policymakers to promote a healthy lifestyle by initiating awareness programmes on the signs, symptoms and risk factors relating to CRC. The implementation of updated screening strategies will help to detect the disease earlier compared with advanced presentations currently seen in hospitals nationwide. The treatment and clinical management of the disease in early stages are much easier and affordable for the patients and their families, and is also less burden to the country's healthcare system.

References

Abbas, T., Keaton, M. A., & Dutta, A. (2013). Genomic instability in cancer. *Cold Spring Harbor Perspectives in Biology*, *5*(3), a012914. https://doi.org/10.1101/cshperspect.a012914.

Abdullah Suhaimi, S. N., Nazri, N., Nani Harlina, M. L., Md Isa, N., & Muhammad, R. (2015). Familial Adenomatous Polyposis-Associated Papillary Thyroid Cancer. *The Malaysian Journal of Medical Sciences, 22*(4), 69–72.

An, S., & Park, S. (2022). Association of Physical Activity and Sedentary Behavior with the Risk of Colorectal Cancer. *Journal of Korean Medical Science*, *37*(19), e158. https://doi.org/10.3346/jkms.2022.37.e158.

Armaghany, T., Wilson, J. D., Chu, Q., & Mills, G. (2012). Genetic alterations in colorectal cancer. *Gastrointestinal Cancer Research*, *5*(1), 19–27.

Arnold, M., Sierra, M. S., Laversanne, M., Soerjomataram, I., Jemal, A., & Bray, F. (2017). Global patterns and trends in colorectal cancer incidence and mortality. *Gut*, *66*(4), 683–691. https://doi.org/10.1136/gutjnl-2015-310912.

Aysal, A., Karnezis, A., Medhi, I., Grenert, J. P., Zaloudek, C. J., & Rabban, J. T. (2012). Ovarian endometrioid adenocarcinoma: incidence and clinical significance of the morphologic and immunohistochemical markers of mismatch repair protein defects and tumor microsatellite instability. *The American Journal of Surgical Pathology*, *36*(2), 163–172. https://doi.org/10.1097/PAS.0b013e31823bc434.

Chen, E., Xu, X., & Liu, T. (2018). Hereditary Nonpolyposis Colorectal Cancer and Cancer Syndromes: Recent Basic and Clinical Discoveries. *Journal of Oncology*, *2018*, 3979135. https://doi.org/10.1155/2018/3979135.

de Oliveira, M. F. A., & Rodrigues, M. A. M. (2021). Peutz-Jeghers syndrome: an unusual autopsy finding in pregnancy. *Autopsy & case reports*, *11*, e2021279. https://doi.org/10.4322/acr.2021.279.

Dragoo, D. D., Taher, A., Wong, V. K., Elsaiey, A., Consul, N., Mahmoud, H. S., Mujtaba, B., Stanietzky, N., & Elsayes, K. M. (2021). PTEN Hamartoma Tumor Syndrome/Cowden Syndrome: Genomics, Oncogenesis, and Imaging Review for Associated Lesions and Malignancy. *Cancers*, *13*(13), 3120. https://doi.org/10.3390/cancers13133120.

Duraturo, F., Liccardo, R., De Rosa, M., & Izzo, P. (2019). Genetics, diagnosis and treatment of Lynch syndrome: Old lessons and current challenges. *Oncology letters*, *17*(3), 3048–3054. https://doi.org/10.3892/ol.2019.9945.

Gao, X. H., Li, J., Zhao, Z. Y., Xu, X. D., Du, Y. Q., Yan, H. L., Liu, L. J., Bai, C. G., & Zhang, W. (2020). Juvenile polyposis syndrome might be misdiagnosed as familial adenomatous polyposis: a case report and literature review. *BMC Gastroenterology*, *20*(1), 167. https://doi.org/10.1186/s12876-020-01238-7.

Ibrahim, A., Barnes, D. R., Dunlop, J., Barrowdale, D., Antoniou, A. C., & Berg, J. N. (2014). Attenuated familial adenomatous polyposis manifests as autosomal dominant late-onset colorectal cancer. *European journal of human genetics: EJHG*, *22*(11), 1330–1333. https://doi.org/10.1038/ejhg.2014.20.

International Mismatch Repair Consortium (2021). Variation in the risk of colorectal cancer in families with Lynch syndrome: a retrospective cohort study. *The Lancet. Oncology*, *22*(7), 1014–1022. https://doi.org/10.1016/S1470-2045(21)00189-3.

James, A. S., Chisholm, P., Wolin, K. Y., Baxter, M., Kaphingst, K., & Davidson, N. O. (2012). Screening and Health Behaviors among Persons Diagnosed with Familial Adenomatous Polyposis and Their Relatives. *Journal of Cancer Epidemiology*, *2012*, 506410. https://doi.org/10.1155/2012/506410.

Jelsig, A. M., Qvist, N., Brusgaard, K., Nielsen, C. B., Hansen, T. P., & Ousager, L. B. (2014). Hamartomatous polyposis syndromes: a review. *Orphanet journal of rare diseases*, *9*, 101. https://doi.org/10.1186/1750-1172-9-101.

Jochem, C., & Leitzmann, M. (2016). Obesity and Colorectal Cancer. *Recent Results in Cancer Research, 208*, 17–41. https://doi.org/10.1007/978-3-319-42542-9_2.

Leclerc, J., Vermaut, C., & Buisine, M. P. (2021). Diagnosis of Lynch Syndrome and Strategies to Distinguish Lynch-Related Tumors from Sporadic MSI/dMMR Tumors. *Cancers*, *13*(3), 467. https://doi.org/10.3390/cancers13030467.

Lee, Y. R., Yehia, L., Kishikawa, T., Ni, Y., Leach, B., Zhang, J., Panch, N., Liu, J., Wei, W., Eng, C., & Pandolfi, P. P. (2020). WWP1 Gain-of-Function Inactivation of PTEN in Cancer Predisposition. *The New England Journal of Medicine*, *382*(22), 2103–2116. https://doi.org/10.1056/NEJMoa1914919.

Leoz, M. L., Carballal, S., Moreira, L., Ocaña, T., & Balaguer, F. (2015). The genetic basis of familial adenomatous polyposis and its implications for clinical practice and risk management. *The Application of Clinical Genetics*, *8*, 95–107. https://doi.org/10.2147/TACG.S51484.

Liu, Q., Liu, M., Liu, T., & Yu, Y. (2020). Familial juvenile polyposis syndrome with a de novo germline missense variant in BMPR1A gene: a case report. *BMC Medical Genetics*, *21*(1), 196. https://doi.org/10.1186/s12881-020-01135-6.

Liu, Y., Chew, M. H., Goh, X. W., Tan, S. Y., Loi, C. T., Tan, Y. M., Law, H. Y., Koh, P. K., & Tang, C. L. (2014). Systematic study on genetic and epimutational profile of a cohort of Amsterdam criteria-defined Lynch Syndrome in Singapore. *PloS One*, *9*(4), e94170. https://doi.org/10.1371/journal.pone.0094170.

Maharaj, R., Shukla, P. J., Sakpal, S. V., Naraynsingh, V., Dan, D., & Hariharan, S. (2014). The impact of hereditary colorectal cancer on the Indian population. *Indian journal of cancer*, *51*(4), 538–541. https://doi.org/10.4103/0019-509X.175307.

Manchana, T., Ariyasriwatana, C., Triratanachat, S., & Phowthongkum, P. (2021). Lynch Syndrome in Thai Endometrial Cancer Patients. *Asian Pacific Journal of Cancer Prevention*, *22*(5), 1477–1483. https://doi.org/10.31557/APJCP.2021.22.5.1477.

Markkanen, E., Dorn, J., & Hübscher, U. (2013). MUTYH DNA glycosylase: the rationale for removing undamaged bases from the DNA. *Frontiers in Genetics*, *4*, 18. https://doi.org/10.3389/fgene.2013.00018.

Mas-Moya, J., Dudley, B., Brand, R. E., Thull, D., Bahary, N., Nikiforova, M. N., & Pai, R. K. (2015). Clinicopathological comparison of colorectal and endometrial carcinomas in patients with Lynch-like syndrome versus patients with Lynch syndrome. *Human pathology*, *46*(11), 1616–1625. https://doi.org/10.1016/j.humpath.2015.06.022.

McCarthy, A. J., & Chetty, R. (2018). *Smad4/DPC4*. *Journal of Clinical Pathology*, *71*(8), 661–664. https://doi.org/10.1136/jclinpath-2018-205095.

Mohamed, Z., Ahmad, R., Yoke, N. S., Zakaria, Z., Ahmad, H., & Yew, T. H. (2003). A nonsense mutation in exon 8 of the APC gene (Arg283Ter) causes clinically variable FAP in a Malaysian Chinese family. *Cancer Science*, *94*(8), 725–728. https://doi.org/10.1111/j.1349-7006.2003.tb01509.x.

Moriichi, K., Tanabe, H., Ono, Y., Kobayashi, Y., Murakami, Y., Iwama, T., Kunogi, T., Sasaki, T., Takahashi, K., Ando, K., Ueno, N., Kashima, S., Takei, H., Mizukami, Y., Fujiya, M., & Okumura, T. (2020). Serrated adenomas with a BRAF mutation in a young patient with familial adenomatous polyposis. *International Journal of Colorectal Disease*, *35*(10), 1967–1972. https://doi.org/10.1007/s00384-020-03657-0.

National Cancer Registry Department. (2019). Malaysia national cancer registry report (MNCR) 2012-2016. National Cancer Institute, Ministry of Health. Retrieved on February 12, 2023, from https://www.moh.gov.my/moh/resources/Penerbitan/Laporan/Umum/20122016%20(MNCRR)/MNCR_2012-2016_FINAL_(PUBLISHED_2019).pdf.

National Cancer Registry Department (2018). Malaysian Study on Cancer Survival (MySCan) National Cancer Institute, Ministry of Health. Retrieved on February 12, 2023, from https://www.moh.gov.my/moh/resources/Penerbitan/Laporan/Umum/Malaysian_Study_on_Cancer_Survival_MySCan_2018.pdf.

Okada, H., Itagaki, S., Enatsu, K., Kiriu, T., & Ishizawa, M. (2013). Vascular pseudoinvasion in a solitary Peutz-Jeghers polyp in the ileum. *Pathology International*, *63*(3), 188–192. https://doi.org/10.1111/pin.12037.

Rohaizak, M., Jasmi, A. Y., Ismail, M. A., Munchar, M. J., & Meah, F. A. (2003). Thyroid carcinoma in patients with familial adenomatous polyposis. *Asian Journal of Surgery*, *26*(3), 183–185. https://doi.org/10.1016/S1015-9584(09)60381-X.

Saita, C., Yamaguchi, T., Horiguchi, S. I., Yamada, R., Takao, M., Iijima, T., Wakaume, R., Aruga, T., Tabata, T., & Koizumi, K. (2018). Tumor development in Japanese patients with Lynch syndrome. *PloS One*, *13*(4), e0195572. https://doi.org/10.1371/journal.pone.0195572.

Shaco-Levy, R., Jasperson, K. W., Martin, K., Samadder, N. J., Burt, R. W., Ying, J., & Bronner, M. P. (2016). Morphologic characterization of hamartomatous gastrointestinal polyps in Cowden syndrome, Peutz-Jeghers syndrome, and juvenile polyposis syndrome. *Human Pathology*, *49*, 39–48. https://doi.org/10.1016/j.humpath.2015.10.002.

Shah, S. C., & Itzkowitz, S. H. (2022). Colorectal Cancer in Inflammatory Bowel Disease: Mechanisms and Management. *Gastroenterology*, *162*(3), 715–730.e3. https://doi.org/10.1053/j.gastro.2021.10.035.

Tan, M. H., Mester, J. L., Ngeow, J., Rybicki, L. A., Orloff, M. S., & Eng, C. (2012). Lifetime cancer risks in individuals with germline PTEN mutations. *Clinical Cancer Research*, *18*(2), 400–407. https://doi.org/10.1158/1078-0432.CCR-11-2283.

Testa, U., Pelosi, E., & Castelli, G. (2018). Colorectal cancer: genetic abnormalities, tumor progression, tumor heterogeneity, clonal evolution and tumor-initiating cells. *Medical Sciences*, *6*(2), 31. https://doi.org/10.3390/medsci6020031.

Tutlewska, K., Lubinski, J., & Kurzawski, G. (2013). Germline deletions in the EPCAM gene as a cause of Lynch syndrome - literature review. *Hereditary cancer in clinical practice*, *11*(1), 9. https://doi.org/10.1186/1897-4287-11-9.

Visvanathan, R., Thambidorai, C. R., & Myint, H. (1992). Do dysplastic and adenomatous changes in large bowel hamartomas predispose to malignancy? -- A report of two cases. *Annals of the Academy of Medicine, Singapore*, *21*(6), 830–832.

Wan Juhari, W. K., Ahmad Amin Noordin, K. B., Wan Abdul Rahman, W. F., Zakaria, A. D., Mohd Sidek, A. S., Abu Hassan, M. R., Macrae, F., & Zilfalil, B. A. (2018). MLH1 and MSH2 Gene mutations and polymorphisms in six malay families with hereditary nonpolyposis colorectal cancer. *International Medical Journal Malaysia, 17*(1),71–78. https://doi.org/10.31436/imjm.v17i1.304.

Wan Juhari, W. K., Wan Abdul Rahman, W. F., Mohd Sidek, A. S., Abu Hassan, M. R., Ahmad Amin Noordin, K. B., Zakaria, A. D., Macrae, F., & Zilfalil, B. A. (2015). Analysis of Hereditary Nonpolyposis Colorectal Cancer in Malay Cohorts using Immunohistochemical Screening. *Asian Pacific Journal of Cancer Prevention*, *16*(9), 3767–3771. https://doi.org/10.7314/apjcp.2015.16.9.3767.

Yamagishi, H., Kuroda, H., Imai, Y., & Hiraishi, H. (2016). Molecular pathogenesis of sporadic colorectal cancers. *Chinese Journal of Cancer*, *35*, 4. https://doi.org/10.1186/s40880-015-0066-y.

Zahary, M. N., Kaur, G., Hassan, M. R., Sidek, A. S., Singh, H., Yeh, L. Y., & Ankathil, R. (2014). Germline mutation and protein expression analysis of mismatch repair genes MSH6 and PMS2 in Malaysian Lynch syndrome patients. *International Journal of Colorectal Disease*, *29*(2), 261–262. https://doi.org/10.1007/s00384-013-1770-1.

Zahary, M. N., Kaur, G., Abu Hassan, M. R., Singh, H., Naik, V. R., & Ankathil, R. (2012). Germline mutation analysis of MLH1 and MSH2 in Malaysian Lynch syndrome patients. *World Journal of Gastroenterology*, *18*(8), 814–820. https://doi.org/10.3748/wjg.v18.i8.814.

Zhang, Y., Meng, Q., Sun, Q., Xu, Z. X., Zhou, H., & Wang, Y. (2021). LKB1 deficiency-induced metabolic reprogramming in tumorigenesis and non-neoplastic diseases. *Molecular Metabolism*, *44*, 101131. https://doi.org/10.1016/j.molmet.2020.101131.

Chapter 6

BRCA: Gene Mutations in Breast Cancer

Nur Azzalia Kamaruzaman[1,*]
Mazlin Mohideen[2]
Norsyifa Harun[3]
Halilol Rahman Mohamed Khan[2]
and Ana Masara Ahmad Mokhtar[4]

[1]National Poison Centre, Universiti Sains Malaysia, Pulau Pinang, Malaysia
[2]Faculty of Pharmacy and Health Sciences, Universiti Kuala Lumpur-Royal College of Medicine Perak (UniKL-RCMP), Ipoh, Perak, Malaysia
[3]Centre for Drug Research, Universiti Sains Malaysia, Pulau Pinang, Malaysia
[4]School of Industrial Technology, Universiti Sains Malaysia, Pulau Pinang, Malaysia

Abstract

Breast cancer reportedly has the highest incidence in Malaysia, and this is despite the availability of screening facilities nationwide. Many gene mutations have been linked to the hereditary nature of the cancer, and the most common are mutations in BRCA1 and BRCA2 genes. These two have an important role in repairing damaged cells, thus ensuring normal growth of breast, ovarian and other tissues. However, problems arise when these genes mutate and lose their functions, which are then passed down to the offspring, thereby increasing the risk of generational cancers. The risk of developing breast cancer may be as high as 72% in women with BRCA1 or BRCA2 mutations. Conventional treatments for breast cancer include surgery, radiotherapy, chemotherapy and anti-hormone medication. The use of olaparib and talazoparib, which are poly-adenosine diphosphate (ADP)-ribose polymerase (PARP) inhibitors,

* Corresponding Author's Email: azzalia@usm.my.

In: Genetic Disorders and Rare Diseases
Editors: Shazlin Shaharudin, Hisham Atan Edinur and Nor Fazila Che Mat
ISBN: 979-8-88697-953-4

have been studied. The clinical trials of these drugs have reached phase III with improvements seen in patient survival. The main challenge is the development of resistance towards treatment. Therefore, researchers have looked into the combined use of olaparib with standard therapies, as well as the antibiotic Novobiocin either alone or together with PARP inhibitors to reduce the risk of the cancer becoming resistant to treatment. Therefore, a better understanding of the role of BRCA1 and BRCA2 in breast cancer is vital to produce an effective treatment plan.

Keywords: cell growth, chemotherapy, hereditary, resistance, side effects, targeted therapy

Introduction

Breast cancer was among the most prevalent cancer among women worldwide in 2020, with an estimated 685,000 deaths and 2.3 million new cases reported (Sung et al. 2021). According to a GLOBOCAN report, two million women were diagnosed with breast cancer in 2018 alone (equivalent to 32.7% of all cancers). The World Health Organisation (WHO) estimated that the disease has claimed 627,000 lives in 2018, comprising 15% of all cancer deaths in women worldwide that year (Bray et al. 2018).

Recently, breast cancer is becoming common among young women. In the United States, approximately 7% of patients diagnosed with breast cancer are aged below 40 (Brinton et al. 2008, Tichy et al. 2013). In 2017, the American Cancer Society also estimated that 12,150 cases occurred among women under 40 and 26,393 cases were women under 45 (DeSantis et al. 2017). The same trend but with a different profile has also been seen in Asian countries, where most patients are between 40 and 50 years old, compared with between 60 and 70 years old in the West (Leong et al. 2010, Abdullah et al. 2013, Chen et al. 2016). Women are often diagnosed much younger in Indonesia, at a mean age of 37 (11.4%), compared to other Asian countries (Abdullah et al., 2016, Nordin et al., 2018; Anwar et al., 2019). The incidence of breast cancer among young women aged 40 and below in selected Asian populations are 27.9% in Nepal (Thapa et al. 2013), 26% in North India (Nandakumar et al. 2005), 19.1% in Singapore (NRDO, 2017), 16.2% in India (Kakarala et al. 2010) and 13.6% in Malaysia (Ibrahim et al. 2012).

The majority of cancer deaths among women in Malaysia is due to breast cancer (Bray et al. 2018). The age-standardised incidence rate (ASR) is 34.1 per 100,000 populations (Brinton et al. 2008, Ministry of Health Malaysia

2019). Although the rate of breast cancer in developed countries is relatively high and most cases are diagnosed at an advanced age, the trend shows that the prognosis and survival rates are better than developing countries (Leong et al. 2010). Of the women who develop breast cancer, 81% of those diagnosed at stage 2 and 88% of those diagnosed at stage 1 have a 68-month median survival time, as well as five years of overall cancer survival if diagnosed early. Malaysia has the second-highest cancer death rate in Southeast Asia at 18.4 per 100,000 populations, right after Singapore with a rate of 18.5.

Furthermore, the incidence differs between various ethnic groups in Malaysia, with Chinese and Indian women having a rate of 1:22 and 1:23, respectively. In Malay women, the rate is as high as 1:30 (Ministry of Health Malaysia 2019). The incidence is reduced by 60% for stage 3 cancers and by 23% in stage 4. Late presentation of breast cancer which comprises around 48% of Malaysian cases is difficult to treat, and may be reduced through the implementation of preventive measures such as early screening (Al-Amri, 2005, Njor et al. 2012, Massat et al. 2016, Ministry of Health Malaysia 2019a). The prevalence of breast cancer in Malaysian women is 1:19, compared with 1:8 in the United States and Europe (Leong et al. 2010, DeSantis et al. 2017).

Figure 1 states the factors which increase breast cancer risk as well as the interventions which may reduce the risk. Nevertheless, only a 30% reduction in the risk of developing breast cancer would be possible, irrespective of the capacity to control every risk factor that might be modifiable. The existing situation demonstrates that around 50% of cases rise among women who have no identifiable risk factors. Other factors include gender (female) and age (over 40 years). In addition, breast cancer in men only occur at about 0.5-1%, and the treatment for men follows the same management principles for women (Sung et al. 2021).

Breast cancer risk rates increase among those with a family history of this type of cancer, although most breast cancer diagnoses occur in women with no known diseases, especially cancer, in their family history. It is not possible to place women at low risk for cancer simply because their family history information is unavailable (Sung et al. 2021). Family-based inheritance of particular mutations of "high penetrance" genes causes individuals to be more at risk of breast cancer. BRCA1, BRCA2, and PALB-2 gene mutations are the types that occur most frequently. Measures to reduce risk may be considered among women whose genes contain these mutations; for instance, they may elect to have both breasts surgically removed. A minimal proportion of women are affected by this approach, which is highly invasive, so careful evaluations of this and all other options should be undertaken, with time allowed to make the decision.

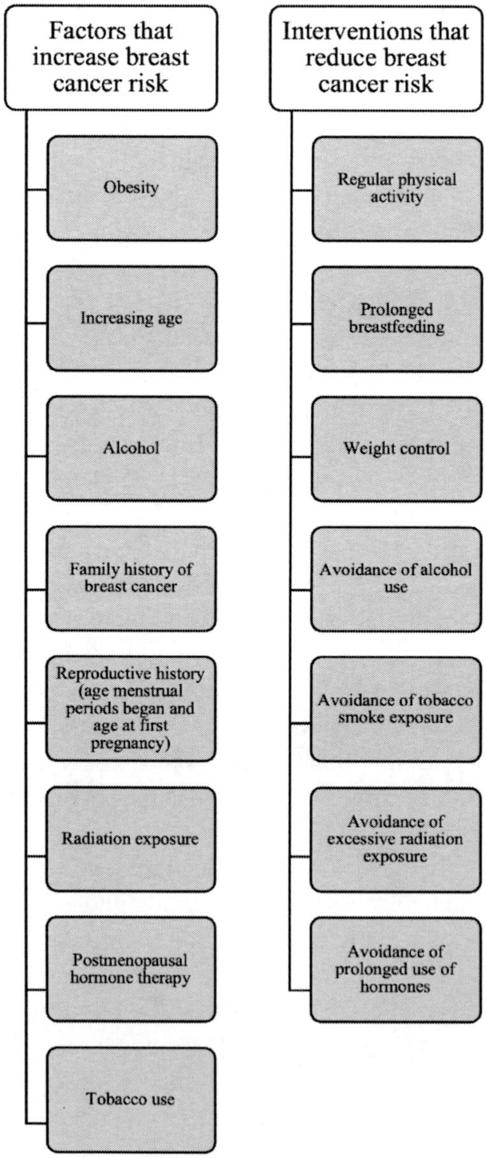

Figure 1. Factors and interventions that increase and reduce the risk of breast cancer including BRCA1 (BReast CAncer gene one) and BRCA2 (BReast CAncer gene two) mutations.

Cancer Control Policies and Strategies in Malaysia

It is imperative to carry out effective policy development to provide early detection services, as well as prevent and improve or control cancer, including breast cancer. Many countries have implemented systematic and/or opportunistic population-based breast cancer screening programs. This implementation is based on established early-stage screening techniques, including ultrasound, mammography, and clinical breast examination (CBE).

The healthcare system in Malaysia consists of public (fully funded by the government) and private healthcare services (Quek, 2014). Government clinics and private hospitals offer opportunistic mammography screening, while the National Population and Family Development Board (NPFDB) Malaysia has stipulated which private healthcare providers can implement subsidized mammogram schemes (Mahmud & Aljunid, 2018).

Progress must be monitored through robust evaluations of the policies and measures to control cancer, from which implementation lessons can be learned and subsequent policy developments guided (Alberg et al., 2013). An integrated cancer-control approach was intended to be implemented through the design of numerous policy document publications; nevertheless, little formal research seems to have been undertaken to evaluate these policies.

The Ministry of Health Malaysia (MOH) established a coordinating team in 2015 comprising doctors, experts in public health, oncologists and policymakers to review the National Cancer Control Action Plan (NCCB) (2008-2015). This review led to the National Strategic Plan for Cancer Control Program (NSP-CCP) 2016-2020. Nine cancer-control aspects are the focus of the NSP-CCP, including screening, traditional medicine, palliative care, primary prevention and research into cancer. Meanwhile, policies are evaluated through a list of specific indicators. Early detection can be determined by offering mammograms, CBE, and MRI (for women at high risk) as forms of screening for breast cancer. By 2020, the aim was to provide a higher rate of 60% for stages 1 and 2, up from 57% in 2011. The Ministry of Education linked with the College of Radiology (Ministry of Health Malaysia 2017), and non-governmental organizations between 2016 and 2020 to implement measures to monitor NSP and evaluate CCP. These included developing screening schemes, monitoring systems to screen cancer and procedures to ensure quality, like the auditing of mammogram centres. Following the guidelines on clinical practice and directions for policy, screening was to be updated to target recommendations for women at high risk and opportunistic screening of the general population via mammograms and

CBE (Ministry of Health Malaysia 2002, Ministry of Health Malaysia 2019a). The NCCB policy (2008-2015) achieved success in 2012 by initiating mammography screening for women at high risk. From 2006 to 2014, there was a rise in the uptake of mammograms from 8% to 24% (Ministry of Health Malaysia 2008) and of CBE from 52% to 65%. Nevertheless, diagnosis at the late stage remains frequent, and between 2011 and 2016, the rate had actually risen from 43% to 48%, according to recent reports from cancer registries (Ministry of Health Malaysia 2016, 2019).

BRCA1 and BRCA2 Mutations

Breast Cancer Susceptibility Genes Type 1 and Type 2 (BRCA1 and BRCA2)

BRCA1 and BRCA2 are the two most prevalent breast cancer susceptibility genes. These genes, referred to as tumour suppressors, are essential in preventing breast cancer because they frequently stop a cell from multiplying and expanding uncontrollably during cell division. However, these BRCA genes may be altered or damaged as a result of mutation, which could cause the cells to multiply uncontrollably, leading to cancer (Karami & Mehdipour, 2013).

Structure of BRCA1 and BRCA2 Genes

The BRCA1 gene encodes a 190-kD protein which is mapped on chromosome 17q21. This 1863-amino-acid protein is composed of 24 exons. The structure of BRCA1 protein comprises several regions (domains), which contain the Really Interesting New Gene (RING) domain at the amino-terminus, a large unstructured region at the centre with nuclear localization signals (NLS) encoded by exon 11, a coiled-coil domain, and followed by tandem BRCA1 carboxy-terminal repeats (BRCTs). The BRCA1 C-terminus, which is conserved in many DNA repair-related proteins, is also present in the structure (Karami & Mehdipour, 2013). Through these domains, BRCA1 interacts with a wide range of proteins and is implicated in a number of cellular processes, including DNA repair, cell-cycle checkpoint activation and transcriptional control (Venkitaraman, 2014).

BRCA2, which is located on chromosome 13q12, encodes the 384-kD BRCA2 protein. It has 27 exons which encompasses about 84.2 kb of genomic DNA (Gorodetska et al. 2019). This BRCA2 protein has an N-terminal transactivation domain, a lengthy exon 11 with a RAD51-specific binding site, and followed by a DNA binding domain near the C-terminus. Additionally, the BRC motif, a BRCT domain found in the core region of BRCA2, interacts with RAD51 and is crucial for controlling DNA damage response functions, such as DNA repair, transcription and cell cycle (Karami & Mehdipour, 2013). BRCA2 has a DNA-binding domain at its C-terminus that includes a helical domain that interacts with the meiosis-specific recombinase DMC1, three oligonucleotide/oligosaccharide-binding (OB) folds, and followed by a tower domain that promotes BRCA2 binding to both single-stranded (ssDNA) and double-stranded DNA (ssDNA) (Loizideou et al. 2007).

DNA Damage Repair Pathways and BRCA Function

There can be tens of thousands of endogenous DNA damage events to genomic DNA due to the presence of toxic chemicals, metabolic wastes, and UV radiation (Lindahl, 1993). Numerous roles for BRCA1 and BRCA2 have been identified, including those in chromatin remodelling and transcription, DNA damage response, and protein ubiquitination (Hall et al. 1990, Powell & Kachnic, 2003, Yarden & Papa, 2006). The two BRCA1 and BRCA2 proteins have varied roles in different phases of DNA damage repair when BRCA1 normally participates in both DNA repair and cell-cycle checkpoint activation, whereas BRCA2 primarily serves as a mediator of the homologous recombination process (Roy et al. 2016).

A few of the most important DNA repair processes include base excision repair, direct repair, nucleotide excision repair (NER), mismatch repair (MMR) and double-strand break (DSB) recombinational repair, which includes both homologous recombinational repair (HRR) and non-homologous end-joining (NHEJ) (Plummer, 2010). DSB is the most threatening type of DNA damage, which can result in chromosome translocation, deletion and mutation if it is not repaired or repaired incorrectly, all of which can result in the development of cancer (Jackson & Bartek, 2009). Basically, the histone H2A family member at H2AX undergoes significant phosphorylation following DNA damage, creating foci at break sites. BRCA1 initiates the repair process when interacting with these foci via its BRCT domain by altering the structure of local chromatin and allowing DNA repair proteins to approach the damaged regions (Paull et al. 2000, Welcsh and King, 2001). BRCA1 carries out the DNA repair functions together with the BRCA1-associated RING domain protein (BARDI). The BRCA1-BARD1 heterodimer serves as an E3 ubiquitin ligase by interacting with other repair proteins at DNA damage (Rebbeck et al. 2015). BRCA1-BARDI complex also assists in cell survival by activating DNA damage checkpoints in the cell cycle. When DNA damage is present, the activated checkpoints eventually halt the cell cycle's progression and prevent it from continuing until the DNA damage has been fully repaired (Sadeghi et al. 2020).

BRCA1 interacts with the bridging protein PALB2 through its coiled-coil domain, linking it to BRCA2, the second important breast cancer suppressor. When the BRCA2 protein binds to RAD51 directly through its BRC repeats and TR2 domain, it enables the loading of RAD51 on ssDNA and seeks for homologous DNA templates, which is a crucial step in the repair of DNA DSBs (Davies et al. 2001). In addition to being essential for homologous recombination (HR), RAD51 also demonstrates tumour-suppressive characteristics of this repair mechanism (Moynahan et al. 2001).

BRCA1 and BRCA2 Gene Mutations

A BRCA mutation occurs when the DNA that makes up the gene sustains some sort of damage. When a BRCA gene is mutated, it may lose the ability to repair DNA damage, which can result in more DNA alterations and mutations and ultimately cause cancer (Mehrgou & Akounchekian, 2016). Therefore, individuals with BRCA gene mutation are substantially more likely than those without mutations to develop breast cancer.

There are around 2,000 distinct mutations in the BRCA1 and BRCA2 genes, including deletions, insertions, and various single nucleotide alterations in either coding or noncoding sequences (Karami & Mehdipour, 2013). An estimated 70–80% of these BRCA1 and BRCA2 nonsense, frameshift and splicing mutations result in truncated proteins, which may cause dysfunctional BRCA proteins or the absence of protein product (Pohlreich et al. 2005, Calo et al. 2010). BRCA1 mutations frequently affect the N-terminal RING domain (Ruffner et al. 2001), which is in charge of the protein's E3 ubiquitin ligase activity (Hashizume et al. 2001). Numerous studies suggest that BRCA1 mutations in the RING domain, which inhibit BRCA1 ubiquitin-protein ligase activity, may increase the risk of cancer development (Ruffner et al. 2001, Nelson & Holt, 2010). Other than the RING domain, the most prevalent

BRCA1 mutations are found in the gene areas corresponding to the BRCT domain and in exons 11 to 13 that encode NLS, which is crucial for BRCA1 functions and serves as binding sites for numerous BRCA1-interacting proteins, such as PALB2, BRCA2 and RAD51 (Clark et al. 2012). Large genomic rearrangements (LGRs), which are typically brought on by homologous recombination between the BRCA1 gene and the same pseudogene sequences, account for around one-third of BRCA1 gene mutations (Zhang et al. 2010). BRCA1 also exhibits a higher incidence of duplication or deletion than BRCA2 (42% and 20%, respectively) due to its high Alu sequence (41.5%) compared to its relatively low density (4.8%) of other repeat sequences (Smith et al. 1996, Thompson and Easten, 2004). In fact, a more severe and highly metastatic subtype of breast cancer called triple-negative breast cancer (TNBC) accounts for over 70% of breast cancers with familial BRCA1 mutations (Nielsen et al. 2004). Thus, individuals with BRCA1 mutations are more likely to acquire breast cancer than those with BRCA2 mutations when BRCA1 mutations reveal a greater lifetime risk of breast cancer, ranging from 57-65%, compared to 45-49% of BRCA2 genes (Antonieu et al. 2003).

Most gene mutations in the BRCA2 protein occur in exons 10 and 11, typically as insertions or deletions that result in missense alterations and premature stop codons, which cause shortened and defective proteins (Fackenthal & Olopade, 2007). The RAD51-binding function of BRCA2 may also be impaired by deletion of its C-terminal region, which would reduce RAD51 recruitment to the damage site and increasing the risk of breast cancers (Lancaster et al. 1996). Additionally, C-terminal truncation of BRCA2 may result in the absence of DSS1-mediated stabilization and BRCA2's rapid degradation, exposing cells to DNA damage (Li et al. 2006, Gudmundsdottir et al. 2004). Furthermore, BRCA2-deficient cells show a diminished ability to repair DNA double-strand breaks (DSBs) and are unable to stimulate the effective resumption of replication forks that have halted (Moynahan et al. 2001).

Some of the mutations in BRCA1 and BRCA2 genes have been identified in numerous studies from various populations, and some of them exhibit a population-specific patterns (Karami & Mehdipour, 2013). The prevalence of BRCA1 and BRCA2 gene mutations differs by ethnicity, geographical regions and may be influenced by lifestyle choices and environmental factors. In Malaysia, about 13.5% of individuals with hereditary breast cancer had BRCA1 and BRCA2 gene mutations (Thirthagiri et al. 2008). Among different ethnicities in Malaysia, BRCA2 mutations were mostly detected in Malays and Chinese, whereas BRCA1 mutations were more common in Indians. This might be because Chinese and Malay populations have far closer genetic relationships than Indian populations, who are more distantly related to Caucasians genetically (Xing et al. 2009, Hatin et al. 2011).

Breast cancer is a multifactorial disease caused by multiple environmental and genetic factors and their interaction (Amini et al. 2021). Consequently, the inherited susceptibility to breast cancer brought on by BRCA1 and BRCA2 mutations is merely a part of a wider picture. In fact, hereditary mutations in the BRCA1 and BRCA2 genes account for only 5% to 10% of all occurrences of breast cancer (Hoang and Gilks, 2018). Most cases are sporadic or non-familial clustering, which may be caused by combinations of multiple, poorly penetrant mutations in a much greater number of genes that may have been impacted by environmental factors (Venkitaraman, 2002).

Sporadic breast cancer is highly associated with somatic loss of BRCA genes when between 50% and 70% of individuals lose a BRCA1 allele and between 30% and 50% lose a BRCA2 allele (Futreal et al. 1994, Cleton-Jansen et al. 1995). Two somatic mutations that affect the alleles on both chromosomes result in the loss of function of two tumour-suppressor genes in sporadic malignancies. There are also sporadic cases when wild-type BRCA have a defective DNA repair pathway, which may have developed as a result of other processes. For instance, non-genetic factors such as promoter methylation, which results in a reduction in gene expression to undetectable levels and loss of heterozygosity, may be responsible for BRCA1 inactivation in sporadic breast tumours (Mylavarapu et al. 2018).

Mutations Involving Other Breast Cancer Contributing Genes

There are also small fractions of the risk of mutations that are attributed to germline mutations in other genes, which are referred to as moderate genetic factors for breast cancer (i.e., PALB2, TP53, CHEK2, PTEN, CDH1, RAD50, ATM etc.) (Yow et al. 2017). PALB2 and TP53 are among the moderate-penetrance pathogenic mutations for breast cancer that are linked to breast cancer susceptibility among Malaysians (Amini et al. 2021).

Direct PALB2 binding to BRCA1 and BRCA2 causes the formation of a complex essential for RAD51-mediated HRR of damaged DNA (Roy et al. 2012). When this interaction is hampered by the functional loss of the PALB2 protein, DNA repair is hindered, which causes the accumulation of mutations in daughter cells throughout cell division (Zhang et al. 2009). While BRCA1 is known to interact with and activate p53 to signal the presence of DNA damage (Ouchi et al. 1998), the functional loss of TP53 protein disrupts the cell cycle arrest. It prevents the cell from moving forward to either allow repair or cause cell death. According to a multi-ethnic study on breast cancer conducted in Malaysia, patients with positive family histories are more likely to have TP53 mutations than BRCA1 or BRCA2 gene alterations (Lee et al. 2012).

Current Diagnosis Methods, Treatments and Preventive Action

Current Diagnosis

BRCA1 and BRCA2 genes are sequenced for mutations in genetic testing for hereditary breast cancer. Blood or saliva samples can be used, and anyone with a deleterious BRCA variant in their tumour would be tested further to determine if the variant is inherited because damaging BRCA variants found in the tumour may be of somatic or germline origin.

Treatment

High penetrance genes BRCA1 and BRCA2 are linked to early-onset breast cancers, as well as an elevated risk of contralateral breast cancer, ovarian cancer, prostate and pancreatic cancer. Hence, patients who are BRCA1 and BRCA2 pathogenic/possibly pathogenic variant carriers are more prone to develop breast, ovarian, and other cancers (Karami & Mehdipour, 2013). Therefore, early thorough screening and preventative measures are warranted for these people. Individuals with pathogenic mutations in BRCA1 or BRCA2 should get post-test counselling that focuses on screening, risk-reducing operations and chemoprevention (Arun et al. 2011, Vallard et al. 2019). In all risk management techniques, a multidisciplinary approach and collaborative decision-making should be utilised.

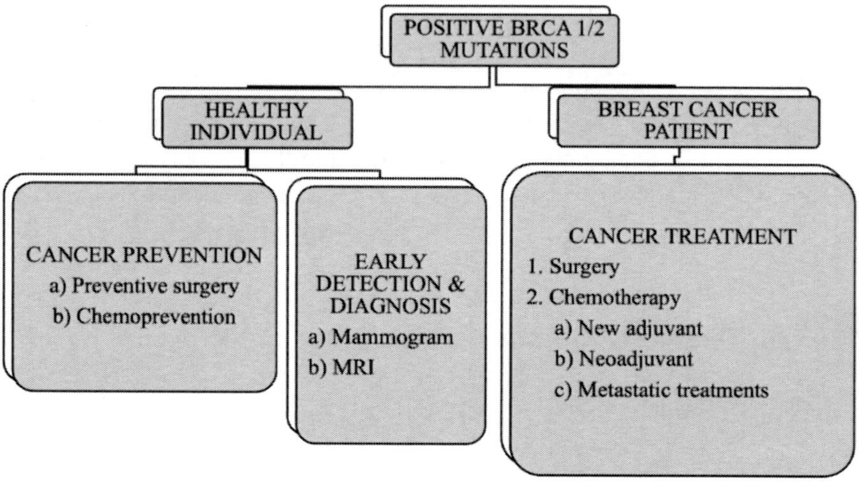

Figure 2. Therapeutic pathways for healthy people and patients with positive BRCA1/2 mutations.

Surgery

A study by Pierce et al. (2010) found that while there was no significant difference in the two groups' overall survival after BCS (breast-conserving surgery/lumpectomy) and mastectomy, although the BCS group had a greater rate of ipsilateral local recurrence than the mastectomy group. The outcome of BCS in BRCA1/2 pathogenic variant breast cancer has been compared with that of sporadic breast cancer in several studies to address this issue (Pierce et al. 2000, Kirova et al. 2010, Valachis et al. 2014, Vallard et al. 2019). A recent meta-analysis showed that there was no difference in overall survival between 526 cases with *BRCA1/2* pathogenic variants and 2,320 sporadic breast cancer cases (Valachis et al. 2014). However, in this study, *BRCA1/2* patients showed higher ipsilateral breast cancer recurrence than sporadic breast cancer patients.

Radiotherapy

Studies have shown that young patients receiving radiation for sporadic breast cancer had an increased chance of developing contralateral breast cancer (Gao et al. 2003). However, a research from the Netherlands failed to find any connection between radiotherapy and the risk of developing contralateral breast cancer (Drooger et al., 2015).

Chemotherapy

BRCA1-positive cells may be more susceptible to taxanes, which block microtubules but may also make them resistant to platinum-based chemotherapeutic treatments (Tassone et al. 2003, Chabalier et al. 2006). Anthracycline and taxane were used in a neoadjuvant chemotherapy regimen, and 46% of BRCA1 mutation carriers experienced a pathological complete response (pCR), compared to only 22% of sporadic breast cancer patients (Arun et al. 2011). A recent meta-analysis research, however, revealed that a taxane-based therapy would be preferable to the anthracycline-taxane combination for patients of advanced breast cancer since taxane is less toxic and both treatments have comparable clinical results (Zheng et al. 2015).

Platinum Agents

Platinum agents directly bind to DNA, forming DNA/platinum adducts that result in double-strand breaks and inter-strand DNA crosslinks. According to a study, cisplatin, a platinum-based agent, caused a substantially higher pCR of 83% in hereditary BRCA1-associated breast cancer than other chemotherapy drugs like doxorubicin and docetaxel, which are taxane-based drugs. The same study also showed that combination therapy of doxorubicin and cyclophosphamide produced a lower pCR (22%) compared with cisplatin alone (Gronwald et al. 2010). Another systematic review and meta-analysis of published studies showed increased pCR when platinum-based agents were used as standard neoadjuvant chemotherapy in treating triple-negative cancers (Saslow et al. 2007).

Poly-Adenosine Diphosphate (ADP)-Ribose Polymerase Inhibitors

The crucial protein known as PARP is responsible for mending single-strand DNA breaks. PARP inhibitors inhibit the protein, causing cell death due to DNA breaks. Olaparib, talazoparib, rucaparib, niraparib and veliparib are five PARP inhibitors currently in the market. In a phase 3 study using olaparib, BRCA1/2 patients who were HER2 negative showed improved progression-free survival rate (Robson et al. 2017). Talazoparib used in EMBRCA trial resulted in a better median progression-free survival compared with conventional chemotherapy (Litton et al. 2018). In a Phase 2 trial in metastatic breast and ovarian BRCA patients, intravenous rucaparib was given, which resulted in 41% of the patients who received it in a state of stable disease status within three months. Promising outcomes were reported in clinical trials using olaparib or talazoparib in ER+ metastatic BRCA1/2 breast cancers (Tutt et al. 2010, Sandhu et al. 2013, Kaufman et al. 2015).

Breast Cancer Prevention in Carriers of BRCA1/BRCA2 Pathogenic Variants

Preventative Surgery

Bilateral Risk-Reducing Mastectomy (Brrm)
Following breast cancer surgery, it has been demonstrated that patients with the BRCA1/2 variation are more likely to develop contralateral breast cancer than patients with sporadic breast cancer (Biglia et al. 2016). The study also demonstrated that bilateral risk-reducing mastectomy decreased both the moderate-risk group and high-risk patients' risk of death.

Bilateral Risk-Reducing Salpingo-Oophorectomy (BRRSO)
By choosing this surgery, women will lower their risk of acquiring ovarian cancer. Premenopausal women also appear to have a lower risk of developing breast cancer in the future (Lostumbo et al. 2010, Domchek et al. 2010), with some earlier studies indicating a risk reduction of approximately 50%. Preventive BRSSO decreased ipsilateral and contralateral breast cancer recurrences in patients with BRCA1/BRCA2 pathogenic mutation (Rebbeck et al. 2002). Furthermore, it significantly decreased breast cancer mortality in individuals with breast cancer caused by a BRCA1/2 pathogenic mutation (Li et al. 2016). BRCA1/2 pathogenic variant carriers have a higher risk, according to recent studies. Recent research has shown that BRCA1/2 pathogenic variant carriers are more likely to develop ovarian cancer, which tends to manifest in BRCA1 pathogenic variant carriers at a younger age than in BRCA2 pathogenic variant carriers (King et al. 2003, Satagopan et al. 2002). According to reports, salpingo-oophorectomy performed as a preventative measure in healthy BRCA1/2 pathogenic variant carriers lowers the risk of ovarian cancer by more than 80% (Kauff et al. 2008, Rebbeck et al. 2009). Based on the aforementioned findings, BRRSO in BRCA1/2 pathogenic variant carriers should be taken into consideration to lower risk of breast cancer as well as to protect against ovarian cancer.

Chemoprevention
It has been proven that the selective oestrogen receptor modulator tamoxifen reduces risk in asymptomatic females by 40–50%. (Howell et al. 2016). These findings suggest that tamoxifen has a very modest protective impact in BRCA1/2 carriers and a marginally better protective effect in BRCA2 carriers.

The study's small sample size (i.e., 8 cases for BRCA1 carriers and 11 cases for BRCA2 carriers, respectively) could account for this restricted effect (King et al. 2001). Tamoxifen's secondary preventive impact was found to reduce the incidence of breast cancer in BRCA1 by 62%, according to a study of 1,583 BRCA1 and 881 BRCA2 pathogenic variant carriers. The second generation SERM raloxifene, used to treat and prevent osteoporosis, has a considerably better side effect profile than tamoxifen, with no rise in endometrial malignancies but an increase in thromboembolic risk. Over an extended follow-up, tamoxifen's risk reduction was inferior (Vogel et al. 2006). Raloxifene is only taken into consideration in postmenopausal patients. Exemestane, an aromatase inhibitor, has been found to provide postmenopausal women at elevated risk with a 65% relative risk reduction with a modest side-effect profile (Goss et al. 2011).

Emerging Research and Therapies

There has been extensive research to understand better treatment strategies for BRCA1/BRCA2 breast cancer patients. BRCA1/2 mutation carriers are at high risk as hereditary breast cancer poses more challenges than sporadic cancer. One research suggested platinum compounds are more effective for treatment as BRCA1/BRCA2 related breast cancer is more susceptible due to defects in homologous recombination. The same study also highlights the importance of combinatorial treatment strategies to ensure a better therapeutic landscape for BRCA1/BRCA2-related breast cancer. This includes combining PARP inhibitors with chemotherapy or immunotherapy for a better prognosis (Pouptsis et al. 2020). To support this work, Tutt et al. (2021) conducted an Olympia trial, whereby top experts of BRCA breast cancer all over the world evaluated 1,836 patients from 420 centres across 23 countries in a double-blind Phase 3 trial. It was found that PARP inhibitor drug olaparib, as adjuvant therapy following completion of standard therapies such as chemotherapy, surgery and radiation, significantly improved the outcome and survival of the patients (Tutt et al. 2021).

In another advanced research in the field of BRCA1/2-related breast cancer, two techniques, which are called cryo-electron microscopy and nuclear magnetic resonance spectroscopy, have been utilised to provide scientists with an understanding of how BRCA1-BARD1 modifies chromatin, which relates to DNA repair mechanism. This study is promising in providing appropriate patient care through variant classification and directing accurate drug development through the generation of 3D structures of BRCA1-BARD1, which could lead to the design of small molecules to inactivate this gene (Hu et al. 2021).

As resistance to PARP inhibitors is an imminent threat to effective treatment, other types of drugs have been identified and studied in the ongoing effort to find the best treatment for BRCA1/2 breast cancer patients. Zhou et al. (2021) found the antibiotic Novobiocin to be most effective in inhibiting DNA polymerase theta, which is important in retaining BRCA cancer cell viability. Inhibiting this protein promotes the death of BRCA cancer cells. The study has shown that Novobiocin, when used alone or in combination with PARP inhibitors, have promising potential in treating BRCA breast cancer. Similarly, another small molecule drug known as ART558 is found to work synergistically with PARP inhibitors to kill BRCA1/2 breast cancer cells while alleviating the adverse side effects associated with it (Zhou et al. 2021).

Other than treatment strategies, other lifestyle factors should also be considered. A study by Galasso et al. (2022) found direct association between physical activity and sleep quality with BRCA carriers. BRCA carriers usually have poor sleep quality due to several factors, such as distress and anxiety over disease diagnosis and in family's future, discomfort from pain and hot flashes as a result of surgery and treatments, and fatigue. The study found that physical activity may promote better sleep quality, and this is essential for a better quality of life as sleep deficiency promotes inflammation, impairs immune response and alters mitochondrial respiratory function and insulin signalling as well as enhances oestrogen secretion, all of which are known to hamper recovery (Galasso et al. 2022).

Conclusion

Breast cancer is an imminent threat to women in Malaysia and worldwide. Various factors increase the risk of breast cancer, but women with mutations in BRCA1 and BRCA2 genes are more susceptible to developing breast cancer. National policies and strategies should focus on supporting and encouraging everyone, especially women, on increasing breast cancer awareness and understand the importance of regular screening. Genetic testing is also recommended for those diagnosed with breast cancer of BRCA1 and BRCA2 gene mutation, as well as their family members. While conventional treatments such as surgery, radiotherapy and chemotherapy are commonly utilised, other strategies may also provide better treatment outcomes, such as combination therapy and improved lifestyle factors.

Acknowledgment

The study is financially supported by the Ministry of Higher Education Malaysia through Fundamental Research Grant Scheme (FRGS) (FRGS/1/2020/STG01/USM/02/9).

References

Abdullah, M. M., Mohamed, A. K. & Foo, Y. C. (2016). Breast cancer survival at a leading cancer centre in Malaysia. *Asian Pacific Journal of Cancer Prevention*, 16(18), 8513-8517. https://doi.org/10.7314/apjcp.2015.16.18.8513

Abdullah, N. A., Mahiyuddin, W. R. W. & Muhammad, N. A. (2013). Survival rate of breast cancer patients in Malaysia: A Population-based Study. *Asian Pacific Journal of Cancer Prevention*, 14(8), 4591-4594. https://doi.org/10.7314/apjcp.2013.14.8.4591.

Al-Amri, A. M. (2005). Prevention of breast cancer. *Journal of Family and Community Medicine*, 12, 71-74.

Alberg, A. J., Cartmell, K. B. and Sterba, K. R. (2013). Outcome evaluation of a state comprehensive cancer control plan: laying the foundation'. *Journal of Public Health Management and Practice*, 19, 300-307. https://doi.org/10.1097/PHH.0b013e31825d208c

Amini, F., Wong, F. H., Ng, E. S. C., Ng, C. Y., Omar, R., Mohd Rejab, S., Mohd Noor, I. W. & Mohd Hussain, B. (2021). Mutation profile of breast cancer in Malaysian patients. *JUMMEC*, *24*(1), 37-44. https://doi.org/10.22452/jummec.vol24no1.6

Antoniou, A., Pharoah, P. D., Narod, S., Risch, H. A., Eyfjord, J. E. & Hopper, J. L. (2003). Average risks of breast and ovarian cancer associated with BRCA1 or BRCA2 mutations detected in case series unselected for family history: A combined analysis of 22 studies. *The American Journal of Human Genetics*, *72*(5), 1117–1130. https://doi.org/10.1086/375033

Anwar, S. L., Raharjo, C. A. & Herviastuti, R. (2019). Pathological profiles and clinical management challenges of breast cancer emerging in young women in Indonesia: A hospital-based study. *BMC Women's Health*, 19(28). 1-8. https://doi.org/10.1186/s12905-019-0724-3

Arun, B., Bayraktar, S., Liu, D. D., Gutierrez Barrera, A. M. & Atchley, D. (2011). Response to neoadjuvant systemic therapy for breast cancer in BRCA mutation carriers and noncarriers: A single-institution experience. *Journal of Clinical Oncology*, 29, 3739-3746. https://doi.org/10.1200/JCO.2011.35.2682

Biglia, N., D'Alonzo, M., Sgro, L. G., Tomasi Cont, N., Bounous, V. & Robba, E. (2016). Breast cancer treatment in mutation carriers: Surgical treatment. *Minerva Ginecology,* 68, 548–556.

Bray, F., Ferlay, J. & Soerjomataram, I. (2018). Global cancer statistics 2018: GLOBOCAN estimates of incidence and mortality worldwide for 36 cancers in 185 countries. *Cancer Journal for Clinicians*, 68(6), 394-424. https://doi.org/10.3322/caac.21492

Brinton, L. A., Sherman, M. E. & Carreon, J. D. (2008). Recent trends in breast cancer among younger women in the United States. *Journal of the National Cancer Institute*, 100(22), 1643-1648. https://doi.org/10.1093/jnci/djn344

Calò, V., Bruno, L., La Paglia, L., Perez, M., Margarese, N., Di Gaudio, F. & Russo A. (2010). The clinical significance of unknown sequence variants in BRCA Genes. *Cancers*, 2(3), 1644–1660. https://doi.org/10.3390/cancers2031644

Chabalier, C., Lamare, C., Racca, C., Privat, M., Valette, A. & Larminat, F. (2006). *BRCA1* downregulation leads to premature inactivation of spindle checkpoint and confers paclitaxel resistance. *Cell Cycle,* 5, 1001–1007. https://doi.org/10.4161/cc.5.9.2726

Chen, C., Sun, S. & Yuan, J-P. (2016). Characteristics of breast cancer in Central China, literature review and comparison with USA. *The Breast*, 30, 208-213. https://doi.org/10.1016/j.breast.2016.01.004

Clark, S. L., Rodriguez, A. M., Snyder, R. R., Hankins, G. D. & Boehning, D. (2012). Structure-function of the tumor suppressor BRCA1. *Computational and Structural Biotechnology Journal*, 1(1), 1-8. https://doi.org/10.5936/csbj.201204005

Cleton-Jansen, A. M., Collins, N., Lakhani, S. R., Weissenbach, J., Devilee, P., Cornelisse, C. J. & Stratton, M. R. (1995). Loss of heterozygosity in sporadic breast tumours at the BRCA2 locus on chromosome 13q12-q13. *British Journal of Cancer*, 72, 1241-1244. https://doi.org/10.1038/bjc.1995.493

Cuzick, J., Sestak, I., Baum, M., Buzdar, A., Howell, A. & Dowsett, M. (2010). Effect of anastrozole and tamoxifen as adjuvant treatment for early-stage breast cancer: 10-year analysis of the ATAC trial. *The Lancet Oncology*, 11(12), 1135-1141. https://doi.org/10.1016/S1470-2045(07)70385-6

Davies, A. A., Masson, J. Y., McIlwraith, M. J., Stasiak, A. Z., Stasiak, A., Venkitaraman, A. R. & West, S. C. (2001) Role of BRCA2 in control of the RAD51 recombination and DNA repair protein. *Molecular Cell*, 7(2), 273-282. https://doi.org/10.1016/s1097-2765(01)00175-7

DeSantis, C. E., Ma, J. & Goding Sauer, A. (2017). Breast cancer statistics, 2017, racial disparity in mortality by state. *Cancer Journal for Clinicians,* 67(6), 439-448. https://doi.org/10.3322/caac.21412

Domchek, S. M., Friebel, T. M., Singer, C. F., Evans, D. G., Lynch, H. T. & Isaacs, C. (2010). Association of risk-reducing surgery in BRCA1 or BRCA2 mutation carriers with cancer risk and mortality. *JAMA*, 304(9), 967-975. https://doi.org/10.3322/caac.21412

Drooger, J., Akdeniz, D., Pignol, J. P., Koppert, L. B., McCool, D. & Seynaeve, C. M. (2015). Adjuvant radiotherapy for primary breast cancer in BRCA1 and BRCA2 mutation carriers and risk of contralateral breast cancer with special attention to patients irradiated at younger age. *Breast Cancer Research and Treatment*, 154(1), 171-180. https://doi.org/10.1001/jama.2010.1237

Fackenthal, J. D. & Olopade, O. I. (2007). Breast cancer risk associated with BRCA1 and BRCA2 in diverse populations. *Nature Reviews Cancer*, 7(12), 937-948. https://doi.org/10.1038/nrc2054

Futreal, P. A., Liu, Q., Shattuck-Eidens, D., Cochran, C., Harshman, K., Tavtigian, S., Bennett, L. M., Haugen-Strano, A., Swensen, J. & Miki, Y. (1994). BRCA1 mutations in primary breast and ovarian carcinomas. *Science*, 266, 120-122. https://doi.org/10.1126/science.7939630

Galasso, L., Castelli, L., Roveda, E., Oliverio, A., Baldassari, I., Esposito, F., Mulè, A., Montaruli, A., Patrizia, P. & Bruno, E. (2022). Physical activity and sleep behaviour in women carrying BRCA1/2 mutations. *Scientific Reports*, 1–7. https://doi.org/10.1038/s41598-022-16687-1

Gao, X., Fisher, S. G. & Emami, B. (2003). Risk of second primary cancer in the contralateral breast in women treated for early-stage breast cancer: A population-based study. International *Journal of Radiation Oncology, Biology, Physics*, 56(4), 1038-1045. https://doi.org/10.1016/s0360-3016(03)00203-7

Gorodetska, I., Kozeretska, I. & Dubrovska, A. (2019). BRCA Genes: The role in genome stability, cancer stemness and therapy resistance. *Journal of Cancer*, 10(9), 2109-2127. https://doi.org/10.7150/jca.30410

Goss, P. E., Ingle, J. N., Ales-Martinez, J. E., Cheung, A. M., Chlebowski, R. T. & Wactawski-Wende, J. (2011). Exemestane for breast-cancer prevention in postmenopausal women. *The New England Journal of Medicine,* 364(25), 2381-2391. https://doi.org/10.1056/NEJMoa1103507

Gronwald, J., Huzarski, T., Grzybowska, E. & Budryk, M. (2010). Pathologic complete response rates in young women with BRCA1-positive breast cancers after neoadjuvant chemotherapy. *Journal of Clinical Oncology,* 28, 375-379. https://doi.org/10.1200/JCO.2008.20.7019

Gudmundsdottir, K., Lord, C. J., Witt, E., Tutt, A. N. & Ashworth, A. (2004). DSS1 is required for RAD51 focus formation and genomic stability in mammalian cells. EMBO Reports, 5(10), 989-993. https://doi.org/10.1038/sj.embor.7400255

Hall, J. M., Lee, M. K., Newman, B., Morrow, J. E., Anderson, L. A. & Huey, B. (1990). Linkage of early-onset familial breast cancer to chromosome 17q21. *Science*, 250 (4988), 1684-1689. https://doi.org/10.1126/science.2270482

Hashizume, R., Fukuda, M. & Maeda, I. (2001). The RING heterodimer BRCA1-BARD1 is a ubiquitin ligase inactivated by a breast cancer-derived mutation. *Journal of Biology Chemistry*, 276(18), 14537–14540. https://doi.org/10.1074/jbc.C000881200

Hatin, W. I., Nur-Shafawati, A. R. & Zahri, M. K. (2011). Population genetic structure of Peninsular Malaysia Malay sub-ethnic groups. *PLoS One,* 6(4), e18312, 1-8. https://doi.org/10.1371/journal.pone.0018312

Hoang, L. N. & Gilks, B. C. (2018). Hereditary breast and ovarian cancer syndrome: moving beyond BRCA1 and BRCA2. *Advances in Anatomic Pathology*, 25(2), 85-95. https://doi.org/10.1097/PAP.0000000000000177

Howell, A., Anderson, A. S., Clarke, R. B., Duffy, S. W., Evans, D. G. & Garcia-Closas, M. (2016). Risk determination and prevention of breast cancer. *Breast Cancer Research,* 16(446), 1-19. https://doi.org/10.1186/s13058-014-0446-2

Hu, Q., Botuyan, M. V., Zhao, D., Cui, G., Mer, E. & Mer, G. (2021). Mechanisms of BRCA1–BARD1 nucleosome recognition and ubiquitylation. *Nature, 596*(7872), 438-443. https://doi.org/10.1038/s41586-021-03716-8

Ibrahim, N. I., Dahlui, M. & Aina, E. N. (2012). Who are the breast cancer survivors in Malaysia? *Asian Pacific Journal of Cancer Prevention*, 13(5), 2213-2218. https://doi.org/10.7314/apjcp.2012.13.5.2213

Jackson, S. P. & Bartek, J. (2009). The DNA-damage response in human biology and disease. *Nature*, 461(7267), 1071-1078. https://doi.org/10.1038/nature08467

Kakarala, M., Rozek, L. & Cote, M. (2010). Breast cancer histology and receptor status characterization in Asian Indian and Pakistani women in the U.S. - A SEER analysis. *BMC Cancer*, 10(191), 1-8. https://doi.org/10.1186/1471-2407-10-191

Karami. F. & Mehdipour, P. (2013). A comprehensive focus on global spectrum of BRCA1 and BRCA2 mutations in breast cancer. *BioMed Research International*, 2013(928562), 1-21. https://doi.org/10.1155/2013/928562

Kauff, N. D., Domchek, S. M., Friebel, T. M., Robson, M. E., Lee, J. & Garber, J. E. (2008). Risk-reducing salpingo-oophorectomy for the prevention of *BRCA1*- and *BRCA2*-associated breast and gynecologic cancer: a multicenter, prospective study. *Journal Clinical Oncology,* 26, 1331-1337. https://doi.org/10.1200/JCO.2007.13.9626

Kaufman, B., Shapira-Frommer, R., Schmutzler, R. K., Audeh, M. W., Friedlander, M. & Balmaña, J. (2015). Olaparib monotherapy in patients with advanced cancer and a germline *BRCA1/2* mutation. *Journal of Clinical Oncology,* 33, 244-250. https://doi.org/10.1200/JCO.2014.56.2728

King, M. C., Marks, J. H., Mandell, J. B. & New York Breast Cancer Study Group (2003). Breast and ovarian cancer risk due to inherited mutations in *BRCA1* and *BRCA2*. *Science,* 302, 643-646. https://doi.org/10.1126/science.1088759

King, M. C., Wieand, S., Hale, K., Lee, M., Walsh, T. & Owens, K. (2001). Tamoxifen and breast cancer incidence among women with inherited mutations in *BRCA1* and *BRCA2*: National Surgical Adjuvant Breast and Bowel Project (NSABP-P1) Breast Cancer Prevention Trial. *JAMA,* 286, 2251-2256. https://doi.org/10.1001/jama.286.18.2251

Kirova, Y. M., Savignoni, A., Sigal-Zafrani, B., de La Rochefordiere, A., Salmon, R. J. & This, P. (2010). Is the breast-conserving treatment with radiotherapy appropriate in *BRCA1/2* mutation carriers? Long-term results and review of the literature. *Breast Cancer Research Treatment,* 120, 119-126. https://doi.org/10.1007/s10549-009-0685-6

Kriege, M., Jager, A., Hooning, M. J., Huijskens, E. & Blom, J. (2012). The efficacy of taxane chemotherapy for metastatic breast cancer in BRCA1 and BRCA2 mutation carriers. *Cancer*, 118, 899-907. https://doi.org/10.1002/cncr.26351

Lancaster, J. M., Wooster, R., Mangion, J., Phelan, C. M., Cochran, C., Gumbs, C., Seal, S., Barfoot, R., Collins, N., Bignell, G., Patel, S., Hamoudi, R., Larsson, C., Wiseman, R. W., Berchuck, A., Iglehart, J. D., Marks, J. R., Ashworth, A., Stratton, M. R. &

Futreal, P. A. (1996). BRCA2 mutations in primary breast and ovarian cancers. *Nature Genetics*, 13, 238-240. https://doi.org/10.1038/ng0696-238

Lee, D. S., Yoon, S. Y., Looi, L. M., Kang, P., Kang, I. N., Sivanandan, K., Ariffin, H., Thong, M. K., Chin, K. F., Mohd Taib, N. A., Yip, C. H. & Teo, S. H. (2012). Comparable frequency of BRCA1, BRCA2 and TP53 germline mutations in a multi-ethnic Asian cohort suggests TP53 screening should be offered together with BRCA1/2 screening to early-onset breast cancer patients. *Breast Cancer Research*, 14(R66), 1-8. https://doi.org/10.1186/bcr3172

Leong, S. P. L., Shen, Z-Z. & Liu, T-J. (2010). Is breast cancer the same disease in Asian and Western countries? *World Journal of Surgery*, 34(10), 2308-2324. https://doi.org/10.1007/s00268-010-0683-1

Li, J., Zou, C., Bai, Y., Wazer, D. E., Band, V. & Gao, Q. (2006). DSS1 is required for the stability of BRCA2. *Oncogene*, 25(8), 1186-1194. https://doi.org/10.1038/sj.embor.7400255

Li, X., You, R., Wang, X., Liu, C., Xu, Z. & Zhou, J. (2016). Effectiveness of prophylactic surgeries in *BRCA1* or *BRCA2* mutation carriers: a meta-analysis and systematic review. *Clinical Cancer Research,* 22, 3971-3981. https://doi.org/10.1158/1078-0432.CCR-15-1465

Lindahl, T. (1993). Instability and decay of the primary structure of DNA. *Nature*, 362(6422), 709-715. https://doi.org/10.1038/362709a0

Liu, Y. & West, S. C. (2002). Distinct functions of BRCA1 and BRCA2 in double-strand break repair. *Breast Cancer Research*, 4(1), 9-13. https://doi.org/10.1186/bcr417

Livraghi, L. & Garber, J. E. (2015). PARP inhibitors in the management of breast cancer: current data and future prospects. *BMC Medicine,* 13(188), 1-16. https://doi.org/10.1186/s12916-015-0425-1

Loizideou, M., Marcou, B., Anastasiadou, V., Newbold, R., Hadjisavvas, A. & Kyriacou, K. (2007). Contribution of BRCA1 and BRCA2 germline mutations to the incidence of early-onset breast cancer in Cyprus. *Clinical Genetics*, 71(2), 165-170. https://doi.org/10.1111/j.1399-0004.2007.00747.x

Lostumbo, L., Carbine, N. E. & Wallace, J. (2010). Prophylactic mastectomy for the prevention of breast cancer. *Cochrane Database of Systematic Reviews*, 11(CD002748), 1465-1858. https://doi.org/10.1002/14651858.CD002748.pub3

Mahmud, A. & Aljunid, S. M. (2018). Availability and accessibility of subsidized mammogram screening program in peninsular Malaysia: A preliminary study using travel impedance approach. *PLoS One,* 13(2), e0191764, 1-15. https://doi.org/10.1371/journal.pone.0191764

Massat, N. J., Dibden, A. & Parmar, D. (2016). Impact of screening on breast cancer mortality: The UK program 20 years on. *Cancer Epidemiology, Biomarkers & Prevention*, 25, 455-462. doi: 10.1158/1055-9965.EPI-15-0803

Mehrgou, A. & Akouchekian, M. (2016). The importance of BRCA1 and BRCA2 genes mutations in breast cancer development. *Medical Journal of the Islamic Republic of Iran*, 30(369), 1-12.

Ministry of Health Malaysia. (2008). *The Third National Health and Morbidity Survey 2006 (NHMS III): Executive Summary*. Retrieved on October 1, 2022, from https://iku.moh.gov.my/images/IKU/Document/REPORT/2006/ExecutiveSummary.pdf

Ministry of Health Malaysia. (2016). *Malaysian National Cancer Registry Report 2007-2011*. Retrieved on December 2, 2022, from https://www.crc.gov.my/wp-content/uploads/documents/report/MNCRRrepor2007-2011.pdf

Ministry of Health Malaysia. (2017). *National Strategic Plan for Cancer Control Programme 2016-2020*. Retrieved on October 10, 2022, from https://www.moh.gov.my/moh/resources/Penerbitan/Rujukan/NCD/Kanser/National_Strategic_Plan_Book_final@25SEPT2017.pdf

Ministry of Health Malaysia. (2019). *Malaysia National Cancer Registry Report (MNCR) 2012-2016*. Retrieved on September 5, 2022, from https://www.moh.gov.my/moh/resources/Penerbitan/Laporan/Umum/2012-2016%20(MNCRR)/MNCR_2012-2016_FINAL_(PUBLISHED_2019).pdf

Ministry of Health Malaysia. (2019a). *Clinical Practice Guidelines: Management of Breast Cancer (Third Edition)*. Retrieved on September 5, 2022, from https://www.moh.gov.my/index.php/dl/554756755a584a6961585268626939445545637653324675633256794c304a795a57467a644342445957356a5a5849765131424858303168626d466e5a57316c626e526662325a66516e4a6c59584e3058304e68626d4e6c636c386f56476870636d5266525752706448c7662696c664b4445704c6e426b5a673d3d.

Moynahan, M. E., Pierce, A. J. & Jasin, M. (2001). BRCA2 is required for homology-directed repair of chromosomal breaks. *Molecular Cell*, 7, 263-272. https://doi.org/10.1016/s1097-2765(01)00174-5

Mylavarapu, S., Das, A. & Roy, M. (2018). Role of BRCA mutations in the modulation of response to platinum therapy. *Frontiers in Oncology*, 8(16), 1-11. https://doi.org/10.3389/fonc.2018.00016

Nandakumar, A., Gupta, P. C. & Gangadharan, P. (2005). Geographic pathology revisited: Development of an atlas of cancer in India. *International Journal of Cancer*, 116(5), 740-754. https://doi.org/10.1002/ijc.21109

Nelson, A. C. & Holt, J. T. (2010). Impact of RING and BRCT domain mutations on BRCA1 protein stability, localization, and recruitment to DNA damage. *Journal of Radiation Research*, 74(1), 1-13. doi: 10.1667/RR1290.1

Nielsen, T. O., Hsu, F. D., Jensen, K., Cheang, M., Karaca, G., Hu, Z., Hernandez-Boussard, T., Livasy, C., Cowan, D., Dressler, L., Akslen, L. A., Ragaz, J., Gown, A. M., Gilks, C. B., van de Rijn, M. & Perou, C. M. (2004). Immunohistochemical and clinical characterization of the basal-like subtype of invasive breast carcinoma. Clinical Cancer Research, 10(16), 5367-5374. https://doi.org/10.1158/1078-0432.CCR-04-0220

Njor, S., Nyström, L. & Moss, S. (2012). Breast cancer mortality in European mammographic screening: a review of incidence-based mortality studies. *Journal of Medical Screening*, 19, 33-41. https://doi.org/10.1258/jms.2012.012080

Nordin, N., Yaacob, N. M. & Abdullah, N. H. (2018). Survival time and prognostic factors for breast cancer among women in North-East Peninsular Malaysia. *Asian Pacific Journal of Cancer Prevention*, 19(2), 497-502. https://doi.org/10.22034/APJCP.2018.19.2.497

NRDO. (2017). *Singapore Cancer Registry Annual Registry Report 2015*. Retrieved on November 1, 2022, from https://www.nrdo.gov.sg/docs/librariesprovider3/Publications-Cancer/cancer-registry-annual-report-2015_web.pdf?sfvrsn=10

O'Donovan, P. J. & Livingston, D. M. (2010). BRCA1 and BRCA2: Breast/ovarian cancer susceptibility gene products and participants in DNA double-strand break repair. *Carcinogenesis*, 31(6), 961-967. https://doi.org/10.1093/carcin/bgq069

Ouchi, T., Monteiro, A. N. A. & August, A. (1998). BRCA1 regulates p53-dependent gene expression. *Proceedings of the National Academy of Sciences of the United States of America*, 95, 2302-2306. https://doi.org/10.1073/pnas.95.5.2302

Paull, T. T., Rogakou, E. P., Yamazaki, V., Kirchgessner, C. U., Gellert, M. & Bonner, W. M. (2000). A critical role for histone H2AX in recruitment of repair factors to nuclear foci after DNA damage. *Current Biology*, 10, 886-895. https://doi.org/10.1016/s0960-9822(00)00610-2

Phillips, K. A., Milne, R. L., Rookus, M. A., Daly, M. B, Antoniou, A. C. & Peock, S. (2013). Tamoxifen and risk of contralateral breast cancer for *BRCA1* and *BRCA2* mutation carriers. *Journal Clinical Oncology,* 31, 3091-3099. https://doi.org/10.1200/JCO.2012.47.8313

Pierce, L. J., Phillips, K. A., Griffith, K. A., Buys, S., Gaffney, D. K. & Moran, M. S. (2010). Local therapy in *BRCA1* and *BRCA2* mutation carriers with operable breast cancer: comparison of breast conservation and mastectomy. *Breast Cancer Research Treatment,* 121, 389-398. https://doi.org/10.1007/s10549-010-0894-z

Plummer, R. (2010). Perspective on the pipeline of drugs being developed with modulation of DNA damage as a target. *Clinical Cancer Research*, 16, 4527-4531. https://doi.org/10.1158/1078-0432.CCR-10-0984

Pohlreich, P., Zikan, M., Stribrna, J., Kleibl, Z., Janatova, M. & Kotlas, J. (2005). High proportion of recurrent germline mutations in the BRCA1 gene in breast and ovarian cancer patients from the Prague area. *Breast Cancer Research*, 7(5), R728-R736. https://doi.org/10.1186/bcr1282

Pouptsis, A., Swafe, L., Patwardhan, M. & Stavraka, C. (2020). Surgical and systemic treatment of hereditary breast cancer: A mini-review with a focus on BRCA1 and BRCA2 mutations. *Frontiers in Oncology*, 10(553080), 1-7. https://doi.org/10.3389/fonc.2020.553080

Powell, S. N. & Kachnic, L. A. (2003). Roles of BRCA1 and BRCA2 in homologous recombination, DNA replication fidelity and the cellular response to ionizing radiation. *Oncogene*, 22(37), 5784–5791. https://doi.org/10.1038/sj.onc.1206678

Quek, D. K. L. (n.d.). *The Malaysian health care system: A review.* [Speaker]. Intensive Workshop on Health Systems in Transition, Kuala Lumpur, Malaysia. Retrieved on October 2022, http://cpds.fep.um.edu.my/events/2009/workshop/29042009/PPT%20&%20full%20paper/session%203/The%20Malaysian%20Health%20Care%20System1-presentation-dr%20david%20quek.pdf

Rebbeck, T. R., Kauff, N. D. & Domchek, S. M. (2009). Meta-analysis of risk reduction estimates associated with risk-reducing salpingo-oophorectomy in *BRCA1* or *BRCA2* mutation carriers. *Journal of the National Cancer Institute,* 101, 80-87. https://doi.org/10.1093/jnci/djn442

Rebbeck, T. R., Lynch, H. T., Neuhausen, S. L., Narod, S. A., Van't Veer, L. & Garber, J. E. (2002). Prophylactic oophorectomy in carriers of BRCA1 or BRCA2 mutations. *The New England Journal of Medicine,* 346(21), 1616-1622. https://doi.org/10.1056/NEJMoa012158

Rebbeck, T. R., Mitra, N., Wan, F., Sinilnikova, O. M., Healey, S. & McGuffog, L. (2015). Association of type and location of BRCA1 and BRCA2 mutations with risk of breast and ovarian cancer. *JAMA*, 313, 1347-1361. https://doi.org/10.1001/jama.2014.5985

Robson, M., Im, S. A., Senkus, E., Xu, B., Domchek, S. M. & Masuda, N. (2017). Olaparib for metastatic breast cancer in patients with a germline BRCA mutation. *The New England Journal of Medicine,* 377(6), 523-533. https://doi.org/10.1056/NEJMoa1706450

Roy, R., Chun, J. & Powell, S. N. (2012). BRCA1 and BRCA2: Different roles in a common pathway of genome protection. *Natural Reviews Cancer,* 12, 68-78. https://doi.org/10.1038/nrc3181

Ruffner, H., Joazeiro, C. A. & Hemmati, D. (2001). Cancer-predisposing mutations within the RING domain of BRCA1: Loss of ubiquitin protein ligase activity and protection from radiation hypersensitivity. *Proceedings of the National Academy of Sciences of the United States*, 98(9), 5134-5139. https://doi.org/10.1073/pnas.081068398

Sadeghi. F., Asgari, M., Matloubi, M., Ranjbar, M., Karkhaneh Yousefi, N., Azari, T. & Zaki Dizaji, M. (2020). Molecular contribution of BRCA1 and BRCA2 to genome instability in breast cancer patients: review of radiosensitivity assays. *Biological Procedures Online*, 22(23), 1-28. https://doi.org/10.1186/s12575-020-00133-5

Sandhu, S. K., Schelman, W. R., Wilding, G., Moreno, V., Baird, R. D. & Miranda, S. (2013). The poly (ADP-ribose) polymerase inhibitor niraparib (MK4827) in *BRCA* mutation carriers and patients with sporadic cancer: A phase 1 dose-escalation trial. *Lancet Oncology,* 14, 882-892. https://doi.org/10.1016/S1470-2045(13)70240-7

Saslow, D., Boetes, C., Burke, W., Harms, S., Leach, M. O. & Lehman, C. D. (2007). American Cancer Society guidelines for breast screening with MRI as an adjunct to mammography. *Cancer Journal for Clinicians,* 57, 75-89. https://doi.org/10.3322/canjclin.57.2.75

Satagopan, J. M., Boyd, J., Kauff, N. D., Robson, M., Scheuer, L. & Narod, S. (2002). Ovarian cancer risk in Ashkenazi Jewish carriers of *BRCA1* and *BRCA2* mutations. *Clinical Cancer Research,* 8, 3776-3781.

Smith, T. M., Lee, M. K., Szabo, C. I., Jerome, N., McEuen, M., Taylor, M., Hood, L. & King, M-C. (1996). Complete genomic sequence and analysis of 117 kb of human DNA containing the gene BRCA1. *Genome Research*, 6, 1029-1049. https://doi.org/10.1101/gr.6.11.1029

Sung, H., Ferlay, J. & Siegel, R. L. (2021). Global cancer statistics 2020: GLOBOCAN estimates of incidence and mortality worldwide for 36 cancers in 185 countries. *Cancer Journal for Clinicians*, 71, 209-249. https://doi.org/10.3322/caac.21660

Tassone, P., Tagliaferri, P., Perricelli, A., Blotta, S., Quaresima, B. & Martelli, M. L. (2003). BRCA1 expression modulates chemosensitivity of BRCA1-defective HCC1937 human breast cancer cells. *British Journal of Cancer,* 88, 1285-1291. https://doi.org/10.1038/sj.bjc.6600859

Thapa, B., Singh, Y. & Sayami, P. (2013). Breast cancer in young women from a low risk population in Nepal. *Asian Pacific Journal of Cancer Prevention,* 14(9), 5095-5099. https://doi.org/10.7314/apjcp.2013.14.9.5095

Thirthagiri, E., Lee, S. Y., Kang, P., Lee, D. S., Toh, G. T., Selamat, S., Yoon, S. Y., Taib, N. A., Thong, M. K., Yip, C. H. & Teo, S. H. (2008). Evaluation of BRCA1 and BRCA2 mutations and risk-prediction models in a typical Asian country (Malaysia) with a relatively low incidence of breast cancer. *Breast Cancer Research*, 10(R59), 1-12. https://doi.org/10.1186/bcr2118

Thompson, D. & Easton, D. (2004). The genetic epidemiology of breast cancer genes. *Journal of Mammary Gland Biology and Neoplasia*, 9(3), 221-236. https://doi.org/10.1023/B:JOMG.0000048770.90334.3b

Tichy, J. R., Lim, E. & Anders, C. K. (2013). Breast cancer in adolescents and young adults: A review with a focus on biology. *National Comprehensive Cancer Network*, 11(9), 1060-1069. https://doi.org/10.6004/jnccn.2013.0128

Tutt, A., Robson, M., Garber, J. E., Domchek, S. M., Audeh, M. W. & Weitzel, J. N. (2010). Oral poly (ADP-ribose) polymerase inhibitor olaparib in patients with *BRCA1* or *BRCA2* mutations and advanced breast cancer: A proof-of-concept trial. *Lancet,* 376, 235-244. https://doi.org/10.1016/S0140-6736(10)60892-6

Tutt, A. N. J., Garber, J. E., Kaufman, B., Viale, G., Fumagalli, D., Rastogi, P., Gelber, R. D., de Azambuja, E., Fielding, A., Balmaña, J., Domchek, S. M., Gelmon, K. A., Hollingsworth, S. J., Korde, L. A., Linderholm, B., Bandos, H., Senkus, E., Suga, J. M., Shao, Z., … & Geyer, C. E. (2021). Adjuvant Olaparib for patients with BRCA1- or BRCA2-mutated breast cancer. *New England Journal of Medicine*, *384*(25), 2394-2405. https://doi.org/10.1056/NEJMoa2105215

Valachis, A., Nearchou, A. D. and Lind, P. (2014). Surgical management of breast cancer in *BRCA*-mutation carriers: a systematic review and meta-analysis. *Breast Cancer Research Treatment,* 144, 443-455. https://doi.org/10.1007/s10549-014-2890-1

Vallard, A., Magné, N., Guy, J. B., Espenel, S., Rancoule, C. & Diao, P. (2019). Is breast-conserving therapy adequate in *BRCA 1/2* mutation carriers? The radiation oncologist's point of view. *British Journal of Radiology,* 92(20170657), 1-9. https://doi.org/10.1259/bjr.20170657

Venkitaraman, A. R. (2002). Cancer susceptibility and the functions of BRCA1 and BRCA2. *Cell*, 108(2),171-182. https://doi.org/10.1016/s0092-8674(02)00615-3

Vogel, V. G., Costantino, J. P., Wickerham, D. L., Cronin, W. M., Cecchini, R. S. & Atkins, J. N. (2006). Effects of tamoxifen vs raloxifene on the risk of developing invasive breast cancer and other disease outcomes: The NSABP Study of Tamoxifen and Raloxifene (STAR) P-2 trial. *JAMA*, 295(23), 2727-2741. https://doi.org/10.1001/jama.295.23.joc60074

Welcsh, P. L. & King, M. C. (2001). BRCA1 and BRCA2 and the genetics of breast and ovarian cancer. *Human Molecular Genetics*, 10(7), 705-713. https://doi.org/10.1093/hmg/10.7.705

Xing, J., Watkins, W. S. & Witherspoon, D. J. (2009). Fine-scaled human genetic structure revealed by SNP microarrays. *Genome Research*, 19(15), 815-825. https://doi.org/10.1101/gr.085589.108

Yarden, R. I. & Papa, M. Z. (2006). BRCA1 at the crossroad of multiple cellular pathways: approaches for therapeutic interventions. *Molecular Cancer Therapeutics*, 5(6), 1396-1404. https://doi.org/10.1158/1535-7163.MCT-05-0471

Yow, W. K., Mahmud, R., Ling, K. H. & Thilakavathy, K. (2017). Breast cancer associated mutations reported among Malaysian Malay, Chinese and Indian patients. *Progress in Bioscience and Bioengineering*, 1(2), 1-11. https://doi.org/10.29269/pbb2017.v1i2.19

Zhang, F., Fan, Q., Ren, K. & Andreassen, P. R. (2009). PALB2 functionally connects the breast cancer susceptibility proteins BRCA1 and BRCA2. *Molecular Cancer Research,* 7(7), 1110-1118. https://doi.org/10.1158/1541-7786.MCR-09-0123

Zhang, J., Fackenthal, J. D., Huo, D., Zheng, Y. & Olopade, O. I. (2010). Searching for large genomic rearrangements of the BRCA1 gene in a Nigerian population. *Breast Cancer Research and Treatment*, 124(2), 573-577. https://doi.org/10.1007/s10549-010-1006-9

Zhou, J., Gelot, C., Pantelidou, C., Li, A., Yücel, H., Davis, R. E., Färkkilä, A., Kochupurakkal, B., Syed, A., Shapiro, G. I., Tainer, J. A., Blagg, B. S. J., Ceccaldi, R. & D'Andrea, A. D. (2021). A first-in-class polymerase theta inhibitor selectively targets homologous-recombination-deficient tumors. *Nature Cancer*, *2*(6), 598-610. https://doi.org/10.1038/s43018-021-00203-x

Zheng, R., Han, S., Duan, C., Chen, K. & You, Z. (2015). Role of taxane and anthracycline combination regimens in the management of advanced breast cancer: A meta-analysis of randomized trials. *Medicine (Baltimore),* 94(17), 1-10. https://doi.org/10.1097/MD.0000000000000803

Chapter 7

von Willebrand Disease: An Inheritable Bleeding Disorder

Noor Haslina Mohd Noor[1,*]
Zefarina Zulkafli[1]
Muhamad Aidil Zahidin[1]
and Hisham Atan Edinur[2]
[1]Hematology Department, School of Medical Sciences, Universiti Sains Malaysia, Kota Bharu, Kelantan, Malaysia
[2]Forensic Programme, School of Health Sciences, Universiti Sains Malaysia, Kota Bharu, Kelantan, Malaysia

Abstract

von Willebrand Disease (vWD) is an inherited bleeding disorder caused by a lack or deficiency of von Willebrand factor (vWF) - a multimeric protein produced by liver sinusoidal cells, megakaryocytes and endothelial cells - which is required for blood clotting. vWF is a large protein comprising 80 subunits with a total size of ≥20,000 kDa. Following damage to blood vessels, it will be released from its inactivated bond with Factor VIII (another protein involved in blood clotting) by thrombin action to facilitate platelet adhesion to sub-endothelia tissues. vWD may arise from qualitative or quantitative defects in vWF. Quantitative defects include low levels of the protein (Type 1) or virtually none in the individual's blood (Type 3). Qualitative defects (Type 2A, 2B, 2M and 2N) occur due to mutated vWF proteins that have lost their function. Inheritance of the disease can either be

* Corresponding Author's Email: drhaslina@usm.my.

In: Genetic Disorders and Rare Diseases
Editors: Shazlin Shaharudin, Hisham Atan Edinur and Nor Fazila Che Mat
ISBN: 979-8-88697-953-4

autosomal dominant or recessive, but females are disproportionately affected. Unlike thalassaemia and other blood disorders, there is large variation in the *vWF* gene and mutations may occur at various points, so much so that gene sequencing is not a good method to diagnose the disease. The replenishment of vWF from donor plasma or recombinant sources remains the cornerstone treatment for affected individuals.

Keywords: bleeding disorder, coagulation, genetic, glycoprotein

Introduction

Dr Erik von Willebrand first observed a defective blood-clotting disease running in families living in the Aland Islands of Finland in 1926 (Zimmerman et al., 1971). This inherited bleeding condition, which was eventually named after him, has poor platelet adhesion and aggregation as its defining features (Bharati and Prashanth, 2011). Many years later, the cause of Von Willebrand Disease (vWD) was narrowed down to quantitative and qualitative defects of a plasma protein known as the Von Willebrand Factor (vWF). In blood, vWF is naturally bound to Factor VIII (FVIII) — an activating protein in the blood coagulation cascade — which ensures haemostasis and prevents the factor from being prematurely degraded (Zimmerman et al., 1971). When bound to FVIII, the inactivated complex is known to have a longer half-life of 12 to 16 hours compared with FVIII in free form, which the half-life is one to two hours only. Following damage to blood vessels, the vWF-FVIII complex will be released from its bond through thrombin action. vWF will facilitate platelet adhesion to the sub-endothelial tissue of the compromised site, while FVIII will activate other factors in the blood coagulation cascade to prevent haemorrhaging.

vWD is one of the most common inherited bleeding disorders. Type 1 and Type 3 of the disease indicate mild to moderate and severe quantitative inadequacies of vWF, respectively. On the other hand, Type 2 is characterised by qualitative impairments in vWF (Ng et al., 2015). The type of inheritance can either be autosomal dominant or recessive, depending on classification. Each subtype of Type 2 vWD involves different types and locations of mutation in the *vWF* gene (Favaloro, 2020).

Epidemiology

vWD affects both men and women equally and can affect up to 1% of the general population. Due to episodes of bleeding during menstruation, pregnancy and after childbirth, women are more likely to experience symptoms of vWD. A United States' Centers for Disease Control and Prevention website stated that more than 14,600 people have been reportedly treated for vWD between 2012 and 2016 at haemophilia centres throughout that country. Of the total, about two-thirds were women and girls (Centers for Disease Control and Prevention, 2020). According to a report on the vWD in Malaysia, 60% of the patients nationwide were females, with Malays making up the majority (63.3%), and 41.3% were aged between 19 and 44 (Periayah et al., 2016). About 15.2% of the patient population was recorded in the state of Sabah. A total of 97.9% of patients nationwide reportedly have Type 1 or Type 2 vWD, whereas only 2.1% of cases were classified as the severe Type 3 disease (Periayah et al., 2016).

Classification

Previously, more than 20 different types of vWD have been identified; however, despite their clear academic significance, these distinctions lacked evidence of therapeutic relevance. Hence, the International Society on Thrombosis and Haemostasis (ISTH) later categorised vWD into six types based on vWF phenotype (Favaloro, 2020). These six vWD classifications corresponded to significant clinical characteristics and treatment needs (Favaloro, 2020). Type 1, which makes up between 70% and 80% of all cases, is identified by a quantitative vWF deficiency (Leebeek & Eikenboom, 2016). Subgroups of Type 2 include the following: 2A, 2B, 2M, and 2N, which account for about 20% of cases. This type is caused by the abnormal function of the vWF protein, which presents as normal or decreased antigen concentration, but a marked drop in facilitating the adhesion of platelets (Bharati & Prashanth, 2011; (Leebeek & Eikenboom, 2016). Patients with Type 2A vWD are classified as having lost the most adhesive vWF forms, which are high-molecular-weight (HMW) multimers. Type 2B distinguishes "hyper-adhesive" vWF forms, which are frequently linked to HMW vWF loss. Type 2N identifies a defective vWF-FVIII binding attributed to a lack of vWF-D domain. Lastly, Type 2M vWD is a rather heterogeneous (residual) set of vWF binding defect that cannot be classified as 2A, 2B or 2N, instead, it reflects vWF dysfunction despite normal levels of HMW vWF multimers (Favaloro, 2020). Only 5% of people worldwide have Type 3 vWD, which is rare. It is the most severe type that results from a lack of circulating vWF (Leebeek & Eikenboom, 2016). Table 1 shows the summary of vWD classifications.

Table 1. von Willebrand disease (vWD) classification

Type	Description
1	Partial quantitative vWF deficiency
2A	Decreased HMW vWF multimer levels and decreased vWF-dependent platelet adhesion
2B	Increased platelet glycoprotein Ib affinity towards vWF
2N	Noticeably reduced affinity towards FVIII binding
2M	Decreased HMW vWF multimer-dependent platelet adhesion without specific multimer deficiency
3	Complete deficiency of vWF in blood (≤5 IU/dL)

vWF- von Willebrand factor, HMW- high-molecular-weight, FVIII- factor VIII.

Pathophysiology

vWF is sizeable and intricate multimeric plasma glycoprotein. It is produced in endothelial cells and stored in granules known as Weibel-Palade bodies, megakaryocytes (precursor of platelets in the bone marrow) and sub-endothelial connective tissue, and plays multiple roles in haemostasis of blood coagulation (Keesler & Flood, 2018). Weibel-Palade bodies contain ultra-large vWF (UL-vWF) multimers, which are the most effective for coagulation at the site of injury. Within the A2 domain, the UL-vWF multimers will undergo proteolytic cleavage by the vWF-cleaving protein (ADAMTS-13) into physiologically active vWF multimers. As a shear sensor, the A2 domain must be folded properly for proteolytic cleavage to occur. Therefore, polymorphisms in the A1 and A2 domains will affect the efficiency of ADAMTS-13 cleavage (Berber, 2012).

With more adhesion sites than lesser types, vWF is built from similar 250 kDa subunits to form disulfide-linked multimers with a total mass of ≥20,000 kDa. This makes the vWF more efficient during haemostasis (Sadler, 1998). A total of 2,050 amino acids make up each monomer of vWF, and different domains within each monomer serve different tasks. In the endoplasmic reticulum, these monomers are N-glycosylated, resulting in the production of dimers. By using disulfide links to cross-link cysteine residues, these dimers are then organised into multimers. The multimers are "packaged" in the Golgi apparatus of cells, each of which has roughly 80 subunits and a molecular weight of 250 kDa. Several cleavage products are also produced because of the development of large multimers. However, only the larger multimers are useful, as opposed to the cleavage products (Bharati & Prashanth, 2011). Dong (2005) provided a potential model of UL-vWF proteolysis by ADAMTS-13 in vivo. ULVWF is anchored to the surface of endothelial cells to form string-like structures under fluid shear stress which facilitates ULVWF cleavage by exposing either the cleavage or binding sites for the metalloprotease. Platelet binding, collagen binding and FVIII binding can be used to explain the three functions of vWF (Keesler & Flood, 2018).

By interacting with glycoprotein 1b (Gp1b) receptors on platelet membranes and components of exposed connective tissue, vWF facilitates the adherence of platelets to sites of vascular damage. Plasma vWF carries blood clotting FVIII, and this interaction is essential for stabilising FVIII, prolonging its half-life, and ensuring its survival in the bloodstream (Keesler & Flood, 2018).

The main function of specific domains present in vWF is to connect with plasma proteins, like FVIII, which aids in haemostasis (Table 2). vWF non-covalently binds to FVIII and protects itself from being degraded by proteolysis (Berber, 2012). vWF binds to collagen when a blood vessel is damaged. The platelet receptors become engaged when coagulation is induced, and vWF will attach to these activated receptors (Bharati & Prashanth, 2011).

Table 2. vWF monomer domains and their functions

Domain in a monomer	**Function**
D/D3	Binds to FVIII
A1	Binds to platelet GPib receptor, heparin, possibly collagen
A2	ADAMTS-13 cleavage
A3	Collagen binding
C1 (RGD domain)	Binds to platelet integrin aIIbβ3 when activated
Cysteine and knot domain	Link with PDGF, TGFβ, βHCG

GP1b- Platelet glycoprotein 1bcomplex, RGD- arginine, glycine, aspartate amino acid sequence in vWF, PDGF- platelet derived growth factor, TGFβ- transforming growth factor β, βHCG- β human chorionic gonadotrophin.

Genetic Inheritance

vWF is expressed from a large gene locus on the short arm of chromosome 12p13.3, with a size of 178 kb and a total of 52 exons. The cDNA is segmented into the D1, D2, D', A1, A2, A3, D4, B1, B, B3, C1, and C2 domains (Smith, 2019). A partial pseudogene is also present on chromosome 22, comprising exons 23–34 (Arshad et al., 2017). There are 2,050 amino acids in a mature vWF. Dominant inheritance is the trait of Types 1, 2A, 2B, and 2M vWD. This means that these disease types may be inherited from a defective gene from one parent. With each pregnancy, there is a 50% chance that the offspring will be born with vWD when one parent possesses the dominant disease type. About 70% of cases with vWD fall under the most prevalent form of the disease, Type 1, which has an autosomal-dominant pattern of inheritance. The most frequent point mutation associated with Type 1 vWD is 42 Y1584C, while other mutations, such as nonsense, missense, minor insertions, splice site and promoter mutations, have also been identified (Berber, 2012, Swami and Kaur, 2017). Missense mutations (75%) can be found in the promoter region 10 to exon 11, 12 and 52 of the vWF. Only a small percentage (5% to 10%) of autosomal dominant patients have more than one mutation contributing to their symptoms, while others have recessive inheritance (Goodeve, 2016).

The second pathogenic mechanism is Type 1C vWD, also known as the rapid vWF clearance. The variants linked with rapid vWF clearance are R1205H (vWD Vicenza), C1130G/F/R, W1144G, I1416N, and S1279F (Berber, 2012). ABO blood types have an impact on vWF clearance as well. Blood group O individuals have shorter vWF half-lives, which may be explained by the quicker vWF clearance from circulation (Goodeve, 2016). About 25% of Type 2 vWD cases are found to have functional or qualitative vWF activity abnormalities. Type 2 is subdivided into 2A, 2B, and 2M based on poor platelet interaction, and 2N is based on faulty FVIII molecule binding (Berber, 2012). In Type 2A vWD, low levels of high- and intermediate-weight multimers result in fewer Gp1b binding sites, thus, equating to poor platelet binding (Berber, 2012). This subtype is a result of frame-shift, insertion, deletion and missense mutations. Exon 28 contains about 73% of these mutations (Berber, 2012). The A2 domain, D3 domain, D2 domain, and CK domains are the locations with the most frequent mutations (Goodeve, 2016).

Type 2B vWD shares an autosomal-dominant inheritance pattern and is characterised by spontaneous and increased vWF affinity to GpIbα receptors on platelets. This happens because of the loss of HMW-vWF multimers in plasma and the pervasive gain-of-function A1 domain mutations (Berber, 2012; Goodeve, 2016). Since large multimers have more GpIb binding sites, it is anticipated that ADAMTS-1's proteolytic action will lead them to leave the plasma sooner. In addition, bound platelets also contribute to the absence of LMWMs in the patient's plasma and conventional thrombocytopenia (Swami & Kaur, 2017). The vWF mutation database receives more than 50 types of mutations. However, only Type 2B variants, 96.0% of which are missense mutations, are detected in exon 28 of the vWF gene, which codes for the A1 domain (Berber, 2012).

Type 2M vWD, a less common variation with autosomal-dominant inheritance and malfunctioning HMW-vWF brought on by vWF gene mutations, exhibits these characteristics (Berber, 2012). Mutations linked to this feature disrupt the vWF-platelet (domain A1) and vWF-collagen (domain A3) interactions. During laboratory testing, there were distinctive multimer pattern and decreased ristocetin-induced platelet aggregation (RIPA) sensitivity. It is important to note that alterations in the vWF domains A1 or A3, which are essential for the interaction between vWF and collagen, may result in decreased vWF collagen binding (vWF:CB) (Swami & Kaur, 2017). Missense mutations make up around 93% of these mutations, and minor in-frame deletions make up about 10% (Berber, 2012). Exon 28 of the vWF gene is where 75% of fully penetrant Type 2M mutations are found.

Type 2N deficiency prevents vWF from binding to FVIII, and it characterises the rare form with an autosomal-recessive inheritance pattern. Mutations in exons 18 to 21 in the D′–D3 domain affect the affinity of vWF towards FVIII, thus, a weak binding will increase the free form of FVIII in plasma and subject it to quick degradation (Goodeve, 2016). Despite a normal multimer profile, laboratory test results of Type 2N individuals will reveal a noticeable decrease in FVIII levels compared with vWF levels (reduced FVIII/vWF:Ag ratio). This is due to a prolonged partial thromboplastic time (PTT) and decreased vWF:FVIII binding (Swami and Kaur, 2017).

Type 3 vWD accounts for less than 5% of vWD occurrences and is characterised by undetectable levels of vWF (≤5 IU/dL) and FVIII (≤10 IU/dL) in the plasma because there is not enough vWF to bind with FVIII and prevent it from degradation (Goodeve, 2016). Exons 2 to 52 of the *vWF* gene contain the coding area for Type 3 mutations, which are autosomal recessive and detected in 80% of cases (Berber, 2012, Swami and Kaur, 2017). Most of the Type 3 gene mutations are nonsense mutations. R1659X, the most prevalent nonsense mutation, is located in exon 28 and is a result of the allele-specific mRNA nonsense-mediated degradation (Berber, 2012). Missense mutation in the D1 and D2 domains comprise the second-most frequent mutation in Type 3 vWD, accounting for roughly 15% to 20% of all mutations. This mutation causes the substitution of cysteine residues, which limits the production of dimers and multimers to ensure vWF production is kept within the endoplasmic reticulum (Berber, 2012, Swami & Kaur, 2017).

Clinical Presentations

The symptoms of vWD vary across patients, depending on disease subtype, the degree of residual vWF activity, and age and gender. Bruising and epistaxis (nose bleed) are common symptoms in affected children, whereas menorrhagia, hematoma and prolonged bleeding after injury are typical in adulthood. In the case of medical and dental treatments, about 60% to 80% of affected individuals may suffer from uncontrolled bleeding following surgery, childbirth and tooth extraction (Leebeek, 2016). More than 70% of women with vWD also reported experiencing menorrhagia and 50% had dysmenorrhoeal bleeding (Bharati and Prashanth, 2011). Type 1 vWD often has mild clinical manifestations compared with Type 2 and 3, which have more severe presentation. The drop in FVIII level generally correlates with severity of bleeding. Haemorrhagic manifestation primarily affects the mucocutaneous tissues, which is a clinical characteristic of vWF deficiency.

Persistent epistaxis, gingival bleeding, menorrhagia and gastrointestinal bleeding are examples of mucocutaneous haemorrhage that may be detrimental to the health of affected individuals, besides reducing their quality of life. Even in patients who have minimal vWF impairment, spontaneous bleeding may still occur at a low incidence. However, Type 1 vWD rarely exhibits severe coagulation deficiency, such as hemarthrosis and deep-muscle hematoma, as the decrease in FVIII protein level is often minimal (Castaman et al., 2013). Gastrointestinal haemorrhage from angiodysplasia is a well-known, severe and possibly fatal condition in vWD patients. Elderly individuals with Type 2 or 3 vWD are more likely to suffer such bleeding and therefore, may require constant monitoring of their condition. Even though it may be a presenting symptom in those with Type 2N or Type 3 illness, intraarticular haemorrhage has not been documented as a significant issue in patients with vWD. The severity of vWD, as well as the level of residual FVIII, has significant impact on the likelihood of joint haemorrhage (Leebeek, 2016). A person with Type 3 vWD may experience significant internal and joint bleeding, but this is extremely uncommon (Bharati & Prashanth, 2011). In

Type 3 vWD, bleeding can occasionally be as severe as mild haemophilia. Patients with low plasma levels of high-molecular weight multimers may experience frequent gastrointestinal bleeding that is challenging to control. In Type 1 vWD individuals, bleeding after childbirth is rare because, in mild cases, the FVIII/vWF level typically return to normal at the end of pregnancy. vWF replacement therapy is frequently necessary to control immediate or delayed postpartum haemorrhage in females with Type 2A, 2B or 3 of the disease. Even in Type 1 vWD individuals showing serious symptoms, post-operative bleeding may not occur, whereas Type 3 patients are always in need of prophylactic treatment (Castaman et al., 2013).

Laboratory Diagnosis

Due to the wide polymorphism of vWF, initial testing for vWD requires a combination of screening procedures because no single test can definitively rule out the presence of a fully functioning protein factor (Castaman et al., 2013). The diagnosis of vWD is usually achieved based on personal and family history of bleeding, in addition to laboratory tests to assess vWF and FVIII activity in the individual's blood (Leebeek, 2016). Since neither Type 1 nor Type 2 individuals exhibit significant bleeding, early diagnosis of their disease is challenging. In contrast, Type 3 individuals often receive an early diagnosis because of their serious bleeding issues since infancy (Bharati & Prashanth, 2011).

Screening for vWD

vWF Antigen (VWF:Ag)

The vWF antigen (VWF:Ag) offers a quantitative assessment of plasma vWF protein. Testing for vWF:Ag may be done automatically using enzyme-linked immunosorbent assay (ELISA) or latex immunoassay (LIA) (Castaman et al., 2010). Although vWF:Ag is a relatively reliable and repeatable marker, it has limitations because it only evaluates the presence or concentration of vWF, and not its activity or function. To assess the functionality of vWF protein, further assays discussed in the following subtopics are performed.

vWF Ristocetin Cofactor Activity (vWF:RCo)

The ability of vWF to bind with GPIbα is one of the biochemical tests used to assess the functionality of vWF through the vWF ristocetin cofactor activity (vWF:RCo). Although the vWF:RCo test is often utilised, its utility is limited by its significant coefficient of variance (Kitchen et al., 2006). Additionally, the efficiency of vWF:RCo may be affected by vWF sequence changes in the A1 domain without changing the vWF function (Flood et al., 2010). However, none of the newly established ristocetin-independent tests that directly assess vWF-GPIbα interactions are commercially available (Favaloro & Mohammed, 2014, Patzke et al., 2014). The necessity of using the vWF:RCo test may potentially be replaced with a more dependable vWF-platelet interaction test and eliminate the need for vWF:Ag in early VWD screening, but it may miss the diagnosis of Type 2M collagen-binding defects.

Factor VIII Activity (FVIII:C)

The first work-up includes FVIII activity (FVIII:C) testing since vWF serves as a carrier for FVIII. The ratio of FVIII:C to vWF:Ag in physiologic equilibrium is about 1. This ratio will be lower in Type 2N of the disease and in Type 3, its activity will be less than 10 IU/dL. Since Type 2N vWD has a unique fault in FVIII binding capability and can emerge with normal vWF:Ag and vWF:RCo, assessment of FVIII:C is crucial in the early work-up for suspected vWD.

VWF:RCo/VWF:Ag Ratio

Evaluation of the vWF:RCo/vWF:Ag ratio prompts further testing for Type 2A, 2B, or 2M vWD, all of which commonly have a vWF:RCo to vWF:Ag ratio of <0.6 (Nichols et al., 2008). However, confirmatory testing is necessary to distinguish between the Type 2 variations. For the summary of vWD screening assays and anticipated outcomes for each category, readers are referred to a publication by Keesler & Flood (2018).

The vWF:GPIbM ratio may be used in lieu of the vWF:RCo ratio in certain assays. vWF:RCo assay using platelets, ristocitin and native GPIb. VWF:GPIbM is a VWF assays using recombinant GPIb mutations reflect VWF:GPIb binding assays similar to VWF:RCo and VWF:GPIbR but that do not employ ristocetin. Another functional VWF assay are collagen binding assay (VWF:CB).

Confirmatory Tests for Von Willebrand Disease

vWF Multimer Distribution

Given that a normal multimer distribution suggests Type 2M vWD, whereas the loss of high molecular weight multimers indicates Type 2A or Type 2B vWD, a decreased vWF:RCo to vWF:Ag ratio should be an indication to examine the vWF multimer distribution. Multimer analysis normally involves gel electrophoresis, but this method is time-consuming and not employed in many laboratories.

vWF Collagen Binding (vWF:CB)

In vWF testing, the binding of collagen serves two roles. It can serve as a substitute for detection of high molecular weight multimers and it have a specific collagen-binding defect in some VWD variants i.e type 2M. Additionally, some vWD variations are labelled as Type 2M vWD because they exhibited a particular collagen-binding deficiency. There are many documented instances of patients who have borderline low vWF:Ag and vWF:RCo, but significant decreases in Type I and/or Type III collagen-binding capabilities.

vWF–Platelet Binding (vWF:PB)

Determination of platelet binding capability, seen as an increase in spontaneous binding of platelets to the damaged site of the blood vessel, is used to confirm Type 2B vWD. This assay, which makes use of patient plasma and commercial platelets, will exhibit improved binding capability in Type 2B vWD individuals, while Type 2A will show lower binding capability. If it is not feasible, low-dose ristocetin-induced platelet aggregation is an alternative.

Low-Dose Ristocetin-Induced Platelet Aggregation (LD-RIPA)

Low-dose ristocetin-induced spontaneous aggregation is seen in Type 2B vWD and platelet-type vWD. It is necessary to differentiate between the vWD variants using genetic testing or vWF:PB. Prescription of desmopressin (DDAVP) — an anti-diuretic used to treat diabetes insipidus, bedwetting, high blood urea and mild forms of bleeding disorders — is typically avoided in patients with Type 2B vWD, but both Type 2A and Type 2B patients will otherwise show patterns of decreased vWF. Type 2B vWD detection is significant due to thc RCo to vWF:Ag ratio and lack of large molecular weight multimers. The need for platelet transfusion during treatment makes the detection of vWD of the platelet type crucial.

vWF-FVIII Binding (vWF:FVIIIB)

VWF:FVIIIB assess the ability of VWF isolated from patient plasma to bind recombinant FVIII. It is used to confirm a diagnosis of type 2N VWD, where a specific defect in FVIII binding exists.

vWF Propeptide (vWFpp)

Type 1C, or clearing faults, and some Type 2 vWD variations have increased vWFpp to vWF:Ag ratios. ELISA is commonly used to determine the quantity of vWFpp. Evaluation of DDAVP response may also reveal clearance deficiencies; for example, after one hour, the vWF:Ag ratio may increase but by the fourth hour following DDAVP administration, vWF levels may return to normal.

vWF Gene Sequencing

Genetic diagnostics are used to a limited extent only in vWD due to the enormous size and high frequency of variations in the *vWF* gene. The high frequency of gene variations found in healthy individuals has thrown into question early descriptions of some sequential changes as mutations. DNA sequencing may be helpful in identifying Type 2 vWD, especially when other clinical testing methods are unavailable or challenging to interpret. In Type 2 vWD, numerous known sequence variants have been recorded.

Sequence changes in Type 2 vWD are confined to the *vWF* region that is defective. It has been found that Type 2B and Type 2M mutations in the A1 domain of *vWF* will interfere with platelet binding. Type 2N has been found to have mutations in the *vWF* D′ and D3 domains, where they have been observed to interfere with FVIII binding. Type 2A defects may be found in either the N- or C-terminal multimerisation domains, the A2 domain (located close to the AD-AMTS13 cleavage site), or both. The *vWF* gene contains defects that cause Type 1 and Type 3 vWD, although not all unique sequence variations are related to vWD. Therefore, caution should be taken when using gene sequencing to confirm a diagnosis.

Treatment

There are several widely accepted and advised therapy recommendations for vWD. The replenishment of vWF protein deficiency forms the cornerstone of all types of available treatment. Options include non-replacement therapy, replacement therapy and others.

Empiric treatment, such as a DDAVP prescription or vWF replacement therapy, are two options to raise vWF levels that can be given to patients who show bleeding symptoms in Type 1 vWD. In the case of heavy menstrual bleeding, additional treatments like hormone therapy or antifibrinolytics may be helpful. As an analogue of vasopressin, DDAVP triggers the rapid release of FVIII and vWF from liver and endothelial cells. Within 30 to 60 minutes of administration, it will cause a two- to four-fold increase in vWF and a three- to six-fold increase in FVIII in the blood of patients. However, DDAVP treatment is not able to stop bleeding symptoms in Type 2 vWD patients because their cells cannot produce functional vWF. Rather, it only increases the level of defective vWF in the blood. On the other hand, individuals with Type 3 vWD cannot produce vWF, hence DDAVP is unable to increase vWF levels in these patients (Swami & Kaur, 2017).

Although DDAVP works for most Type 1 individuals, there are still some who show a lack of response, hence a trial dose is usually administered first. A clearance defect also needs to be taken into consideration if the vWF:Ag is less than 20–30 IU/dL. This may be done by assessing a late time point after DDAVP administration or by analysing the vWF pro-peptide. However, Type 1 vWD patients who have vWF:Ag values of between 10 and 20 IU/dL will still need to be treated with a vWF concentrate as even a three-fold increase in their vWF level is not sufficient to enable surgery.

Type 2 patients will require treatment with a vWF concentrate for most of their bleeding symptoms. This is because DDAVP may increase vWF levels but does not repair the underlying dysfunction. Although Type 2 vWD is considered a relative contraindication to DDAVP treatment, it may still be used to treat mild bleeding like epistaxis if the patient experiences clinical improvement (Keesler & Flood, 2018).

Individuals with insufficient amount or non-functional vWF may be referred for replacement therapy using vWF derived from donated human plasma. Replacement therapy is usually used in emergency treatments such as a life-saving surgery. The vWF from donated plasma, when administered to a patient, must be given time to stabilise with endogenous FVIII levels. Thus, it is usually given to the patient around 12 hours beforehand. The alternative is to administer both vWF and FVIII at once, even though the additional FVIII dosing is unnecessary because endogenous FVIII production is adequate in the context of normal vWF (Keesler & Flood, 2018).

Another replacement therapy option for treating Type 1, 2, and 3 vWD is the utilisation of recombinant vWF (rvWF). Patients with low FVIII levels will require supplemental FVIII medication for emergency therapy because rvWF is not naturally bound to FVIII protein. Both vWF and FVIII are needed in surgery, as well as a preoperative dosage of vWF the day before (Keesler & Flood, 2018).

Conclusion

Type 1 and 2 vWD is an inherited autosomal dominant haemorrhagic disorder, whereas Type 3 is autosomal recessive. However, all disease types arise from defects and/or deficiency in the vWF protein, which is vital for platelet adhesion and initiation of the blood-clotting mechanism. The most common cause of this disease is mutation in the gene that encodes the vWF protein. As bleeding severity may become worse as patients advance in age, there is a need for monitoring and strict treatment planning to reduce the risk of complications and fatality, especially from gastrointestinal bleeding. Replacement therapy using recombinant vWF or those derived from donated human plasma seems the only practical treatment in managing vWD.

References

Arshad, N., Nawaz, S. K., Iqbal, R., Arshad, M., Musheer, F., Naz, A., Mushtaq, I., & Jaleel, S. (2017). Association between genetic polymorphism and risk of von Willebrand disease in Pakistan. *BioMed Research International*, 1070471. https://doi.org/10.1155/2017/1070471

Berber, E. (2012). The molecular genetics of von Willebrand disease. *Turkish Journal Hematology*, *29*(4), 313-324. https://doi.org/10.5505/tjh.2012.39205

Bharati, K. P., & Prashanth, U. R. (2011). Von Willebrand disease: An overview. *Indian Journal of Pharmaceutical Sciences*, *73*(1), 7-16. https://doi.org/10.4103/0250-474X.89751

Castaman, G., Goodeve, A., Eikenboom, J., & European Group on von Willebrand Disease (2013). Principles of care for the diagnosis and treatment of von Willebrand disease. *Haematologica*, 98(5), 667–674. https://doi.org/10.3324/haematol.2012.077263

Castaman, G., Tosetto, A., Cappelletti, A., Goodeve, A., Federici, A. B., Batlle, J., Meyer, D., Goudemand, J., Eikenboom, J. C., Schneppenheim, R., Budde, U., Ingerslev, J., Lethagen, S., Hill, F., Peake, I. R., & Rodeghiero, F. (2010). Validation of a rapid test (VWF-LIA) for the quantitative determination of von Willebrand factor antigen in type 1 von Willebrand disease diagnosis within the European multicenter study MCMDM-1VWD. *Thrombosis Research*, *126*(3), 227-231. https://doi.org/10.1016/j.thromres.2010.06.013

Centers for Disease Control and Prevention (2020). *Data and Statistics on von Willebrand Disease*. Retrieved on October 10, 2022. https://www.cdc.gov/ncbddd/vwd/data.html

Dong J. F. (2005). Cleavage of ultra-large von Willebrand factor by ADAMTS-13 under flow conditions. *Journal of Thrombosis and Haemostasis, 3*(8), 1710-1716. https://doi.org/10.1111/j.1538-7836.2005.01360.x

Favaloro E. J. (2020). Classification of von Willebrand disease in the context of modern contemporary von Willebrand factor testing methodologies. *Research and Practice in Thrombosis and Haemostasis*, *4*(6), 952-957. https://doi.org/10.1002/rth2.12392

Favaloro, E. J., & Mohammed, S. (2014). Towards improved diagnosis of von Willebrand disease: comparative evaluations of several automated von Willebrand factor antigen and activity assays. *Thrombosis Research*, *134*(6), 1292-1300. https://doi.org/10.1016/j.thromres.2014.09.024

Flood, V. H., Gill, J. C., Morateck, P. A., Christopherson, P. A., Friedman, K. D., Haberichter, S. L., Branchford, B. R., Hoffmann, R. G., Abshire, T. C., Di Paola, J. A., Hoots, W. K., Leissinger, C., Lusher, J. M., Ragni, M. V., Shapiro, A. D., & Montgomery, R. R. (2010). Common VWF exon 28 polymorphisms in African Americans affecting the VWF activity assay by ristocetin cofactor. *Blood*, *116*(2), 280–286. https://doi.org/10.1182/blood-2009-10-249102

Leebeek, F. W., & Eikenboom, J. C. (2016). Von Willebrand's Disease. *New England Journal of Medicine*, *375*(21), 2067-2080. https://doi.org/10.1056/NEJMra1601561

Goodeve A. (2016). Diagnosing von Willebrand disease: genetic analysis. *Hematology, 2016*(1), 678-682. https://doi.org/10.1182/asheducation-2016.1.678

Keesler, D. A., & Flood, V. H. (2017). Current issues in diagnosis and treatment of von Willebrand disease. *Research and Practice in Thrombosis and Haemostasis*, *2*(1), 34-41. https://doi.org/10.1002/rth2.12064

Kitchen, S., Jennings, I., Woods, T. A., Kitchen, D. P., Walker, I. D., & Preston, F. E. (2006). Laboratory tests for measurement of von Willebrand factor show poor agreement among different centers: results from the United Kingdom National External Quality Assessment Scheme for Blood Coagulation. *Seminars in Thrombosis and Hemostasis*, *32*(5), 492-498. https://doi.org/10.1055/s-2006-947863

Ng, C., Motto, D. G., & Di Paola, J. (2015). Diagnostic approach to von Willebrand disease. *Blood*, *125*(13), 2029–2037. https://doi.org/10.1182/blood-2014-08-528398

Nichols, W. L., Hultin, M. B., James, A. H., Manco-Johnson, M. J., Montgomery, R. R., Ortel, T. L., Rick, M. E., Sadler, J. E., Weinstein, M., & Yawn, B. P. (2008). von Willebrand disease (VWD): evidence-based diagnosis and management guidelines, the National Heart, Lung, and Blood Institute (NHLBI) Expert Panel report (USA). *Haemophilia*, *14*(2), 171-232. https://doi.org/10.1111/j.1365-2516.2007.01643.x

Patzke, J., Budde, U., Huber, A., Méndez, A., Muth, H., Obser, T., Peerschke, E., Wilkens, M., & Schneppenheim, R. (2014). Performance evaluation and multicentre study of a von Willebrand factor activity assay based on GPIb binding in the absence of ristocetin. *Blood Coagulation and Fibrinolysis*, *25*(8), 860-870. https://doi.org/10.1097/MBC.0000000000000169

Periayah, M. H., Halim, A. S., Saad, A. Z., Yaacob, N. S., & Karim, F. A. (2016). Report on von Willebrand disease in Malaysia. *Open Access Macedonian Journal of Medical Sciences*, *4*(1), 112–117. https://doi.org/10.3889/oamjms.2016.030

Roberts, J. C., & Flood, V. H. (2015). Laboratory diagnosis of von Willebrand disease. *International Journal of Laboratory Hematology*, *37 Suppl 1*(Suppl 1), 11-17. https://doi.org/10.1111/ijlh.12345

Smith, L. J., (2017). Laboratory diagnosis of von Willebrand disease. *American Society for Clinical Laboratory Science*, 30(2), 65-74. https://doi.org/10.29074/ascls.30.2.65

Swami, A., & Kaur, V. (2017). von Willebrand disease: A concise review and update for the practicing physician. *Clinical and Applied Thrombosis/Hemostasis*, *23*(8), 900-910. https://doi.org/10.1177/1076029616675969

Zimmerman, T. S., Ratnoff, O. D., & Powell, A. E. (1971). Immunologic differentiation of classic hemophilia (factor 8 deficiency) and von Willebrand's dissase, with observations on combined deficiencies of antihemophilic factor and proaccelerin (factor V) and on an acquired circulating anticoagulant against antihemophilic factor. *Journal of Clinical Investigation*, *50*(1), 244-254. https://doi.org/10.1172/JCI106480

Chapter 8

α-Thalassaemia: Genetic Variants and Screening Methods

Zefarina Zulkafli[1,2,*]
Noor Haslina Mohd Noor[1,2]
Wan Suriana Wan Ab Rahman[2,4]
and Hisham Atan Edinur[3]

[1]Hematology Department, School of Medical Sciences, Universiti Sains Malaysia, Kota Bharu, Kelantan, Malaysia
[2]Transfusion Medicine Unit, Hospital Universiti Sains Malaysia, Kota Bharu, Kelantan, Malaysia
[3]Forensic Science Programme, School of Health Sciences, Universiti Sains Malaysia, Kota Bharu, Kelantan, Malaysia
[4]School of Dental Sciences, Universiti Sains Malaysia, Kota Bharu, Kelantan, Malaysia

Abstract

α-thalassaemia and its variants are a growing community health problem in the world. Public awareness regarding this condition is imperative to avert the risk of passing down this disease to future generations. As a recessively inherited haemoglobin disorder, there are many types of α-globin gene mutation and deletion that has been characterised. This chapter discusses the genetic disorders in α-thalassaemia, which includes mutations found in a Malaysian population. The prevalence of α-thalassaemia in Malaysia is between 15.8 and 33.6 %. At least 300 mutations and deletions in the α-globin gene have been characterised, and approximately 14 are described in the Malaysian population, including

---

* Corresponding Author's Email: zefarina@usm.my

In: Genetic Disorders and Rare Diseases
Editors: Shazlin Shaharudin, Hisham Atan Edinur and Nor Fazila Che Mat
ISBN: 979-8-88697-953-4

seven deletional and seven non-deletional types. The latest laboratory investigations for screening and diagnoses are also highlighted. Many α-thalassemia traits are asymptomatic and coincidentally discovered during routine analyses like full blood count and full blood picture. It is hoped that this article will not only generate knowledge about the variants of α-thalassaemia and its screening applications, but also raise awareness among clinicians and researchers of this disease. This may inspire ideas for forthcoming research, principally in refining management and prevention of severe manifestations of the disease in Malaysia.

Keywords: α-variants, α- globin gene, deletion, mutation, prevention

Introduction

Haemoglobin abnormalities are the most prevalent inherited monogenic diseases that have become a concern in global health (Williams & Weatherall, 2012; Higgs et al., 2012; Weatherall, 2012). About 7 % of the world population is a carrier of some kind of haemoglobin disease, and 300,000 to 500,000 children are born with severe conditions annually (WHO 1989). If left unchecked, there is high possibility that this disorder will become a liability on the healthcare resources of many countries. This risk is further aggravated by poor disease management and lack of family planning efforts due to insufficient data. Their high prevalence may be attributed to natural selection, high incidence of consanguineous marriages, and epidemiological shifts. Advances in healthcare have also resulted in more children surviving the illnesses and requiring lifelong treatment, especially in developing countries (Williams & Weatherall, 2012; Kattamis et al., 2020).

Haemoglobin (Hb), the primary component of red blood cells (RBC), is responsible for delivering oxygen to tissues in almost all vertebrates. It has a quaternary structure consisting of four iron-containing heme subunits covalently bound to four globin molecules. These heme molecules in RBC will bind with oxygen molecules through ionic forces to form oxyhaemoglobin in the lungs, which will be transported to various tissues and organs. Upon reaching the target tissue, the oxygen molecules will be exchanged with carbon dioxide, which is a product of respiration, to form carbaminohaemoglobin. Carbaminohaemoglobin in RBC will then return to the lungs where the carbon dioxide will be exchanged for oxygen.

Healthy adults should have 12 to 17 g of Hb in every 100 ml of blood, with the majority (95-97 %) comprising haemoglobin A (HbA, heme molecules bound to two alpha (α) and two beta (β) globin chains). The other about 3% is known as haemoglobin A2 (HbA2), which contain two α and two delta (δ) globin chains. For foetal haemoglobin (HbF) < 1%, with two α and two gamma (γ) globin chains.

Two sets of genes encoding two types of α globin chains (HBA1 and HBA2) are located in chromosome 16, whereas the ones encoding the beta (β) globin chains are located in chromosome 11. Genetic flaws in any of the globin genes will result in Hb abnormalities that can be generally categorised as either quantitative or qualitative (Forget and Bunn 2013; Munkongdee et al., 2020). A common example of hereditary Hb disorder with quantitative deficiencies resulting from an unbalanced synthesis of normal globin chains is thalassaemia, specifically α- and β-thalassaemia. They develop when the patients' Hb has fewer or no equivalent α- and β-globin chains. On the other hand, α- and β-globin variants are instances of qualitative haemoglobinopathies produced by structural aberrations (Kohne 2011; Munkongdee et al., 2020).

These inherited Hb disorders reduce the oxygen-binding capacity of RBC and affect its transport throughout the body. The clinical manifestations are varying; some affected individuals will exhibit mild to severe hypochromic anaemia, while others may have life-threatening effects that require lifelong blood transfusion. Multi-organ disruptions, including skeletal and cardiac problems, gallstones and splenomegaly, may also develop in severe patients (Kohne 2011). This chapter will discuss the prevalence of α-thalassaemia and its defective variants in Malaysia in terms of patient demography and type of gene deletion or mutation, besides the routine methods for screening and diagnosis.

Prevalence and Pathogenesis of α - Variants

The prevalence of α-thalassaemia in Malaysia is higher than its β-thalassaemia counterpart, which is between 15.8 and 33.6 % versus 4.5 and 12.8 %, respectively (Wee et al., 2005; Tan et al., 2010). α-thalassaemia is one of the core community health issues in Malaysia's multi-ethnic population, which causes a burden in public healthcare because of complicated treatment and lifelong monitoring of patients (MOH, 2003; Ibrahim et al., 2020). As the most inherited Hb disease worldwide, α-thalassaemia is frequently observed in Southeast Asian, Mediterranean and Middle Eastern populations (Wee et al., 2005; Azma et al., 2014).

Normally, α-globin production is controlled via four α-globin genes; two on each copy of chromosome 16 and this genotype is inscribed as αα/αα. When α-thalassemia occurs, the main basis is the reduction or absence of α-globin chain production, which is required in all types of Hb — the adult HbA (α2β2), fetal HbF (α2⌉2) and minor component HbA2 (α2⌈2) (Harteveld & Higgs, 2010; Galanello & Cao, 2011). α-thalassemia is a recessively inherited disease. A benign trait may occur in an individual carrier who has both normal and defective genes. However, if both parents are carriers of defective genes, the disease will then have higher probability to manifest in their offspring. This is dissimilar for a dominant condition, where only one copy of the gene is needed to manifest symptoms (Old et al., 2012).

Normal individuals have four α-globin genes, with each allele being inherited from each parent. However, if both parents carried at least one defective α-globin allele, their offspring will be at risk of developing thalassaemia intermedia, also known as Haemoglobin H (HbH), or Hb Barts in the worst-case scenario, which will result in foetal fatality. The accurate risk depends on the number of alleles that are defective and which mixture of the HBA1 and HBA2 genes are affected. One (-) or both (--) α-globin gene deletion is a common molecular basis of α-thalassaemia. Point mutations in critical areas will cause non-deletional thalassaemia. Complete mutation/deletion(s) will eradicate chromosomal expression and this condition is known as α^0-thalassaemia. Meanwhile, α^+-thalassaemia is a condition when the mutation/deletion(s) partly downregulates the chromosome expression (Harteveld & Higgs, 2010; Galanello & Cao, 2011).

Furthermore, the quantity of α-globin genes affected by hereditary alterations will determine clinical severity of the disease. Asymptomatic individuals will usually have one or two α-gene deletions or mutations. Those with three gene deletions, on the other hand, will likely present with HbH. Till 2018, 18.26 % of registered α-thalassaemia patients in the Malaysian Thalassaemia Registry (MTR) reportedly had HbH disease. Those with four gene deletions will subsequently develop Hb Barts, which is not compatible with life. Hb Barts affects the foetus, which will usually end up as stillbirth because of hydrops fetalis, unless blood transfusion is carried out (Azma et al., 2014; Ibrahim et al., 2020). Table 1 shows the types of α-thalassaemia and their genotypes, plus the resulting clinical severity.

To date, at least 300 types of mutation and deletion for α-globin gene has been characterised and approximately 14 different types have been described in the Malaysian population, including seven deletional and seven non-deletional types (Table 2). Wide-ranging summaries of the deletions and mutations are stated and updated frequently in various websites, such as http://databases.lovd.nl/shared; http://globin.cse.psu.edu/hbvar/menu.html; http://www.ithanet.eu; http://www.ithanet.eu/db/ithagenes; and http://globin.bx.psu.edu/hbvar/menu.html (Jameela et al., 2011; Rahimah et al., 2012; Azma et al., 2014; Goh et al., 2020).

Table 1. Classification of α-thalassaemia phenotypes, their possible genotypes and clinical severity

Phenotype Classification	Possible Genotype	Clinical severity
Haemoglobin Barts (Hb Bart)	Deletion/inactivation of all four α-globin genes (--/--)	Not compatible with life. Foetus will develop hydrops fetalis and die at birth.
Haemoglobin H (HbH) disease	Deletion/inactivation of three α-globin genes (--/-α)	Moderate to severe anaemia. Some patients may need for lifelong blood transfusion.
α-thalassemia trait/carrier	Deletion/inactivation of two α-globin genes either *in cis* (--/αα, or -α^0 carrier) or *in trans* (-α/-α)	Mild anaemia or asymptomatic
α-thalassemia silent carrier	Deletion/inactivation of one α-globin gene (-α/αα or α^+ carrier)	No symptoms. Offspring will be at risk due to inheritance of defective genes.

Table 2. Types of the α-globin gene deletions and mutations reported in Malaysian populations

Types of deletion	Types of mutation
$-\alpha^{3.7}/\alpha\alpha$	Hb Constant Spring (Hb CS, HBA2: c.427T > C, αCSα/αα)
$-\alpha^{4.2}/\alpha\alpha$	Hb Quong Sze (Hb QS, HBA2: c.377T > C, αQSα/αα,
$—^{MED}/\alpha\alpha$	$\alpha\alpha\alpha^{anti\text{-}3.7}$ triplication
$—^{SEA}/\alpha\alpha$	codon 59 mutation (GGC→GAC)
$—^{THAI}/\alpha\alpha$	initiation codon (ATG→A–G)
$-\alpha^{20.5}/\alpha\alpha$	codon 30
$—^{FIL}/\alpha\alpha$	codon 35

Screening for α-Thalassemia

The clinical manifestation and severity of disease are reliant on the quantity of α-genes affected. Therefore, the clinical phenotype is variable; from normal/asymptomatic to fatal haemolytic anaemia. All affected individuals have varying Hb levels, low level (anaemia), reduced mean corpuscular Hb (MCH/pg), reduced mean corpuscular volume (MCV/fl) and a normal or slightly reduced level of HbA2. In Malaysia, screening methods for thalassemia comprise a full blood count (FBC) and blood smear/ full blood picture (FBP), which are performed as a clinical routine. Molecular methods like gel electrophoresis, high-performance liquid chromatography (HPLC) and capillary electrophoresis (CE) are used to confirm the clinical findings (Azma et al., 2014).

Screening for α-thalassemia is critical for identifying couples at high risk, besides prevention of foetal fatality, severe maternal complications and emotional stress. Majority of α-thalassemia traits in Malaysia are discovered only as coincidental findings during this 2 routine screening haematological analyses which are full blood count (FBC) and full blood picture (FBP).

FBC and FBP

In FBC, the whole blood sample is analysed using an automated blood cell analyser to obtain specific haematological parameters like Hb, haematocrit and RBC count. These parameters are used to calculate RBC indices, such as MCV, MCH and mean corpuscular haemoglobin concentration (MCHC). MCV levels of less than 80 fL and MCH levels of less than 27 pg are used as cut-off values for positive indication of thalassaemia (Azma et al., 2014; Vijian et al., 2021). As for full blood picture (FBP), the morphology of RBC will be assessed under the microscope. The blood smear samples of thalassemic individuals will exhibit microcytic, hypochromic and anisopikilocytosis RBC. If suspected thalassemia cases are detected in FBC and FBP, HPLC and CE will be used to determine the abnormal Hb in the patient and quantify it (Vijian et al., 2021).

High-Performance Liquid Chromatography (HPLC)

HPLC is a separation system that usually uses gas or liquid solvent passed through a charged matrix column to separate components of a sample based on their molecular size. In the case of blood analysis, it splits a net positive charge of Hb into its components. Retention times or the duration a solute occupies a column, separation curve and percentage produced will differ between the types of Hb. The primary benefit of this technique is its precision and sensitivity in the quantification of Hb components with outstanding resolution and reproducibility. HPLC can isolate and measure the quantity of HbA, HbA2, Hb F and abnormal variants like HbH, HbS and Hb Barts in a blood sample. Even though HPLC is automated and proficient in differentiating the types of Hb, it has limitations in identifying and enumerating the percentage between HbH and Hb Barts. It is also not effective in detecting α-globin variants like Hb Constant Spring (CS) (Vijian et al., 2021).

Capillary Electrophoresis (CE)

HbA2, HbE, HbF, HbH, Hb Barts and other variants may be separated and quantified using CE. Packed cells are hemolysed using a hemolysing solution after the plasma is removed. Then, charged particles are detached based on their electrophoretic mobility. At a wavelength of 415 nm, which is ideal for Hb, the subsequent Hb fractions are detected from cathode to anode in the following order: Hb C, A2, E, S, D, F, A, Barts, J and H. The benefits of using CE include quick turnaround, high throughput, small sample volume requirement and low cost. The CE system is also able to measure the level of HbH and Hb Barts, which the HPLC system is unable to perform (Vijian et al., 2021).

Molecular Testing

The usual screening procedures for α-thalassaemia like gel electrophoresis, HPLC and CE cannot be used to determine carrier status. Therefore, molecular analysis is needed to wholly comprehend the clinical characteristics and make an accurate diagnosis. Methods for detecting molecular abnormalities, namely deletional and non-deletional mutations, may be performed using various polymerase chain reaction (PCR) techniques and DNA sequencing. The popular molecular techniques used to explore α-globin gene faults include Multiplex Gap-PCR, multiplex ligation-dependent probe amplification (MLPA) and multiplex amplification refractory mutation system (MARMS) PCR.

Multiplex Gap-PCR

The Multiplex Gap-PCR technique is presently a method of choice to distinguish common α-thalassemia deletion. The primers flanking the deleted region are used to amplify the DNA sequence. Gap-PCR is a rapid technique for detecting the seven most common types of deletion in α-thalassaemia (Vijian et al., 2021).

Multiplex Amplification Refractory Mutation System (MARMS PCR)

MARMS PCR can be used to detect deletion or non-deletion mutations of α-thalassaemia. The allele-specific PCR technique is also known as ARMS PCR (Hassan et al., 2013). Single-tube multiplex ARMS PCR is a method of choice to detect common and non-deletional α-globin gene variants that originate in Southeast Asian populations, including the initiation codon (ATG > A-G; HBA2:c.2delT), codon 30 (HBA2:c.91 93delGAG), codon 35 (SerPro), codon 59 (HBA2 (or HBA1):c.179G > A) (Hb Adana) and (Hb Constant Spring) because it is an efficient and reliable method (Vijian et al., 2021).

Multiplex Ligation-Dependent Probe Amplification (MLPA)

The MLPA procedure is appropriate for both quantitative and rapid analysis of mutations. The MLPA may be used to detect large α-globin gene deletions, both common and uncommon (Wee et al., 2005; Azma et al., 2014; Vijian et al., 2021).

DNA Sequencing

Foremost, DNA sequencing is the only way to identify rare deletion and non-deletion mutations in the α-globin gene. The "next generation sequencing" (NGS) technique is the latest sequencing technology to be introduced (Hassan et al., 2023). It is capable of discovering new and diverse α-thalassaemia variants. However, this technology, although being the most efficient, is also very costly, thus limiting its potential in clinical screening (Vijian et al., 2021).

Conclusion

The diagnosis of α-thalassemia and its variants may sometimes be complex because of a high degree of variability in α-globin gene defects. Hence, the diagnostic methods will be affected by cost, operator expertise and laboratory facilities. Although molecular testing is necessary for conclusive diagnosis, but family history, clinical examination, haematological tests, HPLC and CE remain as "first line" tools to determine thalassemia. With advancements in technology, there are different molecular techniques available for detecting globin gene mutations, and each has its own benefits and drawbacks (Vijian et al., 2021; Old et al., 2014). Scientifically, the knowledge of common and rare mutations is one of the earliest steps for establishment of specific and effective molecular characterisation of the disease, which may be beneficial in genetic counselling and treatment management.

Acknowledgment

This study was funded by the Ministry of Higher Education Malaysia for Fundamental Research Grant Scheme (FRGS/1/2019/SKK06/ USM/02/8).

References

Azma, R. Z., Ainoon, O., Hafiza, A., Azlin, I., Noor Farisah, A. R., Nor Hidayati, S., & Noor Hamidah, H. (2014). Molecular characteristic of alpha thalassaemia among patients diagnosed in UKM Medical Centre. *The Malaysian Journal of Pathology*, *36*(1), 27–32.

Forget, B. G., & Bunn, H. F. (2013). Classification of the disorders of hemoglobin. *Cold Spring Harbor Perspectives in Medicine*, *3*(2), a011684. https://doi.org/10.1101/cshperspect.a011684

Galanello, R., & Cao, A. (2011). Gene test review. Alpha-thalassemia. *Genetics in Medicine*, *13*(2), 83–88. https://doi.org/10.1097/GIM.0b013e3181fcb468

Goh, L. P. W., Chong, E. T. J., & Lee, P. C. (2020). Prevalence of Alpha(α)-Thalassemia in Southeast Asia (2010-2020): A Meta-Analysis Involving 83,674 Subjects. *International Journal of Environmental Research and Public Health*, *17*(20), 7354. https://doi.org/10.3390/ijerph17207354

Hassan, S., Ahmad, R., Zakaria, Z., Zulkafli, Z., & Abdullah, W. Z. (2013). Detection of β-globin Gene Mutations Among β-thalassaemia Carriers and Patients in Malaysia: Application of Multiplex Amplification Refractory Mutation System-Polymerase Chain Reaction. *The Malaysian Journal of Medical Sciences, 20*(1), 13–20.

Hassan, S., Bahar, R., Johan, M. F., Mohamed Hashim, E. K., Abdullah, W. Z., Esa, E., Abdul Hamid, F. S., & Zulkafli, Z. (2023). Next-Generation Sequencing (NGS) and Third-Generation Sequencing (TGS) for the Diagnosis of Thalassemia. *Diagnostics*, *13*(3), 373. https://doi.org/10.3390/diagnostics13030373

Harteveld, C. L., & Higgs, D. R. (2010). Alpha-thalassaemia. *Orphanet Journal of Rare Diseases*, *5*, 13. https://doi.org/10.1186/1750-1172-5-13

Higgs, D. R., Engel, J. D., & Stamatoyannopoulos, G. (2012). Thalassaemia. *Lancet (London, England)*, *379*(9813), 373–383. https://doi.org/10.1016/S0140-6736(11)60283-3

Jameela, S., Sabirah, S. O., Babam, J., Phan, C. L., Visalachy, P., Chang, K. M., Salwana, M. A., Zuraidah, A., Subramanian, Y., & Rahimah, A. (2011). Thalassaemia screening among students in a secondary school in Ampang, Malaysia. *The Medical Journal of Malaysia*, *66*(5), 522–524.

Kattamis, A., Forni, G. L., Aydinok, Y., & Viprakasit, V. (2020). Changing patterns in the epidemiology of β-thalassemia. *European Journal of Haematology*, *105*(6), 692–703. https://doi.org/10.1111/ejh.13512

Kohne E. (2011). Hemoglobinopathies: clinical manifestations, diagnosis, and treatment. *Deutsches Arzteblatt International*, *108*(31-32), 532–540. https://doi.org/10.3238/arztebl.2011.0532

Mohd Ibrahim, H., Muda, Z., Othman, I. S., Mohamed Unni, M. N., Teh, K. H., Thevarajah, A., Gunasagaran, K., Ong, G. B., Yeoh, S. L., Muhammad Rivai, A., Che Mohd Razali, C. H., Din, N. D., Abdul Latiff, Z., Jamal, R., Mohamad, N., Mohd Ariffin, H., & Alias, H. (2020). Observational study on the current status of thalassaemia in Malaysia: a report from the Malaysian Thalassaemia Registry. *BMJ Open*, *10*(6), e037974. https://doi.org/10.1136/bmjopen-2020-037974

Munkongdee, T., Chen, P., Winichagoon, P., Fucharoen, S., & Paiboonsukwong, K. (2020). Update in Laboratory Diagnosis of Thalassemia. *Frontiers in Molecular Biosciences*, *7*, 74. https://doi.org/10.3389/fmolb.2020.00074

Old, J., Harteveld, C. L., Traeger-Synodinos, J., Petrou, M., Angastiniotis, M., & Galanello, R. (2012). *Prevention of Thalassaemias and Other Haemoglobin Disorders: Volume 2: Laboratory Protocols*. (2nd ed.). Thalassaemia International Federation.

Rahimah, A. N., Nisha, S., Safiah, B., Roshida, H., Punithawathy, Y., Nurul, H., Syahzuwan, H., & Zubaidah, Z. (2012). Distribution of alpha thalassaemia in 16 year old Malaysian Students in Penang, Melaka and Sabah. *The Medical Journal of Malaysia*, *67*(6), 565–570.

Tan, J. A., Lee, P. C., Wee, Y. C., Tan, K. L., Mahali, N. F., George, E., & Chua, K. H. (2010). High prevalence of alpha- and beta-thalassemia in the Kadazandusuns in East Malaysia: challenges in providing effective health care for an indigenous group. *Journal of Biomedicine & Biotechnology*, *2010*, 706872. https://doi.org/10.1155/2010/706872

Tamary, H., & Dgany, O. (2005). Alpha-Thalassemia. In M. P. Adam (Eds.) et. al., *GeneReviews®*. University of Washington, Seattle.

Vijian, D., Wan Ab Rahman, W. S., Ponnuraj, K. T., Zulkafli, Z., & Mohd Noor, N. H. (2021). Molecular Detection of Alpha Thalassemia: A Review of Prevalent Techniques. *Medeniyet Medical Journal*, *36*(3), 257–269. https://doi.org/10.5222/MMJ.2021.14603

Weatherall D. J. (2012). The definition and epidemiology of non-transfusion-dependent thalassemia. *Blood Reviews*, *26 Suppl 1*, S3–S6. https://doi.org/10.1016/S0268-960X(12)70003-6

Wee, Y. C., Tan, K. L., Chow, T. W., Yap, S. F., & Tan, J. A. (2005). Heterogeneity in alpha-thalassemia interactions in Malays, Chinese and Indians in Malaysia. *The Journal of Obstetrics and Gynaecology Research*, *31*(6), 540–546. https://doi.org/10.1111/j.1447-0756.2005.00333.x

Williams, T. N., & Weatherall, D. J. (2012). World distribution, population genetics, and health burden of the hemoglobinopathies. *Cold Spring Harbor Perspectives in Medicine*, *2*(9), a011692. https://doi.org/10.1101/cshperspect.a011692

World Health Organization. (1989). Report of the VIth Annual Meeting of the WHO Working Group on the Feasibility Study on Hereditary Disease Community Control Programmes (Hereditary Anaemias, Cagliari (Sardinia, 8-9 April 1989). Retrieved on October 22, 2022. https://apps.who.int/iris/handle/10665/62136

Chapter 9

A Rare Genomic Copy Number Variation in Hypertension-Related Left Ventricular Hypertrophy in the Malaysian Population

Julia Ashazila Mat Jusoh[1,2,*]
Hoh Boon Peng[3,4]
and Khalid Yusoff[3,5]
[1]Institute of Medical Molecular Biotechnology (IMMB), UiTM Sungai Buloh, Selangor, Malaysia
[2]MyGenome Sdn Bhd, Kuala Lumpur, Malaysia
[3]Faculty of Medicine and Health Sciences, UCSI University, Port Dickson, Negeri Sembilan, Malaysia
[4]Division of Applied Biomedical Sciences and Biotechnology, School of Health Sciences, International Medical University, Kuala Lumpur, Malaysia
[5]Faculty of Medicine, UiTM Sungai Buloh Campus, Selangor, Malaysia

Abstract

Cardiovascular disease (CVD) is Malaysia's leading cause of mortality, accounting for 21.65% and 23.79% of all deaths in government and private hospitals in 2018. It is expected to continue rising in the next few decades. Hypertension-related left ventricular hypertrophy (HT-LVH) is an independent risk factor for cardiovascular mortality and morbidity and a substantial predictor of adverse cardiovascular outcomes. Regression of LVH is associated with reduced cardiovascular complications. However, 33.3% only of hypertensive patients in Malaysia benefit from the blood pressure-lowering effects of antihypertensive medication. Therefore, we anticipate a more minor LVH regression among patients

---

* Corresponding Author's Email: juliaashazila@mygenome.asia.

In: Genetic Disorders and Rare Diseases
Editors: Shazlin Shaharudin, Hisham Atan Edinur and Nor Fazila Che Mat
ISBN: 979-8-88697-953-4

in the country. Copy number variation (CNV) has been implicated in the pathogenesis of HT-LVH. A genome-wide analysis study comparing 100 patients with HT-LVH with 200 hypertensive individuals revealed the presence of 208 rare CNVs in the HT-LVH group. The analysis identified several genes for cardiac development and traits, including *IQGAP2, VAV3, F2R*, and *CDH15*. The gene-set was enriched in transcription factors that regulated the "foetal cardiac gene programme" and triggered the hypertrophic cascade by activating pathways associated with Sp1, CREB1, p53, and androgen receptor expression. This shows that controlling pathways associated with foetal cardiac genes may be crucial for LVH treatment. In conclusion, HT-LVH is prevalent among Malaysians, and a rare CNV contributes to its development by disrupting the functional regulation of the foetal cardiac gene programme.

Keywords: blood pressure, cardiovascular disease, heart failure

Introduction

Left ventricular hypertrophy (LVH) is a compensatory response to increased cardiac workload and if not controlled, it can contribute to heart failure. Increased cardiac mass will increase wall thickness, known as cardiac hypertrophy (Harvey & Leinwand, 2011; Saheera & Krishnamurthy, 2020). The leading cause of LVH is hypertension, which is highly prevalent in Malaysia. According to the 2019 Malaysian National Health and Morbidity Survey, 30% of the country's population aged 18 and above had been found to be suffering from hypertension (http://www.iku.gov.my/nhms-2019). By the time of diagnosis, LVH is present in more than one-third of the patients. A total of 24% of hypertensive patients were found to have LVH in an echocardiography study in a primary-care setting (Ching et al., 2012). A community-based survey revealed a 26.6% prevalence of LVH in hypertensive Malaysian men (Jusoh et al., 2022).

Blood pressure and intravascular volume are controlled by the renin-angiotensin-aldosterone system (RAAS), which also plays a crucial role in the development of LVH (Sciarretta et al., 2009). The increased risk of heart failure, atherosclerosis, and other cardiovascular complications has been attributed to LVH (Tin et al., 2002; Zipes & Wellens, 1998). Pathological LVH is a leading cause of death, affecting 36% to 41% of the general population, with rates ranging from 37% to 46.2% in men and 36% to 43.5% in women (Cuspidi et al., 2012; Cuspidi et al., 2012). Age, obesity, diabetes, sodium intake, insulin resistance, and neuro-humoral substances are all risk factors for developing hypertensive LVH (HT-LVH) (Cuspidi et al., 2012). A large portion of Malaysia's HT-LVH cases are found in rural areas, indicating that the patients have lower awareness and limited access to healthcare services to control their hypertension (Jusoh et al., 2022).

There are two types of cardiac hypertrophy: physiological (adaptive) and pathological (maladaptive) (McMullen & Jennings, 2007). Physiological hypertrophy occurs either during pregnancy or after long periods of exercise. In physiological hypertrophy, the heart functions normally, with normal gene expression and there is no evidence of apoptosis or fibrosis (Walsh, 2005). Activation of cell-survival signalling, better energy production and efficiency, mitochondrial quality control, activation of the antioxidant system, and cardiomyocyte proliferation and regeneration are required to sustain adaptive responses (Nakamura & Sadoshima, 2018). On the other hand, pathological LVH is observed when the heart is subjected to pressure or volume overload, like in individuals with aortic stenosis, hypertension, or valvular regurgitation. Interstitial fibrosis, increased expression of foetal genes, myocyte apoptosis and necrosis, and heart dysfunction are common complications in pathological hypertrophy (Walsh, 2005). Adaptive response to wall stress is often the initial phase of this condition, which is necessary to maintain cardiac output (Zhu et al., 2006). Maladaptive responses occur when the stimulus persists for an extended period. The first changes include a shift towards glucose utilisation in anaerobic pathways, which causes the reactivation of foetal genes in the heart tissue (Rajabi et al., 2007; Taegtmeyer et al., 2010). However, the molecular processes that regulate the transition from normal (adaptive) to abnormal (maladaptive) cardiac growth are not well documented.

The risk of cardiovascular disease and major adverse events will increase with the growth of the left ventricular mass index (LVMI), which reduces with the regression of HT-LVH (Bang et al., 2014). HT-LVH regression may be achieved using medication to lower blood pressure to normal levels of below 140/90 mmHg (Ahmed et al., 2020; Mancia et al., 2014; Nakashima et al., 1984). A slight positive correlation has been noted between short-term blood pressure variability and LVMI in a meta-analysis of 12 studies (Madden et al., 2015). In another meta-analysis, it is found that LVH regression may lower the incidence of cardiovascular disease (CVD) by an odds ratio (OR) of 0.41 (Verdecchia et al., 2003). A meta-analysis of 109 studies consisting of 2,357 hypertensive patients showed that LV mass decreased by 15% with the treatment of angiotensin-converting enzyme (ACE) inhibitors, 11% with diuretics, 8% with ß-blockers, and 8.5% with calcium channel blockers

(Dahlof et al., 1992). In a meta-analysis of randomised, double-blind studies, it was found that LVH regression occurred in 13% of patients treated with ACE inhibitors, 9% with calcium channel blockers, 7% with diuretics, and 6% with beta-blockers (Schmieder et al., 1996). Another meta-analysis discovered that angiotensin II receptor blockers, calcium antagonists, ACE inhibitors, diuretics, and beta-blockers could decrease LVMI by 13%, 11%, 10%, 8%, and 6%, respectively (Klingbeil et al., 2003).

However, 37.4% only of patients in Malaysia given anti-hypertensive medication could manage to bring down their blood pressure to below 140/90 mmHg (Majid et al., 2018). There is a lack of information about LVH regression using anti-hypertensive medication among HT-LVH patients in Malaysia. Multiple studies have shown that even with excellent control of blood pressure, LVH regression is not always accomplished (Lonnebakken et al., 2017). Potentially, genetic variants may account for the underlying factors in determining LVH susceptibility and its various responses to anti-hypertensive medication.

Molecular Mechanism of Pathological LVH

G protein-coupled receptors (GPCR) activating tyrosine- and serine/threonine kinase domains, such as gp-130 receptors, play a significant role in the development of pathological hypertrophy in cardiac myocytes. Mechanical stress in the heart causes the release of several autocrine, paracrine, and neurohumoral hormones, including endothelin-1 (ET-1), angiotensin II (Ang II), and noradrenaline. When bound to GPCRs, heterotrimeric G proteins of the Gq/q11 subclass will activate the Phospholipase C (PLC) signalling pathway, hence facilitating the hypertrophy cascade (Weeks & McMullen, 2011). Diacylglycerol (DAG) and 1,4,5-trisphosphate (IP3) are both produced from phosphatidylinositol 4, 5-bisphosphate (PIP2) when PLC signalling is activated. Hypertrophic signalling is promoted by DAG, which activates protein kinase C (PKC) and, in turn, the Map kinase (MAPK) pathway, and by IP3, which binds to sarcoplasmic reticulum (SERCA) receptors, releasing Ca^{2+} ions and activating the calcium-calmodulin or the calcineurin-NFAT (calcium-calmodulin-NFAT) signalling pathways as shown in Figure 1.

Multiple genes are upregulated in pathological hypertrophy. The process frequently involves reactivation of the foetal cardiac gene programme, in which gene expression will revert to a similar pattern in embryonic development (Dirkx et al., 2013). Myosin heavy chain (MHC), skeletal actin, atrial natriuretic peptide (ANP) and brain natriuretic peptide (BNP) are among the foetal genes which are highly expressed during pathological hypertrophy (Du, 2007; Kuwahara et al., 2012). While cardiac α-MHC is elevated after birth, β-MHC predominates during embryonic and foetal phases. After the heart tissue experiences, a blood pressure increase, however, α-MHC will become downregulated, and β-MHC is upregulated within a few hours. Immediate early genes like *c-myc*, *c-jun,* and *c-fos* are expressed after the activation of the foetal gene programme. The transcription factors encoded by these genes control a variety of downstream gene expressions that cause heart cells to grow (Walsh, 2005).

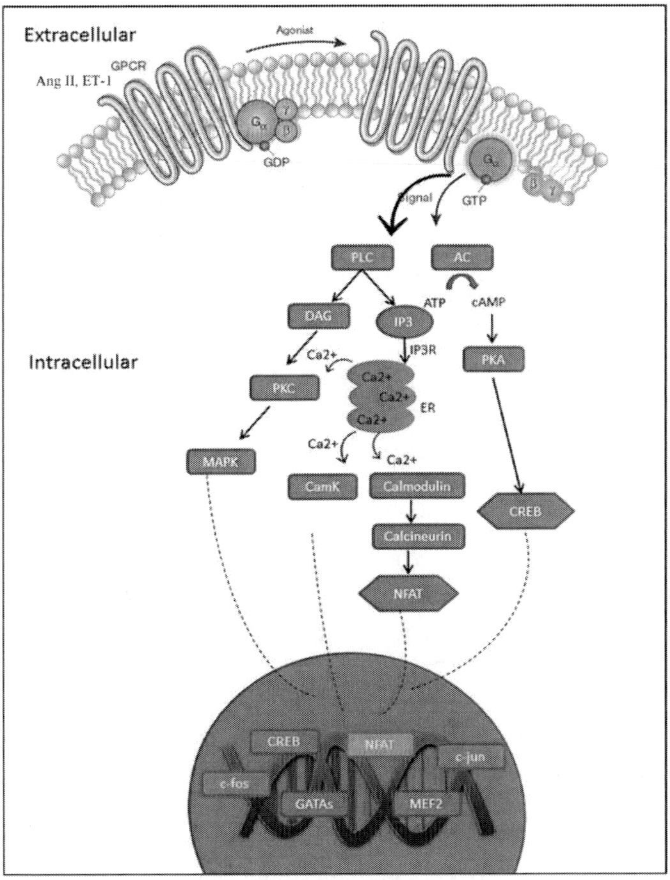

Figure 1. Schematic representation of the G-protein-mediated pathway that leads to activation of foetal gene programme and cardiac hypertrophy.

The Genetic Variation of Left Ventricular Hypertrophy

Genetic variations in the human genome can take a variety of forms, including microscopically visible chromosome aberrations; larger-scale structural variants such as copy number variations (CNVs); microsatellite and minisatellite repeats; fine-scale copy number alterations such as insertions and deletions (INDELS); and, nucleotide changes such as single nucleotide polymorphism (Sharp et al., 2006). The following variants and polymorphisms make up the human genome's architecture and highlight the diversity between individuals at the DNA level. The development of left ventricle hypertrophy is a complicated and multifactorial process. It is linked to interactions between various genes, lifestyle choices, and environmental factors (Schut, 2004). There is no definite inheritance pattern for complex disorders, making it extremely difficult to predict the chances of being affected. Complex diseases are challenging to study and treat since their causes are unclear. Polygenic diseases commonly run-in families, although their inheritance may not follow Mendelian disease patterns. However, this does not rule out the possibility of discovering and studying the genes responsible at some point. For example, in the case of type 1 diabetes, studies have observed that identical twins (who share the same environment and set of genes) have a 30 to 50% risk only in developing the condition together. Meanwhile, dizygotic twins (who share the same environment and only half of each other's' genes) are significantly less concordant (Concannon et al., 2009; Hirschhorn, 2003). Most polygenic diseases like hypertension are also influenced by environmental factors (Cardon & Bell, 2001). LVH has been observed to correlate more to the risk of cardiovascular mortality in African Americans than in Whites, indicating strong interactions among environmental and genetic factors (Havranek et al., 2008), which may account for the ineffectiveness of treatment among African Americans.

The role of RAAS in the pathogenesis of LVH has been proposed by several candidate gene association studies, although this evidence is not yet definitive due to a lack of replication studies reported (Arnett et al., 2009; Shlyakhto et al., 2001). A genetic association analysis by researchers in the United Arab Emirates revealed a link between ACE polymorphism and LVH (Saeed et al., 2005). This is contrary to earlier results indicating that ACE is probably a quantitative trait locus underlying genetic susceptibility to LVH (Lindpaintner et al., 1996). Still, this observation is in agreement with other studies (Schunkert et al., 1994). ACE deletion polymorphism has been linked to LVH in patients with diastolic heart failure in a study involving 176 people

(88 cases and 88 controls) (Bahramali et al., 2016). However, the limited sample size may have caused the study's conflicting results between ACE polymorphism and LVH. Gene-environment interactions may also play a role in these contradictory findings since they may cause some genes to be prevalently expressed in certain populations. It has been found that the AGTR2 +1675G/A polymorphism in angiotensin II type 2 receptor is correlated with the development of LVH (Huber et al., 2010). A genome-wide association study (GWAS) known as the HyperGEN Study failed to find any association between RAAS genes and LVH, but instead, discovered that calcineurin-related genes had a role in causing the disease (Arnett et al., 2009; Huber et al., 2010). A mutation in skeletal muscle Ca^{2+} release channel, also known as ryanodine receptor type 1 (*RYR1*), was found to be associated with LVH in another GWAS. The Korea Association Resource (KARE) study involved analysing the ECG-LVH results of 398 patients and 8,432 controls (Hong et al., 2012). Accordingly, a GWAS conducted on a Japanese population also found no significant association between genetic variations in RAAS and left ventricle mass (LVM), but the high expression of *Tbx3* (a transcription factor linked to the T box gene family) was linked to an increase in LVM (Sano et al., 2016). In another study, patients with arterial hypertension and sustained left ventricular ejection fraction showed a strong correlation between the *CYP17A1* polymorphism rs11191548 and LVMI (Huber et al., 2015). Conclusive evidence suggests that other pathways have more influence on cardiac hypertrophy than RAAS.

One of the key features of LVH is impaired calcium homeostasis. The role of calcium channels in the development of LVH has been the subject of numerous studies. For example, a study of hypertensive patients with and without cardiac hypertrophy (N = 325 and 697) discovered that the G allele of rs238234 calmodulin-binding transcription activator 2 (*CAMTA2*) promotes transcription of genes related to cardiac hypertrophy through its interaction with *Nkx2.5*, and it is a crucial transcription co-activator of cardiac hypertrophy (Song et al., 2016). The genes NRG*1*, *ERI2*, *IL23RAP*, *IL18RAP*, and *ACSM3* are linked to LVH phenotypes in a prospective cohort study of 4,286 women in the United Kingdom (the British Women's Heart and Health Study) (Seoane et al., 2014). In Malaysia, a study has been conducted to determine the role of *KCNB1* in calcineurin signalling in HT-LVH. However, there was no significant association observed between the gene and HT-LVH (Ashazila et al., 2013).

The lack of any gene association observed in genetic studies of LVH may be attributed to:

1. The selection of candidate genes is based solely on the biochemical roles of encoded proteins, leading to the inaccurate selection of candidate genes or SNPs. Therefore, genome-wide screening is recommended to study complex traits such as HT-LVH (Pearson & Manolio, 2008). Gene-environment interactions and haplotypes are also understudied. It is, therefore, possible that the potential biological significance of a particular candidate gene has been concealed.
2. Precise phenotyping. The first GWAS by Wellcome Trust Case-control Consortium (WTCCC) found no significant difference in blood pressure (Burton et al., 2007). As one-fourth of the population-based "controls" were incorrectly classified, the statistical significance was dramatically reduced (McCarthy et al., 2008; Zhang et al., 2010). Instead of phenotypic differences between "case" and "control" groups, it is preferable to categorise the diseases according to their traits, such as, in this case, LV wall thickness or LV mass. Test sensitivity may differ depending on whether LV wall thickness is measured at the 10th and 90th percentile (Rana et al., 2007; Zhang et al., 2010).
3. Common traits like blood pressure and LV wall or mass may be regulated by multiple genes or loci (in one or more pathophysiological pathways), with each gene or locus only contributing a modest amount to the overall genetic impact on the phenotype. Instead of having an immediate detrimental effect on the adverse phenotypes, these frequent changes may result in late-onset of common and complex diseases (Boon Peng & Yusoff, 2013).
4. "Missing heritability" refers to the difference between disease risk explained by genetic loci and overall heritable disease risk based on familial aggregation. The "unexplained reason(s)" for the small fraction of individual disease risk (modest odd ratio of 1.1-1.5) suggests there are missing links in the understanding trait heredity (McCarthy, 2009). Less common (0.5-5%) or rare ($\leq$0.5%) variations with larger effects may have an equal or greater role. Yet, these mutations are frequently too rare to be found by typical molecular methods to demonstrate a statistical association (McCarthy, 2009). Today, the development of new technologies like next-generation sequencing (NGS) has made it possible to identify rare novel variants on a genome-wide scale. These technologies may partially reveal the missing heritability that GWAS on SNP data has overlooked.

5. The impact of other types of genomic changes such as CNV. Since the potential of CNV has not been explored thoroughly, it is unclear how it may affect common disorders like HT-LVH. There have been suggestions, however, that although common CNV may be typable by tag SNP, they represent only a minor risk for disease susceptibility. The complex, segmentally duplicated, and infrequent de novo CNVs, however, are not counted, at least not with the genotyping platform in use today (apart from next-generation sequencing), as they typically do not follow the Mendelian inheritance trait. Moreover, the allelic size of CNVs is frequently not "taggable" by these SNPs. Examples of other diseases affected by CNV are cancer, AIDS (acquired immunodeficiency syndrome) and glomerulonephritis (Aitman et al., 2006; Gonzalez et al., 2005; Mehlotra et al., 2012; Nakajima et al., 2008; Shao et al., 2019).

Copy Number Variation in Hypertension-Related LVH

CNV has been identified as a prevalent type of structural variation in the human genome, making it a significant source of genetic variation (Burton et al., 2007; Conrad & Hurles, 2007; Nowakowska, 2017; Rodriguez-Revenga et al., 2007; Wellenreuther et al., 2019). CNV is defined as a DNA segment of 1 kb or more that is present with variable number of copies relative to the reference genome (Feuk et al., 2006). Genomic regions enriched in segmental duplications are sensitive to chromosomal rearrangements via non-allelic homologous recombination and are recognised as hotspots of genomic instability, therefore susceptible to mutation (Girirajan et al., 2011).

CNV may comprise simple tandem duplications (also known as low copy repeats or segmental duplications), or it may entail more complex arrangements, such as gains or losses of homologous sequences at various genomic locations (Zhang et al., 2009). A considerable amount of the genetic variation is broadly distributed throughout the human genome. This may demonstrate the significance of CNV in genetic diversity and evolution. Iafrate et al., (2004) discovered 200 large-scale copy-number variants (LCVs) in the human genome, 24 of which were found in more than 10% of the studied participants. In a separate study, Redon et al., (2006) looked into 270 subjects of European, African and Asian descent from the HapMap collection and found 1,447 copy number variation regions (CNVRs) that spanned as long as 360 MB (12%) of the human genome, which contained hundreds of genes with important biological activities. CNV has been shown to affect gene expression, phenotypic variation and adaptation by disrupting genes and changing gene dosage, which may result in disease phenotypes or impart vulnerability to complex traits, including psoriasis, pancreatitis, nephritis, lupus, and HIV (Canales & Walz, 2011; Redon et al., 2006). Two examples of CNVs that immediately impact protein levels are the copy number of cyclins B1 in breast cancer patients and the a-synuclein (SNCA) gene in Parkinson's disease (Myhre et al., 2013).

In the International HapMap project, Stranger et al. (2007) studied the relative impact of CNV on gene expression phenotype in 210 unrelated individuals. They found that 17.7% of the detected genetic variation in gene expression is attributed to CNV, which suggested that this variability was not limited to intergenic or intronic regions (Stranger et al., 2007). In line with previous research on mice, Henrichsen et al., (2009) demonstrated that CNVs were responsible for the formation of tissue transcriptomes and, consequently, phenotypic variance. The influence that CNVs have on gene expression inside the CNV area was validated by data on gene expression gathered from the whole genome collected from six main organs. Even though large-scale CNV has a direct effect on disease phenotypes, these variants are common in the genomes of individuals who have normal phenotypes, which suggests that CNVs play an indirect role in the phenotype through position effects or that they predispose to further chromosomal rearrangements in subsequent generations, which may have potentially harmful effects.

Therefore, it has been argued that these genetic markers are a driving factor behind the evolution of the genome and phenotypic variety (Feuk et al., 2006). The deletion of the *RHD* gene, which is responsible for the expression of rhesus negative blood group, is perhaps the best and most straightforward example of copy number variation. *RHD* and *RHCE* are two genes that can be found on chromosome 1p34-36.2. The Rh (Rhesus) blood group antigens are the products of these genes and *RHD* is responsible for expressing the D antigen, one of the most immunogenic blood groups. It is estimated that approximately 40% of Europeans have had their entire *RHD* gene deleted, which is synonymous with their rhesus-negative phenotype and total absence of the D antigen expression (Flegel, 2007).

According to the literature, CNV in the human genome plays a significant role in determining the risk of developing complex diseases, such as:

1. Autoimmune diseases. Variation in copy number of FCGR3A and FCGR3B genes may confer susceptibility to ankylosing spondylitis

and systemic lupus erythematosus (SLE) (Fanciulli et al., 2007; Wang et al., 2016; Yim et al., 2015).

2. HIV infection. CNVs in chemokine ligand 3-like 1 (CCL3L1) and chemokine receptor 5 (CCR5) genes are associated with increased susceptibility to HIV-1 infection (Aklillu et al., 2013; Liu et al., 2010; Usher & McCarroll, 2015).
3. Parkinson's disease. Genomic duplications or triplications of the alpha-synuclein gene (SNCA) may result in early onset Parkinsonism with dementia (Recchia et al., 2004; Keogh et al., 2017).
4. Alzheimer's disease. Duplication of the amyloid precursor protein (APP) has been linked to increased risk of Alzheimer's disease (Hooli et al., 2012).
5. Crohn's disease. Beta-defensin gene CNV is linked to increased risk of developing Crohn's disease (Machado & Ottolini, 2015).

The association between CNV and CVD, particularly HT-LVH, has not been extensively studied and is poorly understood. Most research is focused on monogenic disorders of CVD (Pollex & Hegele, 2007), congenital heart disease (An et al., 2016; Sicko et al., 2016; Zhu et al., 2016) and hypertrophic cardiomyopathy (Lopes et al., 2015). The study by Lopes et al. (2015) involved 505 hypertrophic cardiomyopathy participants who were unrelated, and focused exclusively on 19 genes that had been linked to the disease. These genes were namely *MYBPC3, TPM1, ACTC1, TNNT2, TNNI3, MYH7, MYL2, MYL3, TNNC1, PDLIM3, CSRP3, MYH6, LDB3, VCL, PLN, LMNA, DES, TCAP,* and *RBM20.* They found a significant deletion in *MYBPC3* and *PDLIM3,* a duplication of the whole *TNNT2*, and a substantial duplication in *LMNA* (Lopes et al., 2015).

Even though the copy number of *LPA* has been studied in atherosclerosis, familial hypercholesterolemia (FH), and coronary artery disease, the influence of CNV on non-familial CVD, particularly in HT-LVH, has not been frequently reported (Palacios et al., 2012; Sharma et al., 2012). Marques et al., (2014) attempted to determine the association between CNVs in regions previously associated with blood pressure variation in GWAS and essential hypertension. They discovered that the deletion of CNVs esv27061 and esv2757747 on chromosome 1p13.2 was significantly prevalent in participants with extremely high blood pressure (Marques et al., 2014). This provides evidence that CNV plays a role in essential hypertension. This finding also makes it plausible that CNV is associated with HT-LVH. However, the analysis of the CNV using HT-LVH should not be restricted to just those specific "gene-enriched" CNVs. Studies have revealed that CNVs may affect disease susceptibility through their impact on non-transcribed regions that affect gene expression at a distance (Feuk et al., 2006). Conversely, the potential impact of rare or de novo CNVs should not be disregarded. Thoracic aortic aneurysms and dissections are typical examples of successful treatment (Prakash et al., 2010).

A CNV is generally considered common if found in >1% of the population (Valsesia et al., 2013), but some researchers used higher thresholds of 5 to 10% (Malhotra & Sebat, 2012; McCarroll & Altshuler, 2007). In contrast, rare CNVs are generally considered to be those with <1% population frequency (Consortium, 2008; McCarroll et al., 2008; Soemedi et al., 2012). In the "common disease–common variant (CD-CV)" hypothesis, a disease trait is caused by a combination of common alleles (5% in a population), each providing minor additive effects. A new hypothesis, known as the "missing heritability", proposed that rarer mutations have a higher impact on complex disease risk than previously thought. In a most recent example, a whole genome sequencing-CNV investigation into Alzheimer's disease found an increased prevalence of rare CNVs in patients (Ming et al., 2021). A new strategy was implemented to map the sensitive gene to HT-LVH individuals. This strategy was implemented because some mutations exposed to HT-LVH individuals may be individually rare, highly penetrant, population-specific and of recent origin, even specific to a single case.

Rare CNV in Malaysian Males with HT-LVH

To the best of our knowledge, this is the first study done in Malaysia and Southeast Asia to observe the impact of genetic variation, particularly rare CNVs in HT-LVH (Ashazila, 2020). In the study, a high-resolution SNP array was used to analyse CNVs in 300 hypertensive men, of which 100 had LVH. CNVs found in HT-LVH patients only were classified as rare or private after stringent filtering. Gene ontology and pathway analysis was performed to confirm the involvement of genes; particularly those involved in heart functions and their phenotypes. About 22,337 CNVs were successfully merged with at least two algorithms, or 202.9 CNVs per genome, which was higher than other studies (Glessner et al., 2010; Silversides et al., 2012; Soemedi et al., 2012), but consistent with Pinto et al. (2011), who reported an average of 240 calls per genome using the Illumina 660W platform. Results from this rare CNV analysis revealed interactions between several genes that may increase the risk of developing HT-LVH, suggesting that candidate genes harboured in the rare variations have a more significant role in influencing susceptibility to complex diseases. This study discovered and replicated the novel LVH susceptibility genes *F2R, SUMF1, KCNIP4,* and *IQGAP2.*

It is acknowledged that not all of the reported genes are directly involved in LVH or hypertension. However, the overall results of this study were linked by biological interactions with a large number of genes, many of which are known to play a role in "foetal gene programmes," particularly in the cardiac phenotype (Galindo et al., 2009; Kuwahara et al., 2012; Sack et al., 1997). It is hypothesised that several potential genes may be involved in the development of LVH. Coagulation factor II (F2R), a member of the GPCR family, has been linked to platelet activation, vascular growth and modulation of thrombotic response (http://www.ncbi.nlm.nih.gov/gene/2149). According to earlier studies, IL-6 and F2R may interact to make hypertension patients more susceptible to myocardial infarction and coronary heart disease (Gigante et al., 2010; Gigante et al., 2009). But their function in the inflammatory mechanism of heart hypertrophy is not fully known. The *IQGAP2* gene, located close to *F2R*, connects with *CALM1* (Brill et al., 1996). It is thought to play a role in cardiac development because of its ability to regulate cell morphology and motility via interactions with cytoskeleton components, cell adhesion, and other signalling molecules (http://www.ncbi.nlm.nih.gov/gene/10788). Whole exome sequencing revealed a mutation of *IQGAP2* that causes LVH in a recent study by Zhi et al., (2012). In this replication cohort, both F2R and IQGAP2 were shown to be recurrent. Ischemic heart disease has been linked to *KCNIP4*, a voltage-gated potassium (Kv) channel-interacting protein family (Matarin et al., 2007). A genome-wide association study found the expression of *KCNIP4* related to LVMI increase amongst isolated Amish groups; however, the signal was not significant in subsequent replication studies (Parsa et al., 2011). *KCNIP4* is required for the low repetitive firing and backpropagation of action potential in neurons, as well as the formation of the action potential in the heart (Holmqvist et al., 2002).

The involvement of transcription factors that regulate cell growth, energy metabolism, and apoptosis, specifically Sp1, CREB, and p53, in the development of HT-LVH has been demonstrated by enrichment analysis of rare CNV underlying genes. The ubiquitous transcription factor Sp1 is responsible for regulating the expression of a vast majority of genes, including housekeeping genes, tissue-specific genes, and genes that regulate cell cycle progression. Previous studies have shown that Sp1 had a significant role in the reactivation of foetal cardiac genes and regulation of genes involved in heart metabolism (Flesch, 2001; Ichihara et al., 2006; Lin et al., 2009). The importance of cAMP response element binding protein 1 (CREB1) transcription factor signalling as a cardiac hypertrophy regulator is widely studied (Funakoshi et al., 2002; Muller et al., 2001; Vasan et al., 2009). Phosphorylation of serine 133 in CREB1 by the angiotensin receptor 1 (AGTR1) signalling pathway has been observed to regulate mRNA expression of atrial natriuretic peptide (ANF) (Funakoshi et al., 1999; Funakoshi et al., 2002). It is well established that the expression of p53 may trigger apoptosis in response to numerous stimuli (Fridman & Lowe, 2003). This process is also critically engaged in cardiac hypertrophy (Sano et al., 2007). Myocyte elongation mediated by diastolic dysfunction activates RAAS signalling, resulting in c-terminal p53 phosphorylation. DNA binding takes place at the promoter of the angiotensinogen and AT1 receptor genes, inducing RAAS to produce more Angiotensin II (Leri et al., 2000; Nadal-Ginard et al., 2003).

Androgen receptor signalling may alter cardiac hypertrophy by acting directly on the heart or disrupting the vascular system (English et al., 2001; Hayward et al., 2001; Jones et al., 2004; Kienitz & Quinkler, 2008). However, there is a paucity of information on its function and the underlying molecular mechanism in cardiac hypertrophy since studies are showing inconsistent results (Glessner et al., 2010; Ikeda et al., 2005; Liu et al., 2003; Marsh et al., 1998). Interestingly, the androgen receptor has been demonstrated to interact with the CREB1 transcription factor (Aarnisalo et al., 1998) and is believed to function in the heart's metabolic modulation, increasing ATP synthesis during an increase in cardiac output (Pugh et al., 2000).

Conclusion

LVH may be affected by rare CNVs that alter or disrupt the underlying genes in relevant pathways. In other words, rare CNVs found in this study are not shown to be disease-causing genetic variations. Still, they may contribute as a risk factor in susceptibility to common diseases such as HT-LVH. A separate cohort with more samples is necessary to validate these results. Moreover, functional validation studies defining the function of the genes within these rare CNVs are required to comprehend the mechanisms behind the development of LVH in hypertensive individuals. The findings of this study may eventually lead to additional research on the different responses to anti-hypertensive medication that can prevent the development of HT-LVH.

References

Aarnisalo, P., Palvimo, J. J., & Janne, O. A. (1998). CREB-binding protein in androgen receptor-mediated signaling. *Proceedings of the National Academy of Sciences of the United States of America*, *95*(5), 2122-2127. http://doi.org/10.1073/pnas.95.5.2122

Majid, N. L. A., Omar, M. Z., Khoo, Y. Y., Naidu, B. M., Yn, J. L. M., Hasani, W. S. R., Rifin, H. M., Hamid, H. a. A., Lourdes, T. G. R., & Yusoff, M. F. M. (2018). Prevalence, awareness, treatment and control of hypertension in the Malaysian population: findings from the National Health and Morbidity Survey 2006–2015. *Journal of Human Hypertension*, 32(8–9), 617–624. https://doi.org/10.1038/s41371-018-0082-x

Ahmed, S. N., Jhaj, R., Sadasivam, B., & Joshi, R. (2020). Regression of the left ventricular hypertrophy in patients with essential hypertension on standard drug therapy. *Discoveries (Craiova)*, *8*(3), e115. https://doi.org/10.15190/d.2020.12.

Aitman, T. J., Dong, R., Vyse, T. J., Norsworthy, P. J., Johnson, M. D., Smith, J., Mangion, J., Roberton-Lowe, C., Marshall, A. J., Petretto, E., Hodges, M. D., Bhangal, G., Patel, S. G., Sheehan-Rooney, K., Duda, M., Cook, P. R., Evans, D. J., Domin, J., Flint, J., Boyle, J. J., Pusey, C. D. & Cook, H. T. (2006). Copy number polymorphism in Fcgr3 predisposes to glomerulonephritis in rats and humans. *Nature*, *439*(7078), 851-855. https://doi.org/10.1038/nature04489.

Aklillu, E., Odenthal-Hesse, L., Bowdrey, J., Habtewold, A., Ngaimisi, E., Yimer, G., Amogne, W., Mugusi, S., Minzi, O., Makonnen, E., Janabi, M., Mugusi, F., Aderaye, G., Hardwick, R., Fu, B., Viskaduraki, M., Yang, F., & Hollox, E. J. (2013). CCL3L1 copy number, HIV load, and immune reconstitution in sub-Saharan Africans. *BMC Infectious Diseases*, *13*, 536. https://doi.org/10.1186/1471-2334-13-536.

An, Y., Duan, W., Huang, G., Chen, X., Li, L., Nie, C., Hou, J., Gui, Y., Wu, Y., Zhang, F., Shen, Y., Wu, B., & Wang, H. (2016). Genome-wide copy number variant analysis for congenital ventricular septal defects in Chinese Han population. *BMC Medical Genomics*, *9*, 2. https://doi.org/10.1186/s12920-015-0163-4.

Arnett, D. K., Li, N., Tang, W., Rao, D. C., Devereux, R. B., Claas, S. A., Kraemer, R., & Broeckel, U. (2009). Genome-wide association study identifies single-nucleotide polymorphism in KCNB1 associated with left ventricular mass in humans: the HyperGEN Study. *BMC Medical Genetics*, *10*, 43. https://doi.org/10.1186/1471-2350-10-43.

Bahramali, E., Rajabi, M., Jamshidi, J., Mousavi, S. M., Zarghami, M., Manafi, A., & Firouzabadi, N. (2016). Association of ACE gene D polymorphism with left ventricular hypertrophy in patients with diastolic heart failure: a case-control stud. *BMJ Open*, *6*(2), e010282. https://doi.org/10.1136/bmjopen-2015-010282.

Bang, C. N., Devereux, R. B., & Okin, P. M. (2014). Regression of electrocardiographic left ventricular hypertrophy or strain is associated with lower incidence of cardiovascular morbidity and mortality in hypertensive patients independent of blood pressure reduction - A LIFE review. *Journal of Electrocardiology*, *47*(5), 630-635. https://doi.org/10.1016/j.jelectrocard.2014.07.003.

BoonPeng, H., & Yusoff, K. (2013). The utility of copy number variation (CNV) in studies of hypertension-related left ventricular hypertrophy (LVH): rationale, potential and challenges. *Molecular Cytogenetics*. https://doi.org/10.1186/1755-8166-6-8.

Brill, S., Li, S., Lyman, C. W., Church, D. M., Wasmuth, J. J., Weissbach, L., Bernards, A., & Snijders, A. J. (1996). The Ras GTPase-activating-protein-related human protein *IQGAP2* harbors a potential actin-binding domain and interacts with calmodulin and Rho family GTPases. *Molecular and Cellular Biology*, *16*(9), 4869-4878. https://doi.org/10.1128/MCB.16.9.4869.

Burton, P. R., Clayton, D. G., Cardon, L. R., Craddock, N., Deloukas, P., Duncanson, A., Kwiatkowski, D. P., McCarthy, M. I., Ouwehand, W. H., & Samani, N. J. (2007). Genome-wide association study of 14,000 cases of seven common diseases and 3,000 shared controls. *Nature*, *447*(7145), 661–678. https://doi.org/10.1038/nature05911.

Canales, C. P., & Walz, K. (2011). Copy number variation and susceptibility to complex traits. *Embo Molecular Medicine*, *3*(1), 1-4. https://doi.org/10.1002/emmm.201000111.

Cardon, L. R., & Bell, J. I. (2001). Association study designs for complex diseases. *Nature Reviews Genetics*, 91–99. https://doi.org/10.1038/35052543.

Ching, S., Chia, Y., & Wan Azman, W. (2012). Prevalence and determinants of left ventricular hypertrophy in hypertensive patients at a primary care clinic. *Malaysian Family Physician*, *7*(2-3), 2-9.

Concannon, P., Rich, S. S., & Nepom, G. T. (2009). Genetics of type 1A diabetes. *New England Journal of Medicine*, *360*(16), 1646–1654. https://doi.org/10.1056/nejmra0808284.

Conrad, D. F., & Hurles, M. E. (2007). The population genetics of structural variation. *Nature Genetics*, 39(S7), S30–S36. https://doi.org/10.1038/ng2042.

Cuspidi, C., Meani, S., Sala, C., Valerio, C., Negri, F., & Mancia, G. (2012). Age related prevalence of severe left ventricular hypertrophy in essential hypertension: echocardiographic findings from the ETODH study. *Blood Pressure*, *21*(3), 139-145. https://doi.org/10.3109/08037051.2012.668662.

Cuspidi, C., Sala, C., Negri, F., Mancia, G., Morganti, A., & Italian Society of, H. (2012). Prevalence of left-ventricular hypertrophy in hypertension: an updated review of echocardiographic studies. *Journal of Human Hypertension*, *26*(6), 343-349. https://doi.org/10.1038/jhh.2011.104.

Dahlof, B., Pennert, K., & Hansson, L. (1992). Regression of left ventricular hypertrophy--a meta-analysis [Meta-Analysis]. *Clinical and Experimental Hypertension*, *14*(1-2), 173-180. https://doi.org/10.3109/10641969209036180.

Dirkx, E., da Costa Martins, P. A., & De Windt, L. J. (2013). Regulation of fetal gene expression in heart failure. *Biochimica Et Biophysica Acta: Molecular Basis of Disease*, 1832(12), 2414–2424. https://doi.org/10.1016/j.bbadis.2013.07.023.

Du, X. J. (2007). Divergence of hypertrophic growth and fetal gene profile: the influence of beta-blockers. *British Journal of Pharmacology*, *152*(2), 169-171. https://doi.org/10.1038/sj.bjp.0707353.

English, K. M., Jones, R. D., Jones, T. H., Morice, A. H., & Channer, K. S. (2001). Gender differences in the vasomotor effects of different steroid hormones in rat pulmonary and coronary arteries. *Hormone and Metabolic Research*, *33*(11), 645-652. https://doi.org/10.1055/s-2001-18689.

Fanciulli, M., Norsworthy, P. J., Petretto, E., Dong, R., Harper, L., Kamesh, L., Heward, J. M., Gough, S. C., De Smith, A., & Blakemore, A. I. (2007). FCGR3B copy number variation is associated with susceptibility to systemic, but not organ-specific, autoimmunity. *Nature Genetics*, 39(6), 721–723. https://doi.org/10.1038/ng2046.

Feuk, L., Carson, A. R., & Scherer, S. W. (2006). Structural variation in the human genome. *Nature Reviews Genetics*, 7(2), 85–97. https://doi.org/10.1038/nrg1767.

Flegel, W. A. (2007). The genetics of the Rhesus blood group system. *Vox Sanguinis*. https://doi.org/10.2450/2007.0011-07.

Flesch, M. (2001). On the trail of cardiac specific transcription factors. *Cardiovascular Research*. https://doi.org/10.1016/s0008-6363(01)00218-8.

Fridman, J. S., & Lowe, S. W. (2003). Control of apoptosis by p53. *Oncogene*, *22*(56), 9030-9040. https://doi.org/10.1038/sj.onc.1207116.

Funakoshi, Y., Ichiki, T., Ito, K., & Takeshita, A. (1999). Induction of interleukin-6 expression by angiotensin II in rat vascular smooth muscle cells. *Hypertension*, *34*(1), 118-125. http://doi.org/10.1161/01.hyp.34.1.118.

Funakoshi, Y., Ichiki, T., Takeda, K., Tokuno, T., Iino, N., & Takeshita, A. (2002). Critical role of cAMP-response element-binding protein for angiotensin II-induced hypertrophy of vascular smooth muscle cells. *Journal of Biological Chemistry*, *277*(21), 18710-18717. https://doi.org/10.1074/jbc.M110430200.

Galindo, C. L., Skinner, M. A., Errami, M., Olson, L. D., Watson, D. A., Li, J., McCormick, J. F., McIver, L. J., Kumar, N. M., Pham, T. Q., & Garner, H. R. (2009). Transcriptional profile of isoproterenol-induced cardiomyopathy and comparison to exercise-induced cardiac hypertrophy and human cardiac failure. *BMC Physiology*, *9*, 23. https://doi.org/10.1186/1472-6793-9-23.

Gigante, B., Bennet, A. M., Leander, K., Vikstrom, M., & de Faire, U. (2010). The interaction between coagulation factor 2 receptor and interleukin 6 haplotypes increases the risk of myocardial infarction in men. *PLoS One*, *5*(6), e11300. https://doi.org/10.1371/journal.pone.0011300.

Gigante, B., Vikstrom, M., Meuzelaar, L. S., Chernogubova, E., Silveira, A., Hooft, F. V., Hamsten, A., & de Faire, U. (2009). Variants in the coagulation factor 2 receptor (F2R) gene influence the risk of myocardial infarction in men through an interaction with interleukin 6 serum levels. *Thrombosis and Haemostasis*, 101(05), 943–953. https://doi.org/10.1160/th08-09-0612.

Girirajan, S., Campbell, C. D., & Eichler, E. E. (2011). Human copy number variation and complex genetic disease. *Annual Review of Genetics*, 45(1), 203–226. https://doi.org/10.1146/annurev-genet-102209-163544.

Glessner, J. T., Reilly, M. P., Kim, C. E., Takahashi, N., Albano, A., Hou, C., Bradfield, J. P., Zhang, H., Sleiman, P. M., Flory, J. H., Imielinski, M., Frackelton, E. C., Chiavacci, R., Thomas, K. A., Garris, M., Otieno, F. G., Davidson, M., Weiser, M., Reichenberg, A., Davis, K. L., Friedman, J. I., Cappola, T. P., Margulies, K. B., Rader, D. J., Grant, S. F., Buxbaum, J. D., Gur, R. E. & Hakonarson, H. (2010). Strong synaptic transmission impact by copy number variations in schizophrenia.

Proceedings of the National Academy of Sciences of the United States of America, 107(23), 10584–10589. https://doi.org/10.1073/pnas.1000274107.

Gonzalez, E., Kulkarni, H., Bolivar, H., Mangano, A., Sanchez, R., Catano, G., Nibbs, R. J., Freedman, B. I., Quinones, M. P., Bamshad, M. J., Murthy, K. K., Rovin, B. H., Bradley, W., Clark, R. A., Anderson, S. A., O'Connell R, J., Agan, B. K., Ahuja, S. S., Bologna, R., Sen, L., Dolan, M. J. & Ahuja, S. K. (2005). The influence of CCL3L1 gene-containing segmental duplications on HIV-1/AIDS susceptibility. *Science*, *307*(5714), 1434-1440. https://doi.org/10.1126/science.1101160.

Harvey, P. A., & Leinwand, L. A. (2011). Cellular mechanisms of cardiomyopathy. *Journal of Cell Biology*, 194(3), 355–365. https://doi.org/10.1083/jcb.201101100.

Havranek, E. P., Froshaug, D. B., Emserman, C. D., Hanratty, R., Krantz, M. J., Masoudi, F. A., Dickinson, L. M., & Steiner, J. F. (2008). Left ventricular hypertrophy and cardiovascular mortality by race and ethnicity. *The American Journal of Medicine*, 121(10), 870–875. https://doi.org/10.1016/j.amjmed.2008.05.034.

Hayward, C. S., Webb, C. M., & Collins, P. (2001). Effect of sex hormones on cardiac mass [Research Support, Non-U.S. Gov't Review]. *Lancet*, *357*(9265), 1354-1356. https://doi.org/10.1016/S0140-6736(00)04523-2.

Henrichsen, C. N., Vinckenbosch, N., Zöllner, S., Chaignat, E., Pradervand, S., Schütz, F., Ruedi, M., Kaessmann, H., & Reymond, A. (2009). Segmental copy number variation shapes tissue transcriptomes. *Nature Genetics*, 41(4), 424–429. https://doi.org/10.1038/ng.345.

Hirschhorn, J. N. (2003). Genetic epidemiology of type 1 diabetes. *Pediatric Diabetes*, 4(2), 87–100. https://doi.org/10.1034/j.1399-5448.2001.00013.x.

Holmqvist, M. H., Cao, J., Hernandez-Pineda, R., Jacobson, M. D., Carroll, K. I., Sung, M. A., Betty, M., Ge, P., Gilbride, K. J., Brown, M. E., Jurman, M. E., Lawson, D., Silos-Santiago, I., Xie, Y., Covarrubias, M., Rhodes, K. J., Distefano, P. S., & An, W. F. (2002). Elimination of fast inactivation in Kv4 A-type potassium channels by an auxiliary subunit domain. *Proceedings of the National Academy of Sciences of the United States of America*, 99(2), 1035–1040. https://doi.org/10.1073/pnas.022509299.

Hong, K. W., Shin, D. J., Lee, S. H., Son, N. H., Go, M. J., Lim, J. E., Shin, C., Jang, Y., & Oh, B. (2012). Common variants in RYR1 are associated with left ventricular hypertrophy assessed by electrocardiogram. *European Heart Journal*, 33(10), 1250–1256. https://doi.org/10.1093/eurheartj/ehr267.

Hooli, B., Mohapatra, G., Mattheisen, M., Parrado, A., Roehr, J., Shen, Y., Gusella, J., Moir, R., Saunders, A., & Lange, C. (2012). Role of common and rare APP DNA sequence variants in Alzheimer disease. *Neurology*, 78(16), 1250–1257. https://doi.org/10.1212/wnl.0b013e3182515972.

Huber, M., Lezius, S., Reibis, R., Treszl, A., Kujawinska, D., Jakob, S., Wegscheider, K., Voller, H., & Kreutz, R. (2015). A single nucleotide polymorphism near the CYP17A1 gene is associated with left ventricular mass in hypertensive patients under pharmacotherapy. *International Journal of Molecular Sciences*, 16(8), 17456–17468. https://doi.org/10.3390/ijms160817456.

Huber, M., Voller, H., Jakob, S., Reibis, R., Do, V., Bolbrinker, J., Zergibel, I., Schmieder, R. E., Treszl, A., Wegscheider, K., & Kreutz, R. (2010). Role of the angiotensin II type 2 receptor gene (+1675G/A) polymorphism on left ventricular hypertrophy and geometry in treated hypertensive patients. *Journal of Hypertension*, *28*(6), 1221-1229. https://doi.org/10.1097/HJH.0b013e32833aa356.

Iafrate, A. J., Feuk, L., Rivera, M. N., Listewnik, M. L., Donahoe, P. K., Qi, Y., Scherer, S. W., & Lee, C. (2004). Detection of large-scale variation in the human genome. *Nature Genetics*, 36(9), 949–951. https://doi.org/10.1038/ng1416.

Ichihara, S., Obata, K., Yamada, Y., Nagata, K., Noda, A., Ichihara, G., Yamada, A., Kato, T., Izawa, H., Murohara, T., & Yokota, M. (2006). Inflammation and chronic oxidative stress in radiation-induced late normal tissue injury: therapeutic implications. *Current Medicinal Chemistry*, 16(2), 130–143. https://doi.org/10.2174/092986709787002790.

Ikeda, Y., Aihara, K., Sato, T., Akaike, M., Yoshizumi, M., Suzaki, Y., Izawa, Y., Fujimura, M., Hashizume, S., Kato, M., Yagi, S., Tamaki, T., Kawano, H., Matsumoto, T., Azuma, H., & Kato, S. (2005). Androgen receptor gene knockout male mice exhibit impaired cardiac growth and exacerbation of angiotensin ii-induced cardiac fibrosis. *Journal of Biological Chemistry*, 280(33), 29661–29666. https://doi.org/10.1074/jbc.m411694200.

Jones, R. D., Hugh Jones, T., & Channer, K. S. (2004). The influence of testosterone upon vascular reactivity. *European Journal of Endocrinology*, 29–37. https://doi.org/10.1530/eje.0.1510029.

Mat Jusoh, J. A. (2020). *The prevalence and functional impact of rare genomic copy number variation in hypertension-related left ventricular hypertrophy* (Doctoral dissertation, Universiti Teknologi MARA).

Julia Ashazila, M. J., Danuri, N., Majid, F. A., Peng, H. B., & Yusoff, K. (2013). Genetic association study of KCNB1 gene with the susceptibility of hypertension related LVH (Left Ventricular Hypertrophy) patients in Malaysia. *Journal of Life Sciences*, *7*(4), 341-347.

Jusoh, J. A. M., Rahman, T. H. A., Nasir, N. M., Danuri, N., Majid, F. A., Basir, F., Pare, S. N. A., Boon-Peng, H., & Yusoff, K. (2022). Association of socioeconomic disparities and predisposing factors with higher prevalence of hypertension related left ventricular hypertrophy in males: a Malaysian community-based study. Publish date 2022-04-19 at MedRxiv. https://doi.org/10.1101/2022.04.18.22273987, Cite Date: 2022-10-12.

Keogh, M. J., Wei, W., Wilson, I., Coxhead, J., Ryan, S., Rollinson, S., Griffin, H., Kurzawa-Akanbi, M., Santibanez-Koref, M., Talbot, K., Turner, M. R., McKenzie, C. A., Troakes, C., Attems, J., Smith, C., Al Sarraj, S., Morris, C. M., Ansorge, O., Pickering-Brown, S., Ironside, J. W. & Chinnery, P. F. (2017). Genetic compendium of 1511 human brains available through the UK Medical Research Council Brain Banks Network Resource. *Genome Research*, *27*(1), 165-173. https://doi.org/10.1101/gr.210609.116.

Kienitz, T., & Quinkler, M. (2008). Testosterone and blood pressure regulation [Review]. *Kidney Blood Press Research*, *31*(2), 71-79. https://doi.org/10.1159/000119417.

Klingbeil, A. U., Schneider, M., Martus, P., Messerli, F. H., & Schmieder, R. E. (2003). A meta-analysis of the effects of treatment on left ventricular mass in essential hypertension. *The American Journal of Medicine*, 115(1), 41–46. https://doi.org/10.1016/s0002-9343(03)00158-x.

Kuwahara, K., Nishikimi, T., & Nakao, K. (2012). Transcriptional regulation of the fetal cardiac gene program. *Journal of Pharmacological Sciences*, 119(3), 198–203. https://doi.org/10.1254/jphs.12r04cp.

Leri, A., Fiordaliso, F., Setoguchi, M., Limana, F., Bishopric, N. H., Kajstura, J., Webster, K., & Anversa, P. (2000). Inhibition of p53 function prevents renin-angiotensin system activation and stretch-mediated myocyte apoptosis. *American Journal of Pathology*, 157(3), 843–857. https://doi.org/10.1016/s0002-9440(10)64598-1.

Lin, H., Xiao, J., Luo, X., Chen, G., & Wang, Z. (2009). Transcriptional control of pacemaker channel genes HCN2 and HCN4 by Sp1 and implications in re-expression of these genes in hypertrophied myocytes. *Cellular Physiology and Biochemistry*, *23*(4-6), 317-326. https://doi.org/10.1159/000218178.

Lindpaintner, K., Lee, M., Larson, M. G., Rao, V. S., Pfeffer, M. A., Ordovas, J. M., Schaefer, E. J., Wilson, A. F., Wilson, P. W., & Vasan, R. S. (1996). Absence of association or genetic linkage between the angiotensin-converting–enzyme gene and left ventricular mass. *The New England Journal of Medicine,* 334(16), 1023–1028. https://doi.org/10.1056/nejm199604183341604.

Liu, P. Y., Death, A. K., & Handelsman, D. J. (2003). Androgens and cardiovascular disease. *Endocrine Reviews, 24*(3), 313-340. https://doi.org/10.1210/er.2003-0005.

Liu, S., Yao, L., Ding, D., & Zhu, H. (2010). CCL3L1 Copy number variation and susceptibility to HIV-1 infection: a meta-analysis. *PLOS ONE*, 5(12), e15778. https://doi.org/10.1371/journal.pone.0015778.

Lonnebakken, M. T., Izzo, R., Mancusi, C., Gerdts, E., Losi, M. A., Canciello, G., Giugliano, G., De Luca, N., Trimarco, B., & de Simone, G. (2017). Left ventricular hypertrophy regression during antihypertensive treatment in an outpatient clinic (the Campania Salute Network). *Journal of the American Heart Association, 6(3).* https://doi.org/10.1161/jaha.116.004152.

Lopes, L. R., Murphy, C., Syrris, P., Dalageorgou, C., McKenna, W. J., Elliott, P. M., & Plagnol, V. (2015). Use of high-throughput targeted exome-sequencing to screen for copy number variation in hypertrophic cardiomyopathy. *European Journal of Medical Genetics*, *58*(11), 611-616. https://doi.org/10.1016/j.ejmg.2015.10.001.

Machado, L., & Ottolini, B. (2015). An evolutionary history of defensins: a role for copy number variation in maximizing host innate and adaptive immune responses. *Frontiers in Immunology*, 6. https://doi.org/10.3389/fimmu.2015.00115.

Madden, J. M., O'Flynn, A. M., Fitzgerald, A. P., & Kearney, P. M. (2015). Correlation between short-term blood pressure variability and left-ventricular mass index: a meta-analysis. *Hypertension Research*, 39(3), 171–177. https://doi.org/10.1038/hr.2015.126.

Malhotra, D., & Sebat, J. (2012). Harbingers of a rare variant revolution in psychiatric genetics. *Cell*, 148(6), 1223–1241. https://doi.org/10.1016/j.cell.2012.02.039.

Mancia, G., Fagard, R., Narkiewicz, K., Redon, J., Zanchetti, A., Böhm, M., Christiaens, T., Cifkova, R., De Backer, G., Dominiczak, A. F., Galderisi, M., Grobbee, D. E., Jaarsma, T., Kirchhof, P., Kjeldsen, S. E., Laurent, S., Manolis, A. J., Nilsson, P. M., Ruilope, L. M., Schmieder, R. E., Sirnes, P. A., Sleight, P., Viigimaa, M., Waeber, B. & Zannad, F. (2014). 2013 ESH/ESC practice guidelines for the management of arterial hypertension. *Blood Pressure*, 23(1), 3–16. https://doi.org/10.3109/08037051.2014.868629.

Marques, F. Z., Prestes, P. R., Pinheiro, L. B., Scurrah, K., Emslie, K. R., Tomaszewski, M., Harrap, S. B., & Charchar, F. J. (2014). Measurement of absolute copy number variation reveals association with essential hypertension. *BMC Medical Genomics*, 7(1). https://doi.org/10.1186/1755-8794-7-44.

Marsh, J. D., Lehmann, M. H., Ritchie, R. H., Gwathmey, J. K., Green, G. E., & Schiebinger, R. J. (1998). Androgen receptors mediate hypertrophy in cardiac myocytes. *Circulation*, *98*(3), 256-261. http://www.ncbi.nlm.nih.gov/pubmed/9697826.

Matarin, M., Brown, W. M., Scholz, S., Simon-Sanchez, J., Fung, H. C., Hernandez, D., Gibbs, J. R., De Vrieze, F. W., Crews, C., Britton, A., Langefeld, C. D., Brott, T. G., Brown, R. D., Jr., Worrall, B. B., Frankel, M., Silliman, S., Case, L. D., Singleton, A., Hardy, J. A., Rich, S. S. & Meschia, J. F. (2007). A genome-wide genotyping study in patients with ischaemic stroke: initial analysis and data release. *Lancet Neurology*, *6*(5), 414-420. https://doi.org/10.1016/S1474-4422(07)70081-9.

McCarroll, S. A., & Altshuler, D. M. (2007). Copy-number variation and association studies of human disease. *Nature Genetics*, 39(S7), S37–S42. https://doi.org/10.1038/ng2080.

McCarthy, M. I. (2009). Exploring the unknown: assumptions about allelic architecture and strategies for susceptibility variant discovery. *Genome Medicine*, 1(7), 66. https://doi.org/10.1186/gm66.

McCarthy, M. I., Abecasis, G. R., Cardon, L. R., Goldstein, D. B., Little, J., Ioannidis, J. P., & Hirschhorn, J. N. (2008). Genome-wide association studies for complex traits: consensus, uncertainty and challenges. *Nature Reviews Genetics,* 9(5), 356–369. https://doi.org/10.1038/nrg2344.

McMullen, J. R., & Jennings, G. L. (2007). Differences between pathological and physiological cardiac hypertrophy: novel therapeutic strategies to treat heart failure. *Clinical and Experimental Pharmacology and Physiology*, *34*(4), 255-262. https://doi.org/10.1111/j.1440-1681.2007.04585.x.

Mehlotra, R. K., Dazard, J. E., John, B., Zimmerman, P. A., Weinberg, A., & Jurevic, R. J. (2012). Copy number variation within human beta-defensin gene cluster influences progression to AIDS in the multicenter AIDS cohort study. *Journal of AIDS and Clinical Research*, *3*(10). https://doi.org/10.4172/2155-6113.1000184.

Ming, C., Wang, M., Wang, Q., Neff, R., Wang, E., Shen, Q., Reddy, J. S., Wang, X., Allen, M., Ertekin-Taner, N., De Jager, P. L., Bennett, D. A., Haroutunian, V., Schadt, E., & Zhang, B. (2021). Whole genome sequencing-based copy number variations reveal novel pathways and targets in Alzheimer's disease. *Alzheimers & Dementia*, 18(10), 1846-1867. https://doi.org/10.1002/alz.12507.

Muller, F. U., Boknik, P., Knapp, J., Linck, B., Luss, H., Neumann, J., & Schmitz, W. (2001). Activation and inactivation of cAMP-response element-mediated gene transcription in cardiac myocytes. *Cardiovasc Res*, *52*(1), 95-102. http://www.ncbi.nlm.nih.gov/pubmed/11557237.

Myhre, S., Lingjærde, O. C., Hennessy, B. T., Aure, M. R., Carey, M. S., Alsner, J., Tramm, T., Overgaard, J., Mills, G. B., & Børresen-Dale, A.-L. (2013). Influence of DNA copy number and mRNA levels on the expression of breast cancer related proteins. *Molecular Oncology*, 7(3), 704–718. https://doi.org/10.1016/j.molonc.2013.02.018.

Nadal-Ginard, B., Kajstura, J., Leri, A., & Anversa, P. (2003). Myocyte Death, Growth, and Regeneration in Cardiac Hypertrophy and Failure. *Circulation Research*, 92(2), 139–150. https://doi.org/10.1161/01.res.0000053618.86362.df.

Nakajima, T., Kaur, G., Mehra, N., & Kimura, A. (2008). HIV-1/AIDS susceptibility and copy number variation in CCL3L1, a gene encoding a natural ligand for HIV-1 co-receptor CCR5. *Cytogenetic and Genome Research*, *123*(1-4), 156-160. https://doi.org/10.1159/000184703.

Nakamura, M., & Sadoshima, J. (2018). Mechanisms of physiological and pathological cardiac hypertrophy. *Nature Reviews Cardiology*, 15(7), 387–407. https://doi.org/10.1038/s41569-018-0007-y.

Nakashima, Y., Fouad, F. M., & Tarazi, R. C. (1984). Regression of left ventricular hypertrophy from systemic hypertension by enalapril. *American Journal of Cardiology*, 53(8), 1044–1049. https://doi.org/10.1016/0002-9149(84)90634-9.

Nowakowska, B. (2017). Clinical interpretation of copy number variants in the human genome. *Journal of Applied Genetics,* 58(4), 449–457. https://doi.org/10.1007/s13353-017-0407-4.

Palacios, L., Grandoso, L., Cuevas, N., Olano-Martin, E., Martinez, A., Tejedor, D., & Stef, M. (2012). Molecular characterization of familial hypercholesterolemia in Spain. *Atherosclerosis*, *221*(1), 137-142. https://doi.org/10.1016/j.atherosclerosis.2011.12.021.

Parsa, A., Chang, Y. P., Kelly, R. J., Corretti, M. C., Ryan, K. A., Robinson, S. W., Gottlieb, S. S., Kardia, S. L., Shuldiner, A. R., & Liggett, S. B. (2011). Hypertrophy-associated polymorphisms ascertained in a founder cohort applied to heart failure risk and mortality. *Clinical and Translational Science*, *4*(1), 17-23. https://doi.org/10.1111/j.1752-8062.2010.00251.x.

Pearson, T. A., & Manolio, T. A. (2008). How to interpret a genome-wide association study. *JAMA*, *299*(11), 1335-1344. https://doi.org/10.1001/jama.299.11.1335.

Pinto, D., Darvishi, K., Shi, X., Rajan, D., Rigler, D., Fitzgerald, T., Lionel, A. C., Thiruvahindrapuram, B., Macdonald, J. R., Mills, R., Prasad, A., Noonan, K., Gribble, S., Prigmore, E., Donahoe, P. K., Smith, R. S., Park, J. H., Hurles, M. E., Carter, N. P., Lee, C., Scherer, S. W. & Feuk, L. (2011). Comprehensive assessment of array-based platforms and calling algorithms for detection of copy number variants. *Nature Biotechnology*, 29(6), 512–520. https://doi.org/10.1038/nbt.1852.

Pollex, R. L., & Hegele, R. A. (2007). Copy number variation in the human genome and its implications for cardiovascular disease. *Circulation*, *115*(24), 3130-3138. https://doi.org/10.1161/CIRCULATIONAHA.106.677591.

Prakash, S. K., LeMaire, S. A., Guo, D. C., Russell, L., Regalado, E. S., Golabbakhsh, H., Johnson, R. J., Safi, H. J., Estrera, A. L., Coselli, J. S., Bray, M. S., Leal, S. M., Milewicz, D. M., & Belmont, J. W. (2010). Rare copy number variants disrupt genes regulating vascular smooth muscle cell adhesion and contractility in sporadic thoracic aortic aneurysms and dissections. *American Journal of Human Genetics*, *87*(6), 743-756. https://doi.org/10.1016/j.ajhg.2010.09.015.

Pugh, P. J., English, K. M., Jones, T. H., & Channer, K. S. (2000). Testosterone: a natural tonic for the failing heart? QJM: *An International Journal of Medicine*, 93(10), 689–694. https://doi.org/10.1093/qjmed/93.10.689.

Rajabi, M., Kassiotis, C., Razeghi, P., & Taegtmeyer, H. (2007). Return to the fetal gene program protects the stressed heart: a strong hypothesis. *Heart Failure Reviews*, *12*(3-4), 331-343. https://doi.org/10.1007/s10741-007-9034-1.

Rana, B. K., Insel, P. A., Payne, S. H., Abel, K., Beutler, E., Ziegler, M. G., Schork, N. J., & O'Connor, D. T. (2007). Population-based sample reveals gene–gender interactions in blood pressure in white Americans. *Hypertension,* 49(1), 96–106. https://doi.org/10.1161/01.hyp.0000252029.35106.67.

Recchia, A., Debetto, P., Negro, A., Guidolin, D., Skaper, S. D., & Giusti, P. (2004). α-Synuclein and Parkinson's disease. *The FASEB Journal*, *18*(6), 617-626. https://doi.org/10.1096/fj.03-0338rev

Redon, R., Ishikawa, S., Fitch, K. R., Feuk, L., Perry, G. H., Andrews, T. D., Fiegler, H., Shapero, M. H., Carson, A. R., & Chen, W. (2006). Global variation in copy number in the human genome. *Nature*, 444(7118), 444–454. https://doi.org/10.1038/nature05329.

Rodriguez-Revenga, L., Mila, M., Rosenberg, C., Lamb, A., & Lee, C. (2007). Structural variation in the human genome: the impact of copy number variants on clinical diagnosis. *Genetics in Medicine*, *9*(9), 600-606. https://doi.org/10.1097/gim.0b013e318149e1e3.

Sack, M. N., Disch, D. L., Rockman, H. A., & Kelly, D. P. (1997). A role for Sp and nuclear receptor transcription factors in a cardiac hypertrophic growth program. *Proceedings of the National Academy of Sciences of the United States of America,* 94(12), 6438–6443. https://doi.org/10.1073/pnas.94.12.6438.

Saeed, M., Siddiqui, S., Khan, A., Butt, Z. A., Parvez, S. H., & Frossard, P. M. (2005). Association of ACE polymorphisms with left ventricular hypertrophy. *Neuro Endocrinology Letters*, *26*(4), 393-396.

Saheera, S., & Krishnamurthy, P. (2020). Cardiovascular changes associated with hypertensive heart disease and aging. *Cell Transplant*, *29*, 963689720920830. https://doi.org/10.1177/0963689720920830.

Sano, M., Kamitsuji, S., Kamatani, N., Tabara, Y., Kawaguchi, T., Matsuda, F., Yamagishi, H., & Fukuda, K. (2016). Genome-wide association study of absolute QRS voltage identifies common variants of TBX3 as genetic determinants of left ventricular mass in a healthy Japanese population. *PLOS ONE*, 11(5), e0155550. https://doi.org/10.1371/journal.pone.0155550.

Sano, M., Minamino, T., Toko, H., Miyauchi, H., Orimo, M., Qin, Y., Akazawa, H., Tateno, K., Kayama, Y., Harada, M., Shimizu, I., Asahara, T., Hamada, H., Tomita, S., Molkentin, J. D., Zou, Y., & Komuro, I. (2007). p53-induced inhibition of Hif-1 causes cardiac dysfunction during pressure overload. *Nature*, *446*(7134), 444-448. https://doi.org/10.1038/nature05602.

Schmieder, R. E., Martus, P., & Klingbeil, A. (1996). Reversal of left ventricular hypertrophy in essential hypertension. A meta-analysis of randomized double-blind studies. *JAMA*, *275*(19), 1507-1513. https://doi.org/10.1001/jama.275.19.1507.

Schunkert, H., Hense, H.-W., Holmer, S. R., Stender, M., Perz, S., Keil, U., Lorell, B. H., & Riegger, G. (1994). Association between a deletion polymorphism of the angiotensin-converting-enzyme gene and left ventricular hypertrophy. *New England Journal of Medicine*, *330*(23), 1634-1638. https://doi.org/10.1056/nejm199406093302302.

Schut, A. F. C. (2004, September 29). In search of cardiovascular risk genes. Erasmus University Rotterdam. Retrieved October 19, 2022, from http://hdl.handle.net/1765/7343.

Sciarretta, S., Paneni, F., Palano, F., Chin, D., Tocci, G., Rubattu, S., & Volpe, M. (2009). Role of the renin–angiotensin–aldosterone system and inflammatory processes in the development and progression of diastolic dysfunction. *Clinical Science*, *116*(6), 467–477. https://doi.org/10.1042/cs20080390.

Seoane, J. A., Campbell, C., Day, I. N., Casas, J. P., & Gaunt, T. R. (2014). Canonical correlation analysis for gene-based pleiotropy discovery. *PLOS Computational Biology, 10*(10), e1003876. https://doi.org/10.1371/journal.pcbi.1003876.

Shao, X., Lv, N., Liao, J., Long, J., Xue, R., Ai, N., Xu, D., & Fan, X. (2019). Copy number variation is highly correlated with differential gene expression: a pan-cancer study. *BMC Medical Genetics*, *20*(1), 175. https://doi.org/10.1186/s12881-019-0909-5.

Sharma, P., Boyers, D., Boachie, C., Stewart, F., Miedzybrodzka, Z., Simpson, W., Kilonzo, M., McNamee, P., & Mowatt, G. (2012). Elucigene FH20 and LIPOchip for the diagnosis of familial hypercholesterolaemia: a systematic review and economic evaluation. *Health Technology Assessment.*, *16*(17), 1-266. https://doi.org/10.3310/hta16170.

Sharp, A. J., Cheng, Z., & Eichler, E. E. (2006). Structural variation of the human genome. *Annual Review of Genomics and Human Genetics*, *7*, 407-442. https://doi.org/10.1146/annurev.genom.7.080505.115618.

Shlyakhto, E. V., Shwartz, E. I., Nefedova, Y. B., Zukova, A. V., Vinnic, T. A., & Conrady, A. O. (2001). Lack of association of the renin-angiotensin system genes polymorphisms and left ventricular hypertrophy in hypertension. *Blood Pressure*, *10*(3), 135-141. http://doi.org/10.1080/080370501753182343.

Sicko, R. J., Browne, M. L., Rigler, S. L., Druschel, C. M., Liu, G., Fan, R., Romitti, P. A., Caggana, M., Kay, D. M., Brody, L. C., & Mills, J. L. (2016). Genetic variants in isolated Ebstein anomaly implicated in myocardial development pathways. *PLoS One*, *11*(10), e0165174. https://doi.org/10.1371/journal.pone.0165174.

Silversides, C. K., Lionel, A. C., Costain, G., Merico, D., Migita, O., Liu, B., Yuen, T., Rickaby, J., Thiruvahindrapuram, B., Marshall, C. R., Scherer, S. W., & Bassett, A. S. (2012). Rare copy number variations in adults with tetralogy of Fallot implicate novel risk gene pathways. *PLOS Genetics*, *8*(8), e1002843. https://doi.org/10.1371/journal.pgen.1002843.

Soemedi, R., Wilson, I. J., Bentham, J., Darlay, R., Topf, A., Zelenika, D., Cosgrove, C., Setchfield, K., Thornborough, C., Granados-Riveron, J., Blue, G. M., Breckpot, J., Hellens, S., Zwolinkski, S., Glen, E., Mamasoula, C., Rahman, T. J., Hall, D., Rauch, A., Devriendt, K., Gewillig, M., O' Sullivan, J., Winlaw, D. S., Bu'Lock, F., Brook, J. D., Bhattacharya, S., Lathrop, M., Santibanez-Koref, M., Cordell, H. J., Goodship,

J. A., & Keavney, B. D. (2012). Contribution of global rare copy-number variants to the risk of sporadic congenital heart disease. *American Journal of Human Genetics*, *91*(3), 489-501. https://doi.org/10.1016/j.ajhg.2012.08.003.

Song, W. H., Lin, Y. H., Sun, K., Zhang, Y. H., Song, Y., Hou, L. B., Zhang, C. N., Hui, R. T., & Chen, J. Z. (2016). A functional variant in the coding region of CAMTA2 is associated with left ventricular hypertrophy by affecting the activation of Nkx2.5-dependent transcription. *Journal of Hypertension*, *34*(5), 942-949. https://doi.org/10.1097/HJH.0000000000000873.

Stranger, B. E., Forrest, M. S., Dunning, M., Ingle, C. E., Beazley, C., Thorne, N., Redon, R., Bird, C. P., de Grassi, A., & Lee, C. (2007). Relative impact of nucleotide and copy number variation on gene expression phenotypes. *Science*, 315(5813), 848–853. https://doi.org/10.1126/science.1136678.

Taegtmeyer, H., Sen, S., & Vela, D. (2010). Return to the fetal gene program. *Annals of the New York Academy of Sciences*, 1188(1), 191–198. https://doi.org/10.1111/j.1749-6632.2009.05100.x.

Tin, L. L., Beevers, D. G., & Lip, G. Y. (2002). Hypertension, left ventricular hypertrophy, and sudden death. Current Cardiology Reports, 4(6), 449–457. https://doi.org/10.1007/s11886-002-0105-6.

Usher, C. L., & McCarroll, S. A. (2015). Complex and multi-allelic copy number variation in human disease. *Briefings in Functional Genomics*, 14(5), 329–338. https://doi.org/10.1093/bfgp.

Valsesia, A., Macé, A., Jacquemont, S., Beckmann, J. S., & Kutalik, Z. (2013). The growing importance of CNVs: new insights for detection and clinical interpretation. *Frontiers in Genetics*, 4. https://doi.org/10.3389/fgene.2013.00092.

Vasan, R. S., Glazer, N. L., Felix, J. F., Lieb, W., Wild, P. S., Felix, S. B., Watzinger, N., Larson, M. G., Smith, N. L., Dehghan, A., Grosshennig, A., Schillert, A., Teumer, A., Schmidt, R., Kathiresan, S., Lumley, T., Aulchenko, Y. S., Konig, I. R., Zeller, T., Homuth, G., Struchalin, M., Aragam, J., Bis, J. C., Rivadeneira, F., Erdmann, J., Schnabel, R. B., Dörr, M., Zweiker, R., Lind, L., Rodeheffer, R. J., Greiser, K. H., Levy, D., Haritunians, T., Deckers, J. W., Stritzke, J., Lackner, K. J., Völker, U., Ingelsson, E., Kullo, I., Haerting, J., O'Donnell, C.J., Heckbert, S. R., Stricker, B. H., Ziegler, A., Reffelmann, T., Redfield, M. M., Werdan, K., Mitchell, G. F., Rice, K., Arnett, D. K., Hofman, A., Gottdiener, J. S., Uitterlinden, A.G., Meitinger, T., Blettner, M., Friedrich, N., Wang, T. J., Psaty, B. M., van Duijn, C. M., Wichmann, H. E., Munzel, T. F., Kroemer, H. K., Benjamin, E. J., Rotter, J. I., Witteman, J. C., Schunkert, H., Schmidt, H., Völzke, H., Blankenberg, S. & Blankenberg, S. (2009). Genetic variants associated with cardiac structure and function: a meta-analysis and replication of genome-wide association data. *JAMA*, *302*(2), 168-178. https://doi.org/10.1001/jama.2009.978-a.

Verdecchia, P., Angeli, F., Borgioni, C., Gattobigio, R., de Simone, G., Devereux, R. B., & Porcellati, C. (2003). Changes in cardiovascular risk by reduction of left ventricular mass in hypertension: a meta-analysis. *American Journal of Hypertension*, 16(11), 895–899. https://doi.org/10.1016/s0895-7061(03)01018-5.

Walsh, R. A. (2005). *Molecular Mechanisms of Cardiac Hypertrophy and Failure* Taylor & Francis.

Wang, L., Yang, X., Cai, G., Xin, L., Xia, Q., Zhang, X., Li, X., Wang, M., Wang, K., & Xia, G. (2016). Association study of copy number variants in FCGR3A and FCGR3B gene with risk of ankylosing spondylitis in a Chinese population. *Rheumatology International*, *36*(3), 437-442. https://doi.org/10.1007/s00296-015-3384-0.

Weeks, K. L., & McMullen, J. R. (2011). The athlete's heart vs. the failing heart: can signaling explain the two distinct outcomes? *Physiology*. https://doi.org/10.1152/physiol.00043.2010.

Wellenreuther, M., Mérot, C., Berdan, E., & Bernatchez, L. (2019). Going beyond SNPs: The role of structural genomic variants in adaptive evolution and species diversification. *Molecular Ecology*, 28(6), 1203–1209. https://doi.org/10.1111/mec.15066.

Yim, S. H., Jung, S. H., Chung, B., & Chung, Y. J. (2015). Clinical implications of copy number variations in autoimmune disorders. Korean Journal of Internal Medicine. https://doi.org/10.3904/kjim.2015.30.3.294.

Zhang, F., Gu, W., Hurles, M. E., & Lupski, J. R. (2009). Copy number variation in human health, disease, and evolution. *Annual Review of Genomics and Human Genetics*, 10(1), 451–481. https://doi.org/10.1146/annurev.genom.9.081307.164217.

Zhang, K., Weder, A. B., Eskin, E., & O'Connor, D. T. (2010). Genome-wide case/control studies in hypertension: only the 'tip of the iceberg.' *Journal of Hypertension*, 28(6), 1115–1123. https://doi.org/10.1097/hjh.0b013e328337f6bc.

Zhu, H., Tannous, P., Johnstone, J. L., Kong, Y., Shelton, J. M., Richardson, J. A., Le, V. T. M., Levine, B., Rothermel, B. A., & Hill, J. A. (2007). Cardiac autophagy is a maladaptive response to hemodynamic stress. *Journal of Clinical Investigation*, 117(7), 1782–1793. https://doi.org/10.1172/jci27523.

Zhu, X., Li, J., Ru, T., Wang, Y., Xu, Y., Yang, Y., Wu, X., Cram, D. S., & Hu, Y. (2016). Identification of copy number variations associated with congenital heart disease by chromosomal microarray analysis and next-generation sequencing. *Prenatal Diagnosis*, 36(4), 321–327. https://doi.org/10.1002/pd.4782.

Zipes, D. P., & Wellens, H. J. (1998). Sudden cardiac death. *Circulation*, 98(21), 2334–2351. https://doi.org/10.1161/01.cir.98.21.2334.

Chapter 10

Genetic Susceptibility to Hypertension: A Case for *AGT, CYP11B2* and *ADRB2* Genes

Nur Hasnah Maamor[1,2,*]
and Hoh Boon-Peng[1,3]

[1]Faculty of Medicine and Health Sciences, UCSI University,
Kuala Lumpur, Malaysia
[2]Evidence Based Healthcare sector, National Institute of Health,
Ministry of Health Malaysia, Malaysia
[3]Division of Applied Biomedical Sciences and Biotechnology,
School of Health Sciences, International Medical University, Malaysia

Abstract

Hypertension (HT) causes numerous serious cardiovascular complications such as heart failure and stroke. It is believed to be a consequence of the complex interplay between an individual's genetic make-up and environmental factors. Most HT cases are categorized as primary HT, whereby the identifiable cause is unknown. Renin-angiotensin-aldosterone system (RAAS) and sympathetic nervous system (SNS) are two mechanisms that regulate blood pressure (BP). RAAS regulates sodium and fluid volume homeostasis, while SNS mediates cardiac contractility. The candidate genes that are most studied in these systems include angiotensinogen, *AGT*, and aldosterone synthase, *CYP11B2* (for RAAS); and adrenergic beta 2 receptor *ADRB2* (for SNS). Both are known to influence an individual's susceptibility to primary HT. Although the functionality of the candidate variants for these genes have been reported genetic association studies conducted on different populations have been inconsistent. It is imperative to determine

* Corresponding Author's Email: nurhasnah.m@moh.gov.my.

In: Genetic Disorders and Rare Diseases
Editors: Shazlin Shaharudin, Hisham Atan Edinur and Nor Fazila Che Mat
ISBN: 979-8-88697-953-4

the genetic association between the variants underlying these candidate genes and HT, because they could potentially be used as pharmacogenetic markers to predict a patients' responsiveness to antihypertensive medication. This chapter presents the latest updates on the candidate genetic variants *AGT* (rs699 and rs5051), *CYP11B2* (rs1799998 and rs10087214) and *ADRB2* (rs1042713 and rs1042714) and primary HT across different populations. A recent comprehensive genetic association study conducted on the Malay population from Peninsular Malaysia, as well as a meta-analysis of genetic association study, are also included in this chapter.

Keywords: aldosterone, angiotensin, cardiovascular disease

Introduction of Hypertension

According to International Society of Hypertension (ISH), individual with hypertension (HT) is defined as having (i) an increase in systolic blood pressure, SBP ≥140 mmHg; (ii) an increase in diastolic blood pressure, DBP ≥90 mmHg; (iii) an increase in both SBP and DBP for ≥140/90 mmHg; (iv) to take any form of antihypertensive medication; or (v) been diagnosed with HT by a clinician at least twice in two separate clinic visits with three measurements at 1 minute intervals (Carretero & Oparil, 2000; Ministry of Health, MOH, 2018; Unger et al., 2020; World Health Organization, WHO, 2021). HT is the major driver for cardiovascular disease (CVD) mortality and morbidity (MOH, 2018; Carretero & Oparil, 2000). It has been a major public health threat in most parts of the world, especially in the low-and-middle income countries, affecting more than one billion people annually (WHO, 2021). Table 1 shows the prevalence of HT in Malaysia for adults aged ≥ 18 years based on the classification of HT status.

HT is essentially classified into two types, namely primary and secondary HT. While secondary HT is associated with a defined cause such as renal or endocrinopathy primary HT, which accounts for 95% of all HT cases, is a condition that occurs when an elevation of BP has no clear identifiable cause. The aetiology of primary HT is complicated, involving complex interplays between individual genetic make-up and environmental factors, such as dietary salt intake, obesity, smoking and others (Oparil et al., 2018; Carretero & Oparil, 2000). Genetic heritability accounts for between approximately 30 to 50% of HT in twins and family studies (Ehret & Caulfield, 2013).

Table 1. Classification of BP reading and the prevalence of the classification for adults age ≥ 18 years in Malaysia (MOH, 2018)

Classification*	SBP (mmHg)		DBP (mmHg)	Prevalence of HT in Malaysia[a]
Optimal	<120	And	<80	30.7%
Normal	120–129	And/or	80-84	25.3%
At risk	130-139	And/or	85-89	18.6%
	Hypertension			
Stage I (Mild)	140-159	And/or	90–99	17.3%
Stage II (Moderate)	160–179	And/or	100–109	5.7%
Stage III (Severe)	≥ 180	And/or	≥ 110	2.4%
Isolated Systolic HT	≥ 140	And	<90	11.2%

*Adapted from National Institute for Health and Clinical Excellence (NICE) Hypertension, 2011.
[a] Liana et al., (2018).

Primary HT can be divided into two intermediate phenotypes, i.e., salt-sensitive HT (SS-HT), and salt-resistant HT, based on the BP response to the changes in liberal to restricted salt intake. About 60% of the primary HT are identified as SS-HT (Manosroi & William, 2019). The SS-HT category can be further divided into two sub-intermediate phenotypes based on the plasma renin activity (PRA) response to upright posture and dietary salt restriction, i.e., normal renin, and low renin. The influence of the candidate gene variations is believed to be the driving factor behind the individual proximate phenotype. *AGT* genetic variation is associated with normal renin SS-HT; while *ADRB2* and *CYP11B2* genes are associated with low renin SS-HT (Manosroi & William, 2019).

Prevalence of Hypertension

The global prevalence of HT increases in tandem with economic transitions, modification to individual lifestyles and the acceleration of ageing in the population (Aldiab et al., 2018). Over the past four decades, the prevalence of HT cases has shifted away from high-income countries to low- and middle-income countries such as South and Southeast Asia and Sub-Saharan Africa (Collaboration and NCD Risk Factor Collaboration, 2017) (Figure 1).

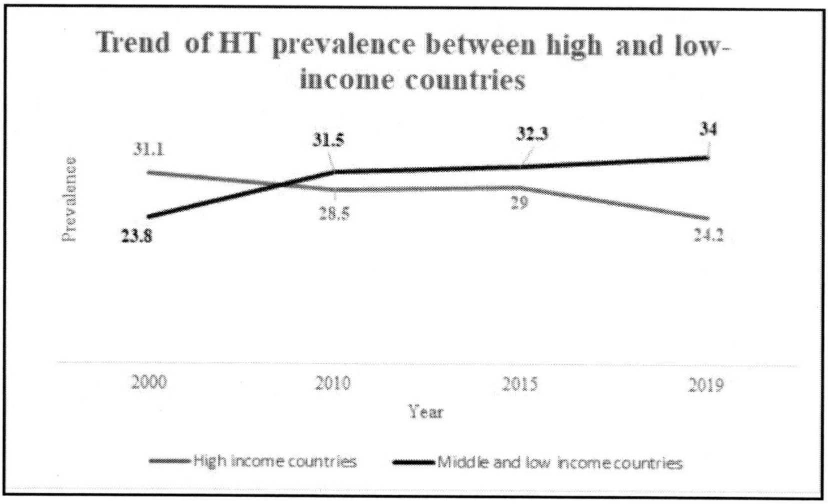

Figure 1. Trend of HT prevalence between high and low-income countries (Lateshia, 2016; Sarki et al., 2015; Beaney et al., 2019; Frayer, 2017; Garies et al., 2019).

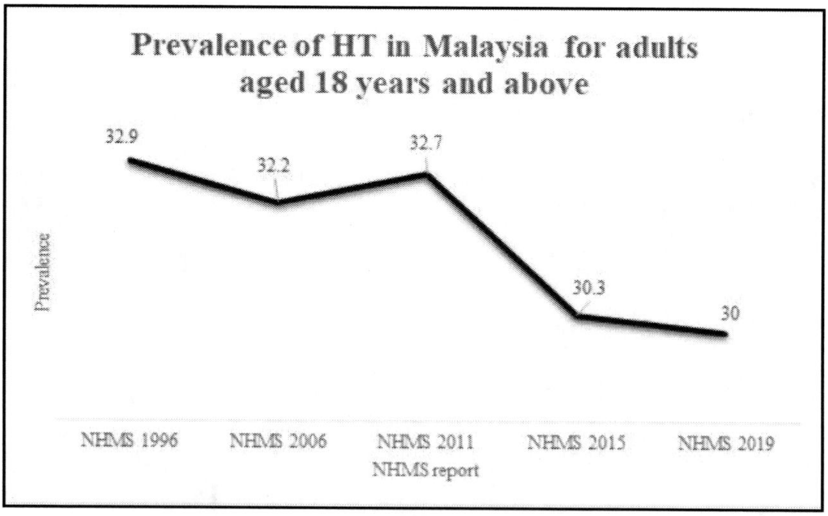

Figure 2. Prevalence of HT in Malaysia for adults aged 18 years and above, report by NHMS 1996 – 2019 (Institute for Public Health, 2008; Institute for Public Health, 2015; Naing et al., 2016; Institute for Public Health, 2020).

In 2010, the global prevalence of HT for population aged 18 years and above was 31.1%, which corresponded to 1.39 billion people (Mills et al., 2016); and subsequently increased to 40.8% in 2017 (Shafi & Shafi, 2017). In Malaysia, National Health and Morbidity Survey (NHMS) documented a slight decrease in the prevalence of HT between 1996 and 2019 among those 18 years and above, the prevalence of HT remains high (Figure 2), and more effort is required to mitigate the prevalence of HT in Malaysia. In Asia, the prevalence of HT for individuals aged 18 years and higher varies across different segments of the population and between countries (Table 2).

Table 2. Prevalence of hypertension for adults 18 years and older in few countries in Asia

Country	Prevalence	Author (Year)
China	37.2%	Lu et al., (2017)
Korea	30.5%	Kang et al., (2019)
Taiwan	24.1%	Cheng et al., (2019)
India	46.0%	Saju et al., (2020)
Nepal	27.3%	Huang et al., (2019)
Bahrain	17.1%	MOH Bahrain (2018)
Iran	44.0%	Fakhri et al., (2020)
Lebanon	31.2%	Cherfan et al., (2018)
Qatar	32.0%	Rashid et al., (2021)
United Arab Emirates	31.1%	Bhagavathula et al., (2021)
Vietnam	21.1%	Meiqari et al., (2019)
Laos	20.0%	Pengpid et al., (2019)
Indonesia	33.4%	Peltzer & Pengpid (2018)
Singapore	23.5%	Tay & Teo (2020)

Pathophysiology of Hypertension

The homeostasis of blood pressure (BP) is dependent on the balance between cardiac output (CO) and peripheral vascular resistance (PVR) (Delong & Sharma 2021): CO X PVR = BP

The increase in CO, PVR, blood volume, sodium and water reabsorption in the kidney leads to an increase in BP (Mayet & Hughes, 2003). Figure 3 shows the pathophysiology of primary HT. On a separate note, over activity of SNS causes the elevated CO, PVR and the retention of both salt and water, which elevates BP levels (Skrzypecki & Ufnal, 2015). In addition, a boost of sympathetic signalling in the SNS results in vasoconstriction and enhances the activity of adrenergic via vascular tone (McCorry, 2007).

BP regulation is a complex mechanism, involving numerous pathways that are interconnected. Some of the pathways that have been well-studied include: (i) natriuretic peptide; (ii) kinin-kallikrein; (iii) chemoreceptor and baroreceptor; (iv) endothelial dysfunction; (v) epithelial sodium channels (ENaCs); (vi) impaired pressure natriuresis; (vii) impaired renal function; (viii) bradykinin; (ix) nitric oxide. The overactivity of these mechanisms results in elevated vascular tone, change in the pressure-natriuresis relationship and sodium as well as water retention, which increases the blood volume in turn (Beevers et al., 2001; Kurtz et al., 2016). Figure 4 illustrates five main mechanisms in BP regulation and the underlying genes of interest in this study.

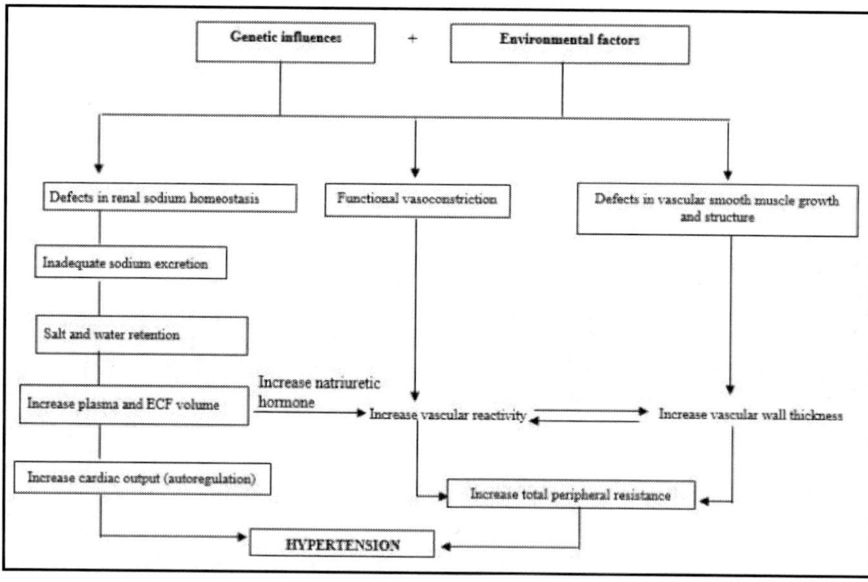

Figure 3. Pathophysiology of hypertension. Abnormal regulation in renal excretion of sodium, functional regulation of vascular tone and structural regulation of vascular calibre. Environmental factors especially increased sodium intake may potentiate the effects of genetic factors. The resultant increases in cardiac output and peripheral resistance contribute to hypertension. ECF = extracellular fluid (Kumar 2005).

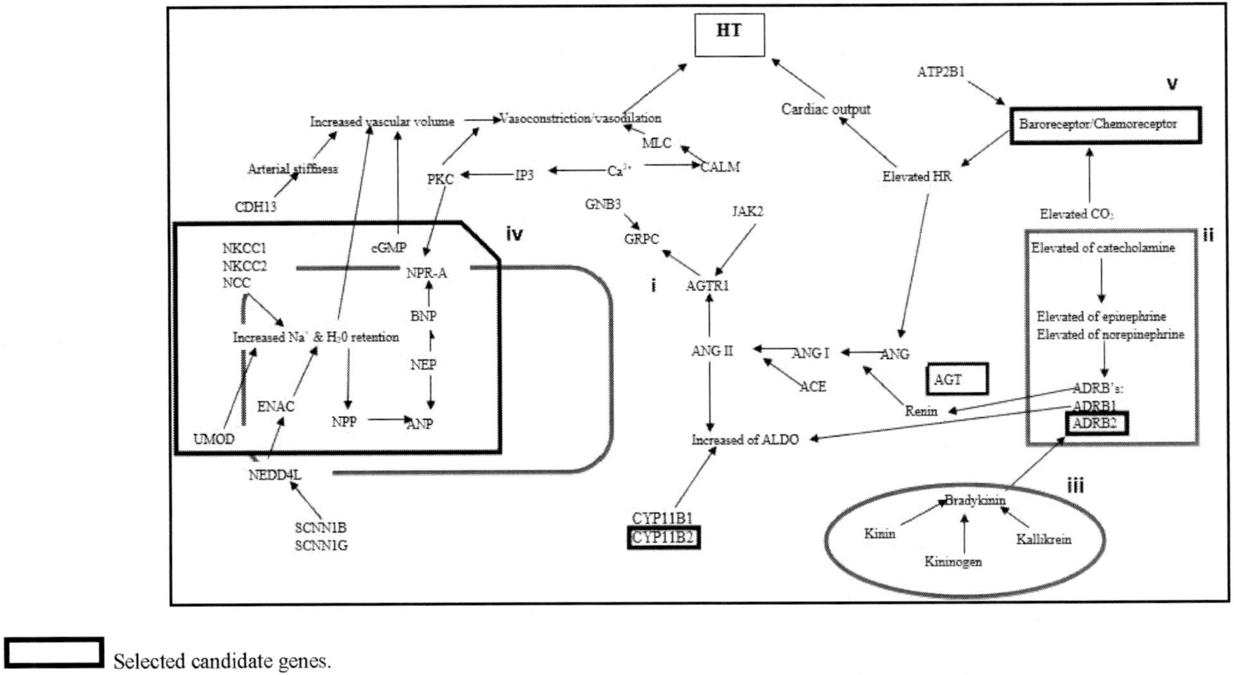

Figure 4. Five main mechanisms in BP regulation. (i) RAAS, (ii) SNS, (iii) kallikrein-kinin, (iv) natriuretic system, and (v) baroreceptor or chemoreceptor sensory. These mechanisms are related to each other and the elevation of few elements in the mechanisms leads to the HT. (i) the increase levels of renin, ALDO and angiotensin II (ANG II); (ii) elevated catecholamine, epinephrine, norepinephrine (NE), ADRB leads to the increased of both renin and ALDO secretion; (iii) activated bradykinin leads to the increased ADRB2 secretion; (iv) increase sodium leads to water retention and increase BP; (v) increases of heart rate and cardiac output. All of these mechanisms leads to the HT (Hoh et al., 2019).

Genetics of Hypertension

HT involves of numerous aetiological mechanisms and interplays between individual's genetic make-up and environmental factors (Touyz, 2014). What is more challenging, is that multiple genes (polygenic) are involved in shaping the HT phenotypes, each with only modest effects, coupled with multiple gene-to-gene interactions and pleiotropic effects (Shih & O'Connar, 2008) leading to the undetermined aetiology of HT. Genetic factors are thought to contribute approximately 30–60% of BP variation. However, known genetic factors explain only 3% of BP variance, underscoring the fact that many genetic variants have yet to be discovered (Munroe et al., 2013; Ahn & Gupta 2017) or in short implying much remained in the black box. There is almost no single prime system that is primarily involved in regulating BP (Patel et al., 2017).

Candidate gene study designs based on specific gene(s) of interest that are targeted within the physiological mechanisms, the specific function of the candidate genes, or biochemical pathways that are known to be associated with BP variations (Corvol et al., 1999). The study design is useful in understanding the genetic component of BP variation across the different sections of the population in different countries at a relatively low genotyping cost (Delles & Padmanabhan, 2012). However, this approach has some pitfalls: (i) it is less likely to be reproduced (Tanira & Balushi, 2004); (ii) the contribution of a single gene to BP variation may be much less effective; and (iii) the selection candidate genes is based on the known BP regulation pathway and not completely informative of the variability within the gene (Delles & Padmanabhan, 2012). Despite the limitations, the design of this study remains one of the cornerstones in the genetic HT research and has been implemented extensively (Delles & Padmanabhan, 2012).

Genome-wide association studies (GWAS) is performed using chip-based microarray technology and is designed to identify genetic associations with observable traits (Pearson & Manolio, 2008). GWAS is a hypothesis neutral approach, designed to identify whole genome associations with observable traits (Pearson & Manolio, 2008). GWAS uncovers common variants with small effect sizes that are often missed by candidate gene and family linkage analysis (Basson et al., 2012). HT is among the first complex trait studied using GWAS (Wellcome Trust Case Control Consortium, 2007). However, attempts to investigate the genetic variants associated with BP have been challenging. In 2007, the GWAS study that acquired a case-control study design was performed by Wellcome Trust Case Control Consortium

(WTCCC) on the populations with European ancestry, however no statistically significant association with HT was identified (WTCCC, 2007). The WTCC Consortium was established in 2000 and this consortium was a collaboration between 50 research groups from the United Kingdom conducted an investigation with the aim of conducting GWAS to shed light on the genetic architecture of common human diseases (WTCCC, 2018). Similarly, Framingham Heart Study found no association signal that reached genome-wide significance level (Levy et al., 2007). As technology advanced, higher density of genotyping technology was available and the genotyping cost is more affordable. Table 3 lists a few GWAS studies that observed an association between single-nucleotide polymorphisms (SNPs) and BP ($p<5x10^{-8}$). SNPs is a single genetic code variation, usually biallelic (two alternative bases occur) with the minimum frequency (>1%) in the population (i.e., polymorphism) (Wang et al., 1998). SNP is the most common form of variation in the genome that may contribute to changes in the genomic sequence, either in promoter, exons or introns regions (Van Dijk et al., 2014; Ahmad et al., 2018). SNP is extensively used to study genetic differences between individuals and populations (Vallejos-Vidal et al., 2020). Nonetheless, GWAS of HT for the native groups in Malaysia, notably the Malays has never been reported on.

Table 3. List of GWAS studies that observed an association between the SNPs and BP

No	Author (Year)	Population	Number of subjects	No of SNPs associated with BP
1	Levy et al., (2009)	CHARGE Consortium (European)	29,136	33
2	Adeyemo et al., (2009)	African American	1,017	0
3	Hong et al., (2010)	Korean	7,551	14
4	Ehret et al., (2011)	European	200,000	29
5	Fox et al., (2011)	African American	7,473	14
6	Guo et al., (2012)	Chinese	328	9
7	Evangelou et al., (2018)	European	1,000,000	535
8	Takeuchi et al., (2018)	Japanese	130,777	15
9	Chen et al., (2021)	Chinese	380 (in twin)	0
10	Kolifarhood et al., (2021)	Iran	7,694	10

Angiotensinogen (*AGT*) and Hypertension

Angiotensinogen (AGT) is the natural substrate of RAAS that is synthesised in the liver (Dhanachandra et al., 2014). *AGT* is located at chromosome 1q42-43. This gene is 12,068 bp in length and contains five exons (Zhen et al., 2020). *AGT* was the first candidate gene associated with human HT (Jeunemaitre et al., 1992). The SNP rs699, or more commonly known as M235T is one of the most widely studied *AGT* variant in HT (Purkait et al., 2017). M235T changes the nucleotide A to G (at nucleotide position 704, located in the second exon of the gene). The nucleotide substitution alters the amino acid methionine (M) to threonine (T) at codon 235. Higher plasma AGT concentration was observed in individuals who carried the T amino acid (corresponding to G nucleotide) (Jeunemaitre et al., 1992). It was found that the normotensive white American children who were homozygous GG had an approximately 13% higher plasma AGT concentration than those who carried AA genotype (Bloem et al., 1995). T amino acid was associated with elevated AGT concentration and affects the expression level of AGT (Norat et al., 2008) in Caucasians, African-Caribbean, and Asia populations (Inoue et al., 1997). Another SNP namely, rs5051, or more commonly known as A-6G, is located in the promoter region, upstream of the initiation transcript regulatory region. This substitution is thought to affect the transcriptional activity of *AGT* (Gong et al., 2019). The -6A variant leads to the elevation of gene transcription and one trans-acting nuclear factor in the angiotensinogen promoter, as demonstrated by their influence on the basal transcription rate (Goracy et al., 2021). The excessed expression of the -6A variant is observed to be associated with the elevated BP and aldosterone (ALDO) level (Nakajima et al., 2004).

The two candidate SNPs rs5051 and rs699 are in strong linkage disequilibrium (LD). LD refers to the non-random association of alleles at two or more loci in a general population. LD is used to investigate the association between two or more alleles within similar blocks, which may relate to the time of the mutation events, genetic distance, and population history (Goode, 2017). It may improve the power of the genetic association studies (Slatkin, 2008). Strong LD is defined as association with markers pairs of SNPs within the similar block, which can be observed based on the r^2 or D' (Slatkin, 2008). If r^2 or D' value is ≥ 0.8 the LD is considered as strong LD (Kerna et al., 2013).

In line with the findings of previous studies, our research paper on the mainstream Malay population in Malaysia also found a strong LD between these SNPs (Maamor et al., 2023a, under review). Intriguingly, the association of rs699 and rs5051 with HT is inconsistent across the global populations

(Kunz et al., 1997). A genetic association with HT was observed in populations from North America, Australia, Japan, Europe, Slovak, Tibet, and Taiwan (Hata et al., 1994; Kamitani et al., 1994; Kui et al., 2012; Krizanova et al., 1997; Nakajima et al., 2004; Conlin, 2008); but not in the Africa or the Caribbean (Dickson & Sigmund 2006; Barley et al., 1995; Bloem et al., 1995; Hingorani et al., 1996).

In Malaysia, research on candidate SNPs and HT is limited (Say et al., 2005; Ghazali et al., 2008). One study found a significant association between the rs699 and primary HT (Say et al., 2005). However, the study was carried out by pooling the major ethnicities in Malaysia namely the Malay, Chinese and Indians in one analysis. Owing to the fact that these populations are known to have different genetic ancestries and genetic makeup and as a result have unique phenotypic features, pooling these ethnic groups together in a genetic association analysis may have resulted in a statistical bias type I error. Contradictory studies suggested no significant association between rs699 and HT among the Malays (Ghazali et al., 2008). However, these studies were hindered by limited sample sizes. Interestingly, utilising a much larger sample size, our study revealed similar findings among the HT Malay (Maamor et al., 2023a, under review). These variants remained no appreciative associations when associating with alteration of SBP, DBP and mean arterial pressure, MAP) (Maamor et al., 2023b, under review).

Aldosterone Synthase (*CYP11B2*) and Hypertension

ALDO synthase gene (*CYP11B2)* is a member of cytochrome *P450* superfamily of enzymes (steroid 18-hydroxylase, 18 oxidases, and 11 β hydroxylases), located at chromosome *8q1*. It consists of nine exons, and is 7,284 bp in length. *CYP11B2* catalyses the terminal steps of steroid biosynthesis (*11-deoxycorticosterone*) in the final stage of ALDO biosynthesis (Hlubocka et al., 2009). This gene is expressed in the adrenal gland and fasciculate and is responsible for ALDO production (Sookoian et al., 2007).

The variant of *rs1799998* (or commonly known as *-344A/G*) is a commonly studied SNP in *CYP11B2*. This variant is located at the position *-344* of the promoter region. The G allele was associated with an elevated ALDO plasma level (Pojaga et al., 1998), and the development of low renin HT (Tsukada et al., 2002). The carrier of G allele was associated with decreased baroreflex sensitivity (Tsukada et al., 2002), which effects the BP level that in turn leads to an increased risk of HT. Another SNP, *rs10087214*, its association with primary HT is less investigated. Only one study reported in the Han Chinese population, but no significant association was observed (Zhang et al., 2017).

Contradicting results were reported on the association between rs1799998 and primary HT. This variant was associated with HT in populations from northwest of China (Li et al., 2016), Japan (Takeuchi et al., 2012), India (Vamsi et al., 2016), Iraq (Ameer et al., 2015) and African American (Henderson et al., 2004), but not Han Chinese (Niu et al., 2010; Sun et al., 2011). Moreover, there are conflicting reports as to whether the G or T allele is the risk allele for HT. The G allele had been reported to have a higher risk to HT in Japan, European and Han Chinese (Li et al., 2006; Pojoga et al., 1998; Cheng & Xu, 2009) whereas another study reported that the T allele was significantly associated with HT in French and Scottish populations (Barbato et al., 2004).

The reason of this contradictory finding is uncertain, however, several explanations are plausible. Firstly, heterogeneity of the population being studied. Most of the studies were population based and not controlled. Secondly, the phenotype for genes involved in sodium/volume homeostasis, in this case *CYP11B2*, low renin and BP levels are likely dependent on environmental factors (Ghafar et al., 2019). Thirdly, different minor and major alleles between different populations may have complicated or skewed the findings (Adeyemo & Rotimi, 2010).

The genetic association between *CYP11B2* and primary HT in Malaysia has not been reported before. Therefore, this study conducted a genetic association analysis on the two candidate SNPs of interest (*rs1799998* and *rs10087214*) with the causes and prevalence of primary HT in individuals of Malay decent or ancestry (N = 918), and found that the *rs10087214-GG* genotype was significantly associated with HT (p = 0.027). When assessing the effect of this variant on the changes of BP among hypertensive individuals, the *rs10087214-G* allele was found to significantly elevate SBP (p = 0.049), DBP (p = 0.024) and MAP (p = 0.013) among HT Malay males; but not females. Further analysis revealed that the risk haplotype (consisting of a single chromosome set in their somatic cells) *rs1799998-G/rs10087214-A* and diplotype (consist of a two-chromosome set in their somatic cells) exhibited an even stronger effect of BP elevation among the males – an elevation of ~7 mm/Hg MAP on average. The fact that this study observed no appreciative effect of BP elevation among the female risk allele carriers could plausibly be explained in part by the effects of oestrogen hormones that may have protected the females from increased BP, HT and associated risks (Paresh et al., 2019). The SNPs *rs1799998* and *rs10087214* are in strong LD ($r^2 = 0.75 - 0.94$) in mainstream Malay populations (Maamor et al., 2023a, under review).

Adrenergic Beta 2 Receptor (*ADRB2*) and Hypertension

The *ADRB2* gene is expressed in various tissues types including fat, vascular, heart, and smooth muscle (Hoit et al., 2000). This gene is a member of the G-protein coupled receptor superfamily, and it is located at chromosome *5q31-32*, with 2,033 bp in length. This gene is intron-less, and encodes for 413 amino acids (Maciejewska-Skrendo et al., 2019).

ADRB2 plays a role in vascular tone and regulates vascular smooth muscle (Pacanowski et al., 2008). It affects volume homeostasis via elevation of renin secretion and altered vasodilation function (Sun et al., 2010) in vascular smooth muscle, cause vessel resistance (Lang et al., 1995) and agonist-mediated receptor downregulation in salt-sensitive HT individuals during the increase of salt intake (Pojaga et al., 2006).

The variant rs1042713, also known as Gly16Arg or 46G>A, and rs1042714, also known as Gln27Glu or 79C>G, are the most studied SNPs in *ADRB2* gene. These variants cause attenuated vasodilation, increased peripheral resistance, BP (Atia et al., 2012), associated with the decreased renin level and increased ALDO secretion (Pojoga et al., 2006).

Both *ADRB2* SNPs had been associated with HT in several populations including Japanese (Misono et al., 2009), Chinese Singaporean (Lee et al., 2004), Han Chinese (Ge et al., 2005), African-Caribbean (Kotanko et al., 1997), Caucasian-Americans (Hoit et al., 2000) and Norwegian (Timmermann et al., 1998); but not in European (Hermann et al., 2002), Italian (Galletti et al., 2004), Africans (Candy et al., 2000) and the American-blacks (Xie et al., 2000). However, Pojoga et al., (2006) observed 46AA/79CC diplotype is associated with the HT.

The genetic association study of *ADRB2* and HT in Malaysia has been rather limited: only two publications were found (Atia et al., 2012; Komara et al., 2014). Atia et al. (2012) reported no significant association observed between both variants and essential HT; but Komara et al. (2014) claimed the opposite. The major pitfalls that may affect the results for these two studies could be (i) small sample size recruited; (ii) the heterogeneity of populations used as they consisted samples of Malay, Chinese and Indian ancestries. We replicated the genetic association with close to 1,000 samples of Malay ancestry, and revealed no significant association between both variants and primary HT in Malay populations (Maamor et al., 2023b, under review). Interestingly, when assessing the effect of these SNPs on the alteration of BP among the HT individuals, females rs1042714-CC risk genotype carriers had a decreased the BP as opposed to the non-risk genotype. The analysis performed in young females showed a significant different MAP between rs1042714 risk genotype carriers and those non-risk genotype carriers ($p = 0.042$); whereas among the older females, carriers for rs1042714 risk genotype showed a significant difference in DBP ($p = 0.012$) and MAP ($p = 0.011$) as opposed to the non-risk genotype (Maamor et al., 2023a, under review). This finding is slightly different from the finding published by Pojaga et al., (2006) that revealed greater increase in MAP among individuals who carried 46AA/79CC diplotype. However, this finding did not mention which gender is more effected to the increased of BP in MAP (Pojoga et al., 2006).

The higher level of oestrogen in the female may likely be one explanation. This hormone has shown to attenuate RAAS by decreasing angiotensin 1 receptor (AT1R) and ACE expression, leading to the decrease of ANG II thence the BP (Maranon & Reckhelhoff, 2013). Another possible reason that may explain the effects of rs1042714-CC on HT females is the presence of the higher oestrogen level increases endothelial adrenoreceptor expression, which upon adrenergic stimulation leads to secretion of nitric oxide (NO). This causes the vasodilation in vessel and decrease the BP in females (Riedel et al., 2019). Interestingly, while populations of European ancestry show moderate to strong LD between the two candidate SNPs (Pojoga et al., 2006; Al-Balushi et al., 2015), we found that these SNPs exhibit a very weak linkage among the mainstream Malay population (r^2 between 0.06 - 0.09). Owing to this finding, we therefore postulate that these SNPs may act independently in regulating the BP among the HT females (Farheen et al., 2011).

Meta-Analysis

Judging from the inconclusive findings as elaborated in the earlier sections, a meta-analysis was performed to summarize the finding regarding to the genetic associations between the selected candidate SNPs with HT. Four SNPs namely, *AGT*-rs699, *ADRB2*-rs1042713, *ADRB2*-rs1042714 and *CYP11B2*-rs1799998, were investigated after the following inclusion and exclusion criteria were applied. Owing to the notion that populations from different ancestries carry different genetic makeup, which may confound the statistical analysis in a genetic association study (Yako et al., 2018), the datasets of the meta-analysis performed (Maamor et al., 2023b, under review) categorized the publications based on known genetic ancestries, and/or geographical populations: (i) European, (ii) Southern Chinese, (iii) East Asian (consisting of Northern Chinese and Japanese), (iv) Southern Indian, (v) Northern Indian, (vi) Latin American (vii) African (viii) the Middle East. A comprehensive systematic literature search was conducted in three databases: PubMed, National Centre for Biotechnology Information (NCBI), Cochrane, and Science Direct with the specific keywords (listed at Table 4) as well as following the inclusion and exclusion criteria (Maamor et al., 2023b, under review).

Table 4. Keywords that used when performing meta-analysis

Genes	Keywords
AGT-rs699	(i) hypertension, (ii) AGT, (iii) Angiotensinogen, (iv) rs699, (v) M235T, (vi) M268T and (v) Hypertension AND (vi) AGT OR Angiotensinogen AND rs699 OR M235T OR M26T.
CYP11B2-rs1799998	(i) hypertension, (ii) CYP11B2, (iii) Aldosterone synthase, (iv) rs1799998, (v) -344T/C and (vi) Hypertension AND (vii) CYP11B2 OR Aldosterone synthase AND rs1799998 OR -344T/C.
ADRB2	(i) hypertension, (ii) ADRB2, (iii) B2AR, (iv) beta 2-adrenergic receptor, (v) rs1042713, (vi) rs1042714, (vii) Gln27Glu, (viii) Arg16Gly, (ix) A46G, (x) C79G, (xi) Q27E and (xii) Hypertension AND (xiii) ADRB2 OR B2AR OR beta-adrenergic receptor AND rs1042713 OR Arg16Gly OR A46G AND rs1042714 OR Gln27Glu OR C79G OR Q27E.

Inclusion criteria during articles' search:

- Article written in English
- Full text article
- Case-control design study
- Subject's age: adult 18 years and above
- Essential/primary HT
- Available genotype number for HT
- Normotensive (NT)
- HT defined as BP ≥140 in systolic blood pressure (SBP) or ≥90 diastolic blood pressure (DBP) mmHg or both or on anti-hypertensive medication
- NT defined as BP <140/90 mmHg

Exclusion criteria:

- Publication from review articles, meta-analysis, abstracts and meeting reports
- Duplicating first authors, corresponding authors, affiliations, suspected genotyping error (reported frequencies significantly deviated from expected or potential in genotyping error potentially due to flipping strand issue)

The journals were manually inspected for the possibility of overlapping data or journal by observing the author's name and institute. The eligible articles included in this study are listed in Table 5. The quality of the articles was assessed using an adapted version of the Newcastle-Ottawa Quality Assessment Scale (NOS). Articles with score 7 stars and more are identified as high quality. The summary and the flow applied during searching is shown in Figure 5. The sample information included in the meta-analysis is summarized in Table 6.

Table 5. List of publications or articles included in the meta-analysis for *AGT*-rs699, *CYP11B2*-rs1799998, *ADRB2*-rs1042713 and *ADRB2*-rs1042714)

Gene/ ID	**NO**	**Ethnicity**	**First author (year)**	**Case no.**	**Control no.**	**HT diagnosis standard**	**Quality score of NOS**
AGT/ rs699							
	1	Asia	Kishimoto (2001)	201	201	SBP≥160, DBP≥95	Good
	2	Asia	Kario (1997)	235	103	SBP≥140, DBP≥90	Good
	3	Asia	Iso (2000)	229	229	SBP≥160, DBP≥95	Good
	4	Asia	Sato (2000)	180	195	SBP≥160, DBP≥95 or on treatment	Good
	5	Asia	Kato (2000)	838	631	SBP≥160, DBP≥95 or on treatment	Good
	6	Asia	Kato (1999)	717	515	SBP≥160, DBP≥95 or on treatment	Good
	7	Asia	Morise (1995)	80	100	SBP≥160, DBP≥95	Good
	8	Asia	Hata (1994)	105	81	SBP≥160, DBP≥95	Good
	9	Asia	Wang (2014)	1076	687	SBP≥140, DBP≥90	Good
	10	Asia	Li (2014)	652	780	SBP≥140, DBP≥90	Good
	11	Asia	Hu (2014)	100	97	SBP≥140, DBP≥90 or on treatment	Good

Gene/ ID	NO	Ethnicity	First author (year)	Case no.	Control no.	HT diagnosis standard	Quality score of NOS
	12	Asia	Najatizadeh (2008)	450	360	SBP≥140, DBP≥90	Good
	13	Asia	Kohli (2016)	545	400	SBP≥140, DBP≥90	Good
	14	Asia	Ramu (2011)	462	444	SBP≥140, DBP≥90	Good
	15	Asia	Padma (2015)	215	230	SBP≥140, DBP≥90 or o treatment	Good
	16	Asia	Charita (2012)	241	242	SBP≥140, DBP≥90 or on treatment	Good
	17	Asia	Mohana (2012)	279	200	SBP≥140, DBP≥90 or on treatment	Good
	18	Asia	Dhanachandra (2014)	211	211	SBP≥140, DBP≥90 or on treatment	Good
	19	Asia	Srivastava (2012)	250	248	SBP≥140, DBP≥90 or on treatment	Good
	20	Asia	Thomas (2000)	232	178	SBP≥140, DBP≥90	Good
	21	Asia	Cheung (1998)	101	103	SBP>160, DBP>90	Good
	22	Asia	Fang (2010)	178	256	SBP>160, DBP>90	Good
	23	Asia	Wu (2004)	453	325	SBP≥140, DBP≥90 or on treatment	Good
	24	Asia	Agachan (2003)	100	74	SBP≥140, DBP≥90 or on treatment	Good
	25	Asia	Saab (2011)	124	146	SBP≥140, DBP≥90 or on treatment	Good
	26	Asia	Frossard (1998)	135	61	SBP>160, DBP>95	Good
	27	Europe	Hingorani (1996)	223	187	SBP≥160, DBP≥95	Good
	28	Europe	Fernández (1998)	75	75	SBP>160, DBP>100	Good
	29	Europe	Mondorf (1998)	112	124	SBP>160, DBP>100	Good
	30	Europe	Kiema (1996)	508	523	SBP≥160, DBP≥95	Good
	31	Europe	Rodriguez (2000)	237	242	SBP>140, DBP>90	Good
	32	Europe	Barbalić (2006)	107	122	SBP>140, DBP>90	Good
	33	Europe	Vas'ku (2002)	206	192	SBP>140, DBP>90	Good
	34	Europe	Kolovou (2015)	83	83	SBP>140, DBP>90	Good
	35	Europe	Procopcuic (2002)	38	21	SBP>140, DBP>95	Good
	36	Europe	Bengra (2002)	60	60	SBP>140, DBP>90	Good
	37	Europe	Jeunemaitre (1993)	136	90	SBP≥160, DBP≥95	Good

Table 5. (Continued)

Gene/ ID	NO	Ethnicity	First author (year)	Case no.	Control no.	HT diagnosis standard	Quality score of NOS
	38	Europe	Caulfield (1994)	63	64	DBP≥120 or on treatment	Good
	39	Europe	Berocki (1997)	299	284	SBP>140, DBP>90	Good
	40	Europe	Berocki (1997)	129	126	SBP>140, DBP>90	Good
	41	Europe	Sunder (2002)	182	182	DBP≥120	Good
	42	Europe	Vasku (1998)	173	176	SBP>140, DBP>90	Good
	43	Europe	Barley (1994)	80	74	SBP>140, DBP>90	Good
	44	Europe	Jeunemaitre (1997)	477	415	DBP≥95	Good
	45	Latin America	Freitas (2007)	82	78	SBP≥140, DBP≥90	Good
	46	Latin America	Bautista (2008)	255	231	SBP≥140, DBP≥90 or on treatment	Good
	47	Latin America	Fardella (1998)	64	62	SBP>140, DBP>90	Good
CYP11 B2/rs17 99998							
	1	Europe	Zhu (2003)	138	97	SBP≥140, DBP≥90	Good
	2	Europe	Hlubocka (2009)	213	156	SBP≥140, DBP≥90 or on treatment	Good
	3	Europe	Castellano (2003)	1778	583	DBP ≥ 100	Good
	4	Europe	Staessen (2001)	339	1122	SBP>140, DBP>90 or on treatment	Good
	5	Europe	Bengra (2002)	60	60	SBP>140, DBP>90	Good
	6	Asia	Chen (2011)	510	510	SBP≥140, DBP≥90	Good
	7	Asia	Niu (2010)	475	475	SBP>140, DBP>90 or on treatment	Good
	8	Asia	Li (2011)	1059	1120	SBP≥140, DBP≥90	Good
	9	Asia	Wang (2014)	700	1090	SBP≥140, DBP≥90	Good
	10	Asia	Li (2016)	390	424	SBP≥140, DBP≥90 or on treatment	Good
	11	Asia	Ji (2015)	345	157	SBP≥140, DBP≥90	Good
	12	Asia	Gu (2004)	503	503	SBP>140, DBP>90 or on treatment	Good
	13	Asia	Sun (2011)	310	310	SBP>140, DBP>90	Good
	14	Asia	Tsujita (2001)	1502	2496	SBP>140, DBP>90 or on treatment	Good
	15	Asia	Tsukada (2002)	250	221	SBP≥140, DBP≥90	Good

Gene/ ID	NO	Ethnicity	First author (year)	Case no.	Control no.	HT diagnosis standard	Quality score of NOS
	16	Asia	Komiya (2000)	73	134	SBP>160, DBP>95	Good
	17	Asia	Kato (2000)	841	633	SBP≥160, DBP≥95 or on treatment	Good
	18	Asia	Patnaik (2014)	246	274	SBP>140, DBP>90 or on treatment	Good
	19	Asia	Rajput (2005)	100	190	SBP>140	Good
	20	Asia	Nejatizadeh (2010)	450	360	SBP≥140, DBP≥90	Good
	21	Asia	Rajan (2010)	406	424	SBP>140, DBP>90	Good
	22	Asia	Vamsi (2016)	279	200	SBP≥140, DBP≥90 or on treatment	Good
ADRB2 /rs1042 713							
	1	Europe	Jia (2000)	298	298	SBP≥140, DBP≥90	Good
	2	Europe	Timmermann (1998)	18	16	SBP≥140, DBP≥90	Good
	3	Europe	Xie (2000)	201	179	SBP≥140, DBP≥90	Good
	4	Europe	Filigheddu (2004)	517	184	SBP≥140, DBP≥90	Good
	5	Europe	Bartels (2007)	258	171	SBP≥140, DBP≥90 or on treatment	Good
	6	Europe	Poojaga (2006)	280	65	DBP ≥ 100 (not on treatment) DBP ≥ 90 (on treatment)	Good
	7	Europe	Sunder (2002)	182	182	DBP ≥ 120	Good
	8	Europe	Castellano (2003)	324	247	SBP≥140, DBP≥90 or on treatment	Good
	9	Europe	Hermann (2002)	690	277	DBP≥100	Good
	10	Europe	Herrmann (2000)	36	101	SBP≥140, DBP≥90	Good
	11	Europe	Tang (2003)	118	124	SBP>160, DBP>100 or on treatment	Good
	12	Africa America	Xie (2000)	155	128	SBP≥140, DBP≥90	Good
	13	Africa America	Herrmann (2000)	40	56	SBP≥140, DBP≥90	Good
	14	Africa America	Tang (2003)	134	143	SBP≥160, DBP≥100 or on treatment	Good

Table 5. (Continued)

Gene/ ID	NO	Ethnicity	First author (year)	Case no.	Control no.	HT diagnosis standard	Quality score of NOS
	15	Asia	Lou (2011)	747	390	SBP≥140, DBP≥90 or on treatment	Good
	16	Asia	Shan-Fa (2008)	58	58	SBP≥140, DBP≥90 or on treatment	Good
	17	Asia	Kato (2001)	839	631	SBP ≥160, DBP≥95 or on treatment	Good
	18	Asia	Misono (2009)	194	208	SBP≥140, DBP≥90	Good
ADRB2 /rs1042 714							
	1	Europe	Jia (2000)	298	298	SBP≥140, DBP≥90	Good
	2	Europe	Bartels (2007)	258	171	SBP≥140, DBP≥90 or on treatment	Good
	3	Europe	Pojaga (2006)	280	65	DBP ≥ 100 (not on treatment) DBP ≥ 90 (on treatment)	Good
	4	Europe	Castellano (2003)	324	247	SBP≥140, DBP≥90 or on treatment	Good
	5	Europe	Sunder (2002)	182	182	DBP ≥ 120	Good
	6	Europe	Hermann (2002)	690	277	DBP≥100	Good
	7	Europe	Xie (2000)	155	128	SBP≥140, DBP≥90	Good
	8	Asia	Lou (2011)	747	390	SBP≥140, DBP≥90 or on treatment	Good
	9	Asia	Shan-Fa (2008)	58	58	SBP≥140, DBP≥90 or on treatment	Good
	10	Asia	Ge (2005)	503	504	SBP≥160, DBP≥100	Good
	11	Asia	Kato (2001)	839	631	SBP ≥160, DBP≥95 or on treatment	Good
	12	Asia	Mo (2007)	288	149	SBP≥140, DBP≥90	Good

The meta-analysis was performed using MetaGenyo, an online programme for meta-analysis of genetic association study (https://meta genyo.genyo.es/). The association between the candidate variants and HT were assessed using an odds ratio (OR) with a 95% confidence interval (Cl).

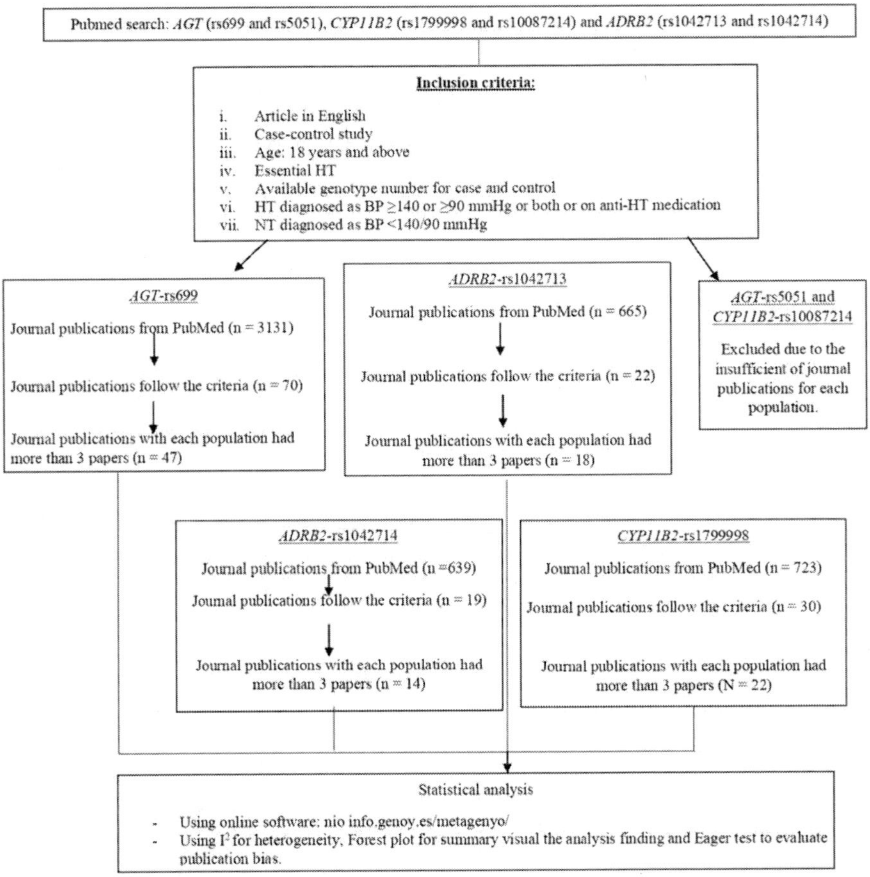

Figure 5. Summary of the search process for *AGT*-rs699, *CYP11B2*-rs1799998 and *ADRB2*-rs1042713 and rs1042714.

Fixed or random-effect models was acquired in this study, based on the significance of inter-study heterogeineity ($p < 0.05$). The fixed-effect model was calculated using the Mantel-Haenszel method by assuming that study sampled had the same effect size with the study weights adjusted according to the in-study variance ($p_{homogeneity} > 0.1$). On a separate note, random-effect model was calculated using DerSimonian and Laird model by assuming that the effect size of the studied sample varied and calculating study weights both from within-study and between-study variances with consideration of the extent of heterogeneity ($p_{heterogeneity} < 0.10$) (Martorell-Marugan et al., 2017). A funnel plot was generated and evaluated using Egger's test to assess possible publication bias. The standard error of the log (OR) of each plot was plotted against its OR in the funnel plot. Egger's test with a $p < 0.05$ shows the possibility of publication bias. A sensitivity test was generated in the forest plot for a selected genetic model to examine the robustness of the meta-analysis. This analysis was carried out several times, each time by excluding one of the articles in order to observe and assess the effect of each study on the overall statistics.

AGT-rs699

Overall, 3,131 publications were retrieved: PubMed (n = 3,064 publications), Cochrane (n = 23 publications) and Science Direct (n = 44 publications). Sixty-eight articles met the criteria set. Eighteen were subsequently excluded from further analyses because there were fewer than three publications on the populations classified, as required by MetaGenyo to perform the Egger's test to assess publication bias. Subsequently, upon manual inspection, three more publications were excluded because the reported genotype and allele frequencies were unusually deviated from other publications, implying potential either sampling error, or genotyping error in the said publications. After the stringent filtering criteria, 47 publications remained. A total of 11,923 HT and 10,380 NT individuals were involved in this analysis. The sample information included in the meta-analysis is summarized in Table 6.

Eight subgroup analyses were included in the meta-analysis, which revealed a modest but significant association between rs699-G and HT among the Indian population (South + North) in allele (P = 0.03, OR = 1.37, 95% CI 1.03 – 1.82, $P_{heterogeneity}$= 0.0001) and dominant inheritance (GG + GA vs AA) (P = 0.009, OR = 1.45, 95% CI 1.09 – 1.91, $P_{heterogeneity}$ = 0.0086), under random model effect, considering interstudy heterogeneity detected in the analysis (Table 7).

Table 6. Sample information (hypertensive, HT and normotensive, NT) included in the meta-analysis for (i) *AGT*-rs699; (ii) *CYP11B2*-rs1799998; (iii) *ADRB2*-rs1042713 and (iv) *ADRB2*-rs1042714

Genes	Population	HT	NT
(i) *AGT*-rs699	Asian		
	East Asian (Northern Han Chinese and Japanese)	4,313	3,565
	Southern Han Chinese	1,063	959
	Southern Indian	1,196	1,131
	Northern Indian	1,244	1,009
	Middle East	359	281
	Europe	3,188	2,865
	Latin America	401	371
(ii) *CYP11B2*-rs1799998	European	3,037	2,018
	Northern Han Chinese	4,603	4,113
	Japanese	2,666	3,502
	Indian	1,439	1,381
(iii) *ADRB2*-rs1042713	European	2,922	1,844
	African American	329	336
	East Asian	2,128	1,501
(iv) *ADRB2*-rs1042714	European	2,250	1,435
	Northern Han Chinese	1,298	936
	East Asian		
	Northern Han Chinese	1,298	936
	Southern Chinese	288	149
	Japanese	1,120	839

Table 7. Meta-analysis of genetic association for (i) AGT-rs699, (ii) *CYP11B2*-rs1799998, (iii) *ADRB2*-rs1042713, and (iv) *ADRB2*-rs1042714

i. Meta-analysis of genetic association for *AGT*-rs699									
Country	**Model**	**No. publication**	**OR**	**95% CI**	**p-value**	**Model**	**p-heterogeneity**	**I^2**	**Egger's test p-value**
European	Allele	18	1.08	[0.96; 1.21]	0.22	Random	0.001	0.58	0.72
	Recessive	18	1.1	[0.93; 1.32]	0.25	Random	0.038	0.41	0.95
	Dominant	18	1.1	[0.94; 1.29]	0.24	Random	0.013	0.48	0.50
Japanese	Allele	8	1.23	[0.95; 1.51]	0.11	Random	0.002	0.75	0.12
	Recessive	8	1.27	[0.94; 1.71]	0.11	Random	0.001	0.79	0.05
	Dominant	8	1.28	[0/93; 1.74]	0.11	Fixed	0.64	0	0.74
East Asian	Allele	10	1.15	[0.98; 1.36]	0.07	Random	0.0004	0.70	0.27
	Recessive	10	1.23	[0.98; 1.54]	0.06	Random	0	0.78	0.36
	Dominant	10	0.98	[0.77; 1.23]	0.87	Fixed	0.13	0.34	0.092
Southern Han Chinese	Allele	5	1.04	[0.88; 1.23]	0.09	Fixed	0.54	0	0.50
	Recessive	5	1.09	[0.90; 1.32]	0.59	Fixed	0.45	0	0.05
	Dominant	5	0.85	[0.50; 1.44]	0.36	Fixed	0.70	0	0.10
Southern Indian	Allele	4	1.10	[0.97; 1.24]	0.56	Fixed	0.30	0.17	0.28
	Recessive	4	1.12	[0.94; 1.32]	0.19	Fixed	9.17	0.39	0.62
	Dominant	4	1.14	[0.88; 1.38]	0.37	Fixed	0.84	0	0.57
Northern + Southern Indian	Allele	6	1.37	[1.03; 1.82]	0.03*	Random	0.0001	0.90	0.11
	Recessive	6	1.61	[0.98; 2.67]	0.06	Random	0.0001	0.92	0.76
	Dominant	6	1.45	[1.09; 1.91]	0.009*	Random	0.0086	0.68	0.15
Middle Eastern	Allele	3	1.06	[0.63; 1.77]	0.82	Random	0.0078	0.79	0.0008
	Recessive	3	1.38	[0.31; 6.17]	0.67	Random	0.0001	0.9024	0.4254
	Dominant	3	1.07	[0.75; 1.53]	0.71	fixed	0.49	0	0.39

i. Meta-analysis of genetic association for *AGT*-rs699									
Country	**Model**	**No. publication**	**OR**	**95% CI**	**p-value**	**Model**	**p-heterogeneity**	**I^2**	**Egger's test p-value**
Latin American	Allele	3	1.08	[0.86; 1.36]	0.51	fixed	0.18	0.42	0.14
	Recessive	3	1.36	[0.76; 2.42]	0.30	random	0.08	0.61	0.1
	Dominant	3	1.07	[0.54; 2.1]	0.84	fixed	0.31	0.15	0.05
ii. Meta-analysis of genetic association for *CYP11B2*-rs1799998									
European	Allele	5	0.82	[0.75; 0.91]	0.00012*	Fixed	0.55	0	0.77
	Recessive	5	0.72	[0.61; 0.85]	0.0019*	Fixed	0.18	0.37	0.91
	Dominant	4	0.81	[0.70; 0.94]	0.008*	Fixed	0.96	0	0.78
European**	Allele	4	0.82	[0.74; 0.90]	6.9E-05*	Fixed	0.69	0	0.37
	Recessive	4	0.70	[0.59; 0.83]	6.38E-05*	Fixed	0.29	0.18	0.27
	Dominant	4	0.81	[0.70; 0.94]	0.008	Fixed	0.96	0	0.50
Northern Han Chinese	Allele	8	1.09	[0.95; 1.21]	0.20	Random	0.003	0.67	0.80
	Recessive	8	1.10	[0.88; 1.39]	0.37	Random	0.03	0.52	0.86
	Dominant	8	1.10	[0.96; 1.26]	0.17	Random	0.01	0.58	0.51
Japanese	Allele	4	1.03	[0.88; 1.20]	0.64	Random	0.06	0.59	0.72
	Recessive	4	0.97	[0.82; 1.15]	0.76	Fixed	0.79	0	0.75
	Dominant	4	1.08	[0.86; 1.37]	0.47	Random	0.02	0.68	0.63
East Asian#	Allele	12	1.06	[0.97; 1.16]	0.16	Random	0.0014	0.64	0.48
	Recessive	12	1.05	[0.98; 1.23]	0.12	Random	0.098	0.37	0.92
	Dominant	12	1.09	[0.97; 1.23]	0.47	Random	0.0043	0.60	0.29
Indian***	Allele	5	1.11	[0.79; 1.56]	0.52	Random	0.0001	0.88	0.08
	Recessive	5	1.28	[0.82; 2.00]	0.26	Random	0.001	0.68	0.01
	Dominant	5	1.02	[0.64; 1.60]	0.92	Random	0.0001	0.87	0.29

Table 7. (Continued)

Country	Model	No. publication	OR	95% CI	p-value	Model	p-heterogeneity	I^2	Egger's test p-value
iii. Meta-analysis of genetic association for *ADRB2*-rs1042713									
European	Allele	11	0.98	[0.89; 1.07]	0.66	fixed	0.25	0.20	0.37
	Recessive	11	1.03	[0.91; 1.16]	0.68	fixed	0.68	0	0.49
	Dominant	11	0.90	[0.76; 1.06]	0.21	fixed	0.38	0.05	0.63
East Asian#	Allele	4	1.26	[1.05; 1.51]	0.01*	random	0.05	0.61	0.13
	Recessive	4	1.36	[1.01; 1.83]	0.04*	random	0.07	0.58	0.46
	Dominant	4	1.34	[0.99; 1.83]	0.06	random	0.02	0.68	0.32
African American	Allele	3	0.84	[0.68; 1.05]	0.12	fixed	0.56	0	0.71
	Recessive	3	0.95	[0.67; 1.35]	0.76	fixed	0.13	0.51	0.52
	Dominant	3	0.68	[0.48; 0.97]	0.03*	fixed	0.84	0	0.02
iv. Meta-analysis of genetic association for *ADRB2*-rs1042714									
European	Allele	7	0.95	[0.86; 1.05]	0.29	Fixed	0.96	0	0.44
	Recessive	7	0.97	[0.81; 1.15]	0.70	Fixed	0.87	0	0.66
	Dominant	7	0.91	[0.79; 1.05]	0.21	Fixed	0.99	0	0.24
Northern Han Chinese	Allele	3	1.01	[0.50; 2.04]	0.98	random	0.0003	0.88	0.79
	Recessive	3	0.91	[0.43; 1.88]	0.79	Fixed	0.23	0.33	0.53
	Dominant	3	0.98	[0.42; 2.29]	0.96	random	0.0001	0.90	0.87
East Asian#	Allele	5	1.00	[0.68; 1.48]	0.99	random	0.0004	0.80	0.41
	Recessive	5	0.90	[0.50; 1.62]	0.73	Fixed	0.41	0	0.133
	Dominant	5	0.98	[0.63; 1.54]	0.94	random	0.0001	0.83	0.56

*, significantly associated with HT, **exclude one study (Bengra et al., 2002) due to unusual genotyping frequencies; # East Asian: Northern Han Chinese and Japan; *** Indian: Eastern, Northern and Southern Indian; I^2 = Index of heterogeneity.

- *AGT*-rs699: allele model (G vs A), recessive model (GG vs GA + AA) and dominant model (GG + GA vs AA).
- *CYP11B2*-rs1799998: allele model (G vs A), recessive model (GG vs GA + AA) and dominant model (GG + GA vs AA).
- *ADRB2*-rs1042713: allele model (G vs A), recessive model (GG vs GA + AA) and dominant model (GG + GA vs AA).

CYP11B2-rs1799998

A total of 723 publications were retrieved for *CYP11B2*-rs1799998: PubMed (n = 635), Cochrane (n = 49) and Science Direct (n = 39). Only 30 publications met the criteria set. Eight publications were further excluded from analysis as there were less than three publications for the selected populations classified. Only 22 publications remained in subsequent analysis: Japanese (4 publications), European (5 publications), Indian (5 publications), and Northern Chinese (8 publications). Overall, 11,745 HT and 11,014 NT. The sample information included in the meta-analysis is summarized in Table 6.

Meta-analysis revealed a significant association between *CYP11B2* rs1799998-G and HT among the European population (P = 0.00012, OR = 1.21, 95% CI 1.10 – 1.33, $P_{heterogeneity}$ = 0.55), in both recessive (GG + GA vs AA) (P = 0.008, OR = 1.22, 95% CI 1.05 – 1.42, $P_{heterogeneity}$ = 0.97), and dominant mode of inheritance (GG vs GA + AA) (P = 0.00019, OR = 1.38, 95% CI 1.16 – 1.62, $P_{heterogeneity}$ = 0.18), under the fixed-effect model. Subsequently we observed an unusually different allele frequencies reported by Bengra et al., (2002) as opposed to the other articles in this study, therefore this publication was excluded and the data was re-analyse. Apparently, the association effect was stronger when the article published by Bengra et al., (2002) was excluded. Analysis showed significant association between HT and the allele G (P = 6.9E^{-05}, OR = 1.22, 95% CI 1.10 – 1.34, $P_{heterogeneity}$ = 0.69), in recessive (GG + GA vs AA) (P = 0.008, OR = 1.22, 95% CI 1.05 – 1.42, $P_{heterogeneity}$ = 0.97) and dominant mode of inheritance (GG vs GA + AA) (P = 6.8E-05, OR = 1.42, 95% CI 1.19 –1.68, $P_{heterogeneity}$ = 0.30) under the fixed effect model. No significant association between rs1799998 and HT was observed in Northern Han Chinese, Japanese, and East Asian (Northern Han Chinese + Japanese) and Indian populations (Table 7).

ADRB2-rs1042713

A total of 665 publications were retrieved: PubMed (n = 608), Cochrane (n = 4 publications) and Science Direct (n = 53 publications), of which only 22 met the criteria set in this study. Additionally, four more publications were excluded from further analyses because there were less than three publications on the categorized populations. As a result, 18 publications representing three populations were remained: European (11 publications), African-American (3 publications) and East Asian (4 publications; covering 2 publications for

Northern Chinese and 2 populations for Japanese). Overall, 5,739 HT and 3,681 NT subjects were included. The sample information included in the meta-analysis is summarized in Table 6.

Meta-analysis results revealed a significant association between HT among the East Asian (Northern Han and Japan) in rs1042713-G allele (P = 0.01, OR = 1.26, 95% CI 1.05 – 1.51, $P_{heterogeneity} = 0.05$), and recessive mode of inheritance (GG + GA vs AA) (P = 0.04, OR = 1.36, 95% CI 1.01 – 1.83, $P_{heterogeneity} = 0.07$), under the random model effect. No significant association between rs1042713 and HT was observed in the European (Table 7).

ADRB2-rs1042714

Overall, 639 publications were retrieved: PubMed (n = 558 publications), Cochrane (n = 4 publications) and Science Direct (n = 77 publications), of which only 19 publications met the requirements. Eight publications were further excluded from the analysis as there were less than three publications on the selected populations. As a result, 12 publications remained: European (7 publications); and East Asian (5 publications; covering two populations from Southern Chinese and two populations for Japanese. Overall, 4,953 HT and 3,359 NT individuals were included. The sample information included in the meta-analysis is summarized in Table 6. No appreciative association between *ADRB2*-rs1042714 and HT was observed in both European and East Asian populations (Table 7).

Summary for Meta-Analysis

Overall, the meta-analysis reveals that the genetic association between the candidate SNPs of interest and primary HT vary across different populations. Based on the analysis carried out, significant association between HT and (i) *AGT*-rs699 G risk allele was observed among the Indian population (Southern and Northern Indian) for both allele and dominant mode of inheritance; (ii) *CYP11B2*-rs1799998 G risk allele among the European population for allele, dominant and recessive mode of inheritance under fixed model; and (iii) *ADRB2*-rs1042713 G risk allele observed among the East Asian population (Chinese and Japanese) for both allele and recessive mode of inheritance under random model. Surprisingly no significant association was observed between *ADRB2*-rs1042714 and HT across all populations tested.

The meta-analysis revealed that *AGT* rs699-G conferred 1.37 (in allele model) and 1.45 (dominant model) increased risk of HT in in the Indian population (Northern and Southern India). On a separate note, due to insufficient number of journal publications in African American and Southeast Asian in *AGT*-rs699, meta-analysis for these populations is not available. The analysis programme acquired requires at least three publications to be included in the analysis. Surprisingly, no association was obtained between *AGT*-rs699 and HT in European population although the European populations had greater number of HT samples than the Indian. This may due to the recruitment of small sample size in the publications for European studies in this meta-analysis and potentially resulted in sampling error (Lin, 2018). Study by Cheung et al., (2019) stated that when the sample size is large, the sampling variance of the effect size can be assumed to be approximately known and normal (Cheung et al., 2019). On a separate note, at least 500 HT individuals should be acquired in each publication to increase the power of meta-analyses (Li & Lou 2014), as small number could result in insufficient statistical power to estimate the effect of the variant on the disease (Zhang et al., 2013; Lin, 2018). Unfortunately, most studies, especially those earlier ones, had sample size lower than required. Besides that, the allele frequencies may appear heterogenous solely due to the nature of sampling variability when the trial sizes are relatively small (Kato et al., 1999). This meta-analysis was conducted with an attempt to the maximize number of publications included in the analysis, hence the effect of heterogeneity may have been compromised and therefore, sample size per publication was not restricted in this study (minimum study sample size that set for this meta-analysis is, N = 30 per group). Furthermore, most of the published articles of the selected candidate genes in this study had less than 500 HT individuals. Besides that, the involvement of intermediate phenotypes for HT, such as salt sensitivity. It has been documented that regulation of BP in the presence or absence of salt sensitivity varies considerably among individuals within and between populations (Rust & Ekmekcioglu, 2016). This may contribute to the lack of consistent association between genes and HT that reported by many studies (Yako et al., 2017).

The *CYP11B2*-rs1799998 conferred 1.21 – 1.38 higher risk of HT development in the European population. In contrast to this study, previous publication reported significant association between *CYP11B2*-rs1799998 and HT in a Chinese population (Li & Liu, 2014). The discrepancy may be due to different publication selection criteria, thence leading to different sample size included in the meta-analysis. Li & Liu (2014) included 29 publications (8,482 HT and 8,560 NT) whereas this study only contained 8 publications (4,292 HT and 4,589 NT). However, the association remains inconclusive because Li & Liu (2014) included not only Han Chinese populations, but other minority groups in China including Hani, Yi and Kazaks as well. Whether the inclusion of these minority groups would result in population stratification in the analysis of genetic association has not been tested. Further population genetic analyses would be required to confirm the effects of admixed populations to genetic association study.

Significant association for *ADRB2* rs1042713-G was shown in the East Asian (under recessive model) but not in European population, which is concordant with the earlier meta-analysis study by Lou et al., (2011). The difference in the heterogeneity of allelic frequencies among the populations may cause inconsistent outcome in the case-control analysis and effect meta-analysis study finding (Lou et al., 2011). Owing to the insufficient number of journal publications, the meta-analysis for African populations could not be performed. In addition, previous meta-analysis for this variant by Lou et al., (2011) excluded the minority non-Han Chinese populations from China to avoid the potential population stratification and analysis bias as they may have a different genetic makeup than the majority Han Chinese population (Lou et al., 2011). On a separate note, there was no overall or ethnicity-specific association in *ADRB2*-rs1042714 in any models (allele, dominant and recessive), which contradicts to the prior meta-analysis on the Northern Han China HT population (Lou et al., 2011) as the significant association between the variant and HT was observed in the severe HT individuals, SBP $\geq$ 160 and DBP $\geq$ 100 mmHg. This differential phenotyping criterion could have caused the discrepancy in analysis results.

Conclusion

In summary, the genetic association study for *AGT*-rs699 and rs5051, *CYP11B2*-rs1799998 and rs10087214, and *ADRB2*-rs1042713 and rs104714 with HT vary across different populations globally. Based on our analysis on the mainstream Malay populations form Malaysia, the primary HT susceptibility could be attributed to sex, as have been proposed by earlier reports. Several lines of supporting evidence: (i) *CYP11B2* SNPs are associated with primary HT in the Malay males; (ii) *ADRB2*-rs1042714 is associated with primary HT in the Malay females; (iii) Older females, which presumably having lower level of oestrogen, showed similar genetic susceptibility to primary HT as in the males. Provided a proper designed clinical trial is conducted to confirm its informativeness, these variants may be considered as a putative pharmacogenetic marker for anti-HT medication among the patients from Southeast Asia region, such as angiotensin receptor blocker and aldosterone receptor antagonists.

The meta-analysis provides an update and summary of the genetic association between the selected SNPs and HT across the different populations. Despite the number of samples, which is likely the major reason, one postulation that could explain the variability of HT susceptibility across different populations, is the different aetiologies of HT in these populations owing to varying exposure to climate, diet, lifestyle and local adaptation (Nakajima et al., 2004; Di Rienzo & Hudson 2005). Understanding the reason of different susceptibility of HT is important to provide essential insights toward selecting appropriate gene marker(s) and designing precision medicine approach for HT management. This study is believed to be the first meta-analysis genetic association study of the HT and the candidate genes and performed based on population genetic ancestries. Further meta-analyses will be required to warrant the findings of this study.

Acknowledgment

We would like to thank the Director General of Health Malaysia for his permission to publish this article and Ministry of Higher Education Malaysia under REDISCOVER grant.

Ethical Approval/Methodology

Ethical approval for this study was obtained from the Medical Research and Ethics Committee (MREC), Ministry of Health Malaysia.

Funding

This study is funded by the Ministry of Higher Education Malaysia under Long Term Research Grant Scheme (Grant code: 600-RMI/LRGS 5/3 (2/2011)-2).

Conflict of Interest

There is no conflict of interest between the authors.

References

Adeyemo, A., Gerry, N., Chen, G., Herbert, A., Doumatey, A., Huang, H., Zhou, J., Lashley, K., Chen, Y., Christman, M, & Rotimi, C. (2009). A genome-wide association study of hypertension and blood pressure in African Americans. *PLoS Genetics, 5(7),* e1000564. https://doi.org/10.1371/journal.pgen.1000564.

Adeyemo, A., & Rotimi, C. (2010). Genetic variants associated with complex human diseases show wide variation across multiple populations. *Public Health Genomics, 13(2),* 72-79. https://doi.org/10.1159/000218711.

Agachan, B., Isbir, T., Yilmaz, H., & Akoglu, E. (2003). Angiotensin converting enzyme I/D, angiotensinogen T174M-M235T and angiotensin II type 1 receptor A1166C gene polymorphisms in Turkish hypertensive patients. *Experimental & Molecular Medicine, 35(6),* 545-549. https://doi.org/10.1038/emm.2003.71.

Ahmad, T., Valentovic, M. A., & Rankin, G. O. (2018). Effects of cytochrome P450 single nucleotide polymorphisms on methadone metabolism and pharmacodynamics. *Biochemical Pharmacology, 153,* 196-204. https://doi.org/10.1016/j.bcp.2018.02.020.

Ahn, S. Y., & Gupta, C. (2018). Genetic programming of hypertension. *Frontiers in Pediatrics, 5,* 285. https://doi.org/10.3389/fped.2017.00285.

Al-Balushi, K., Zadjali, F., Al-Sinani, S., Al-Zadjali, A. M., & Bayoumi, R. (2015). Frequencies of the Arg16Gly, Gln27Glu and Thr164Ile Adrenoceptor β2 Polymorphisms among Omanis. *Sultan Qaboos University Medical Journal, 15(4),* e486. https://doi.org/10.18295/squmj.2015.15.04.007.

Aldiab, A., Shubair, M. M., Al-Zahrani, J. M., Aldossari, K. K., Al-Ghamdi, S., Househ, M., Razzak, H. A., El-Metwally, A., & Jradi, H. (2018). Prevalence of hypertension and prehypertension and its associated cardioembolic risk factors; a population based cross-sectional study in Alkharj, Saudi Arabia. *BMC Public Health, 18(1),* 1-9. https://doi.org/10.1186/s12889-018-6216-9.

Ameer, Q. A. A., Aziz, I. H., & Salo, W. H. (2014). Genetic polymorphism of (CYP11B2) gene in high blood pressure Iraqi patients. *Blood Pressure, 2015,* 50.

Barbalić, M., karić-Jurić, T., Cambien, F., Barbaux, S., Poirier, O., Turek, S., Vrhovski-Hebrang, D., Cubrilo-Turek, M., Rudan, I., Rudan, P. & Narančić, N. S. (2006). Gene polymorphisms of the renin-angiotensin system and early development of hypertension. *American Journal of Hypertension, 19(8),* 837-842. https://doi.org/10.1016/j.amjhyper.2006.01.004.

Barbato, A., Russo, P., Siani, A., Folkerd, E. J., Miller, M. A., Venezia, A., Grimaldi, C., Strazzullo, P., & Cappuccio, F. P. (2004). Aldosterone synthase gene (CYP11B2) C-344T polymorphism, plasma aldosterone, renin activity and blood pressure in a multi-ethnic population. *Journal of Hypertension, 22(10),* 1895-1901. https://doi.org/10.1097/00004872-200410000-00011.

Barley, J., Blackwood, A., Sagnella, G., Markandu, N., MacGregor, G., & Carter, N. (1994). Angiotensinogen Met235--> Thr polymorphism in a London normotensive and hypertensive black and white population. *Journal of Human Hypertension, 8(8),* 639-640.

Bartels, N. K., Börgel, J., Wieczorek, S., Büchner, N., Hanefeld, C., Bulut, D., Mügge, A., Rump, L. C., Sanner, B. M., & Epplen, J. T. (2007). Risk factors and myocardial infarction in patients with obstructive sleep apnea: impact of β2-adrenergic receptor polymorphisms. *BMC Medicine, 5(1),* 1-8. https://doi.org/10.1186/1741-7015-5-1.

Basson, J., Simino, J., & Rao, D. C. (2012). Between candidate genes and whole genomes: time for alternative approaches in blood pressure genetics. *Current Hypertension Reports, 14(1),* 46-61. https://doi.org/10.1007/s11906-011-0241-8.

Bautista, L. E., Vargas, C. I., Oróstegui, M., & Gamarra, G. (2008). Population-based case-control study of renin-angiotensin system genes polymorphisms and hypertension among Hispanics. *Hypertension Research, 31(3),* 401-408. https://doi.org/10.1291/hypres.31.401.

Beaney, T., Schutte, A. E., Stergiou, G. S., Borghi, C., Burger, D., Charchar, F., Cro, S., Diaz, A., Damasceno, A., Espeche, W., Jose, A. P., Khan, N., Kokubo, Y., Maheshwari, A., Marin, M. J., More, A., Neupane, D., Nilsson, P., Patil, M., Prabhakaran, D., Ramirez, A., Rodriguez, P., Schlaich, M., Steckelings, U. M., Tomaszewski, M., Unger, T., Wainford, R., Wang, J., Williams, B., Poulter, N. R; & MMM Investigators. (2020). May Measurement Month 2019: the global blood pressure screening campaign of the International Society of Hypertension. *Hypertension, 76(2),* 333-341. https://doi.org/10.1161/HYPERTENSIONAHA.120.14874.

Beevers, G., Lip, G. Y., & O'Brien, E. (2001). The pathophysiology of hypertension. *BMJ (Clinical research ed.), 322(7291),* 912–916. https://doi.org/10.1136/bmj.322.7291.912.

Bengra, C., Mifflin, T. E., Khripin, Y., Manunta, P., Williams, S. M., Jose, P. A., & Felder, R. A. (2002). Genotyping of essential hypertension single-nucleotide polymorphisms by a homogeneous PCR method with universal energy transfer primers. *Clinical Chemistry, 48(12),* 2131-2140. http://doi.org/10.1093/clinchem/48.12.2131.

Bhagavathula, A. S., Shah, S. M., & Aburawi, E. H. (2021). Prevalence, awareness, treatment, and control of hypertension in the United Arab Emirates: a systematic review and meta-analysis. *International Journal of Environmental Research and Public Health, 18(23),* 12693. https://doi.org/10.3390/ijerph182312693.

Bloem, L. J., Manatunga, A. K., Tewksbury, D. A., & Pratt, J. H. (1995). The serum angiotensinogen concentration and variants of the angiotensinogen gene in white and black children. *The Journal of Clinical Investigation, 95(3),* 948-953. https://doi.org/10.1172/JCI117803.

Borecki, I. B., Province, M. A., Ludwig, E. H., Ellison, R. C., Folsom, A. R., Heiss, G., Lalouel, J. M., Higgins, M., & Rao, D. C. (1997). Associations of candidate loci angiotensinogen and angiotensin-converting enzyme with severe hypertension: The NHLBI Family Heart Study. *Annals of epidemiology, 7(1),* 13-21. https://doi.org/10.1016/s1047-2797(97)00155-5.

Carretero, O. A., & Oparil, S. (2000). Essential hypertension: part I: definition and etiology. *Circulation, 101(3),* 329-335. https://doi.org/10.1161/01.cir.101.3.329.

Castellano, M., Rossi, F., Giacchè, M., Perani, C., Rivadossi, F., Muiesan, M. L., Salvetti, M., Beschi, M., Rizzoni, D., & Agabiti-Rosei, E. (2003). β2-Adrenergic receptor gene polymorphism, age, and cardiovascular phenotypes. *Hypertension (Dallas, Tex.: 1979), 41(2),* 361–367. https://doi.org/10.1161/01.hyp.0000052831.85600.79.

Caulfield, M., Lavender, P., Farrall, M., Munroe, P., Lawson, M., Turner, P., & Clark, A. (1994). Linkage of the angiotensinogen gene to essential hypertension. *New England Journal of Medicine, 330(23),* 1629-1633. https://doi.org/10.1056/NEJM199406093302301.

Charita, B., Padma, G., Sushma, P., Deepak, P., & Padma, T. (2012). Estimation of risk and interaction of single nucleotide polymorphisms at angiotensinogen locus causing susceptibility to essential hypertension: a case control study. *Journal of the Renin-Angiotensin-Aldosterone System, 13(4),* 461–471. https://doi.org/10.1177/1470320312444650.

Chen, B., Nie, S., Luo, S., Zhang, W., & Xiao, C. (2011). Association of the human CYP11B2 gene and essential hypertension in southwest Han Chinese population: a haplotype-based case-control study. *Clinical and experimental hypertension* (New York, N.Y.: 1993), *33(2),* 106–112. https://doi.org/10.3109/10641963.2010.531835.

Chen, J., Wang, W., Li, Z., Xu, C., Tian, X., & Zhang, D. (2021). Heritability and genome-wide association study of blood pressure in Chinese adult twins. *Molecular Genetics & Genomic Medicine, 9(11),* e1828. https://doi.org/10.1002/mgg3.1828.

Cheng, H. M., Lin, H. J., Wang, T. D., & Chen, C. H. (2020). Asian management of hypertension: Current status, home blood pressure, and specific concerns in Taiwan. *Journal of Clinical Hypertension, 22(3),* 511–514. https://doi.org/10.1111/jch.13747.

Cheng, X., & Xu, G. (2009). Association between aldosterone synthase CYP11B2 polymorphism and essential hypertension in Chinese: a meta-analysis. *Kidney & Blood Pressure Research, 32(2),* 128–140. https://doi.org/10.1159/000215738.

Cheung, B. M., Leung, R., Shiu, S., Tan, K. C., Lau, C. P., & Kumana, C. R. (1998). M235T polymorphism of the angiotensinogen gene and hypertension in Chinese. *Journal of Hypertension, 16(8),* 1137–1140. https://doi.org/10.1097/00004872-199816080-00009.

Cherfan, M., Blacher, J., Asmar, R., Chahine, M. N., Zeidan, R. K., Farah, R., & Salameh, P. (2018). Prevalence and risk factors of hypertension: a nationwide cross-sectional study in Lebanon. *Journal of Clinical Hypertension, 20(5),* 867–879. https://doi.org/10.1111/jch.13268.

Conlin, P. R. (2008). Genes and environment in blood pressure control—salt intake again shows its importance. *The American Journal of Clinical Nutrition, 88(2),* 255–256. https://doi.org/10.1093/ajcn/88.2.255.

Corvol, P., Persu, A., Gimenez-Roqueplo, A. P., & Jeunemaitre, X. (1999). Seven lessons from two candidate genes in human essential hypertension: angiotensinogen and epithelial sodium channel. *Hypertension, 33(6),* 1324–1331. https://doi.org/10.1161/01.hyp.33.6.1324.

Di Rienzo, A., & Hudson, R. R. (2005). An evolutionary framework for common diseases: the ancestral-susceptibility model. *Trends in Genetics, 21(11),* 596–601. https://doi.org/10.1016/j.tig.2005.08.007.

Delles, C., & Padmanabhan, S. (2012). Genetics and hypertension: is it time to change my practice? *The Canadian Journal of Cardiology, 28(3),* 296–304. https://doi.org/10.1016/j.cjca.2012.02.004.

Delong, C., & Sharma, S. (2019). Physiology, peripheral vascular resistance. Treasure Island (FL): StatPearls Publishing. https://www.ncbi.nlm.nih.gov/books/NBK538308/ [Accessed on July 15 2021].

Dhanachandra Singh, K., Jajodia, A., Kaur, H., Kukreti, R., & Karthikeyan, M. (2014). Gender specific association of RAS gene polymorphism with essential hypertension: a case-control study. *BioMed Research International, 2014,* 538053. https://doi.org/10.1155/2014/538053.

Dickson, M. E., & Sigmund, C. D. (2006). Genetic basis of hypertension: revisiting angiotensinogen. *Hypertension, 48(1),* 14–20. https://doi.org/10.1161/01.HYP.0000227932.13687.60.

International Consortium for Blood Pressure Genome-Wide Association Studies; Ehret G. B., Munroe P. B., Rice K. M., Bochud M., Johnson A. D., Chasman D. I., Smith A. V., Tobin M. D., Verwoert G. C., Hwang S. J., Pihur V., Vollenweider P., O'Reilly P. F., Amin N., Bragg-Gresham J. L., Teumer A., Glazer N. L., Launer L., Zhao J. H., Aulchenko Y., Heath S., Sõber S., Parsa A., Luan J., Arora P., Dehghan A., Zhang F., Lucas G., Hicks A. A., Jackson A. U., Peden J. F., Tanaka T., Wild S. H., Rudan I., Igl W., Milaneschi Y., Parker A. N., Fava C., Chambers J. C., Fox E. R., Kumari M., Go M. J., van der Harst P., Kao W. H., Sjögren M., Vinay D. G., Alexander M., Tabara Y., Shaw-Hawkins S., Whincup P. H., Liu Y., Shi G., Kuusisto J., Tayo B., Seielstad M., Sim X., Nguyen K. D., Lehtimäki T., Matullo G., Wu Y., Gaunt T. R., Onland-Moret N. C., Cooper M. N., Platou C. G., Org E., Hardy R., Dahgam S., Palmen J., Vitart V., Braund P. S., Kuznetsova T., Uiterwaal C. S., Adeyemo A., Palmas W., Campbell H., Ludwig B., Tomaszewski M., Tzoulaki I., Palmer N. D.; CARDIoGRAM consortium; CKDGen Consortium; KidneyGen Consortium; EchoGen consortium; CHARGE-HF consortium; Aspelund T., Garcia M., Chang Y. P., O'Connell J. R., Steinle N. I., Grobbee D. E., Arking D. E., Kardia S. L., Morrison A. C., Hernandez D., Najjar S., McArdle W. L., Hadley D., Brown M. J., Connell J. M., Hingorani A. D., Day I. N., Lawlor D. A., Beilby J. P., Lawrence R. W., Clarke R., Hopewell J. C., Ongen H., Dreisbach A. W., Li Y., Young J. H., Bis J. C., Kähönen M., Viikari J., Adair L. S., Lee N. R., Chen M. H., Olden M., Pattaro C., Bolton J. A., Köttgen A., Bergmann S., Mooser V., Chaturvedi N., Frayling T. M., Islam M., Jafar T. H., Erdmann J., Kulkarni S. R., Bornstein S. R., Grässler J., Groop L., Voight B.

F., Kettunen J., Howard P., Taylor A., Guarrera S., Ricceri F., Emilsson V., Plump A., Barroso I., Khaw K. T., Weder A. B., Hunt S. C., Sun Y. V., Bergman R. N., Collins F. S., Bonnycastle L. L., Scott L. J., Stringham H. M., Peltonen L., Perola M., Vartiainen E., Brand S. M., Staessen J. A., Wang T. J., Burton P. R., Soler Artigas M., Dong Y., Snieder H., Wang X., Zhu H., Lohman K. K., Rudock M. E., Heckbert S. R., Smith N. L., Wiggins K. L., Doumatey A., Shriner D., Veldre G., Viigimaa M., Kinra S., Prabhakaran D., Tripathy V., Langefeld C. D., Rosengren A., Thelle D. S., Corsi A. M., Singleton A., Forrester T., Hilton G., McKenzie C. A., Salako T., Iwai N., Kita Y., Ogihara T., Ohkubo T., Okamura T., Ueshima H., Umemura S., Eyheramendy S., Meitinger T., Wichmann H. E., Cho Y. S., Kim H. L., Lee J. Y., Scott J., Sehmi J. S., Zhang W., Hedblad B., Nilsson P., Smith G. D., Wong A., Narisu N., Stančáková A., Raffel L. J., Yao J., Kathiresan S., O'Donnell C. J., Schwartz S. M., Ikram M. A., Longstreth W. T. Jr., Mosley T. H., Seshadri S., Shrine N. R., Wain L. V., Morken M. A., Swift A. J., Laitinen J., Prokopenko I., Zitting P., Cooper J. A., Humphries S. E., Danesh J., Rasheed A., Goel A., Hamsten A., Watkins H., Bakker S. J., van Gilst W. H., Janipalli C. S., Mani K. R., Yajnik C. S., Hofman A., Mattace-Raso F. U., Oostra B. A., Demirkan A., Isaacs A., Rivadeneira F., Lakatta E. G., Orru M., Scuteri A., Ala-Korpela M., Kangas A. J., Lyytikäinen L. P., Soininen P., Tukiainen T., Würtz P., Ong R. T., Dörr M., Kroemer H. K., Völker U., Völzke H., Galan P., Hercberg S., Lathrop M., Zelenika D., Deloukas P., Mangino M., Spector T. D., Zhai G., Meschia J. F., Nalls M. A., Sharma P., Terzic J., Kumar M. V., Denniff M., Zukowska-Szczechowska E., Wagenknecht L. E., Fowkes F. G., Charchar F. J., Schwarz P. E., Hayward C., Guo X., Rotimi C., Bots M. L., Brand E., Samani N. J., Polasek O., Talmud P. J., Nyberg F., Kuh D., Laan M., Hveem K., Palmer L. J., van der Schouw Y. T., Casas J. P., Mohlke K. L., Vineis P., Raitakari O., Ganesh S. K., Wong T. Y., Tai E. S., Cooper R. S., Laakso M., Rao D. C., Harris T. B., Morris R. W., Dominiczak A. F., Kivimaki M., Marmot M. G., Miki T., Saleheen D., Chandak G. R., Coresh J., Navis G., Salomaa V., Han B. G., Zhu X., Kooner J. S., Melander O., Ridker P. M., Bandinelli S., Gyllensten U. B., Wright A. F., Wilson J. F., Ferrucci L., Farrall M., Tuomilehto J., Pramstaller P. P., Elosua R., Soranzo N., Sijbrands E. J., Altshuler D., Loos R. J., Shuldiner A. R., Gieger C., Meneton P., Uitterlinden A. G., Wareham N. J., Gudnason V., Rotter J. I., Rettig R., Uda M., Strachan D. P., Witteman J. C., Hartikainen A. L., Beckmann J. S., Boerwinkle E., Vasan R. S., Boehnke M., Larson M. G., Järvelin M. R., Psaty B. M., Abecasis G. R., Chakravarti A., Elliott P., van Duijn C. M., Newton-Cheh C., Levy D., Caulfield M. J., Johnson T. (2011). Genetic variants in novel pathways influence blood pressure and cardiovascular disease risk. *Nature,* 478(7367), 103-109. https://doi.org/10.1038/nature10405.

Ehret, G. B., & Caulfield, M. J. (2013). Genes for blood pressure: an opportunity to understand hypertension. *European Heart Journal, 34(13),* 951–961. https://doi.org/10.1093/eurheartj/ehs455.

Evangelou E., Warren H. R., Mosen-Ansorena D., Mifsud B., Pazoki R., Gao H., Ntritsos G., Dimou N., Cabrera C. P., Karaman I., Ng F. L., Evangelou M., Witkowska K., Tzanis E., Hellwege J. N., Giri A., Velez Edwards D. R., Sun Y. V., Cho K., Gaziano J. M., Wilson P. W. F., Tsao P. S., Kovesdy C. P., Esko T., Mägi R., Milani L., Almgren P., Boutin T., Debette S., Ding J., Giulianini F., Holliday E. G., Jackson A.

U., Li-Gao R., Lin W. Y., Luan J., Mangino M., Oldmeadow C., Prins B. P., Qian Y., Sargurupremraj M., Shah N., Surendran P., Thériault S., Verweij N., Willems S. M., Zhao J. H., Amouyel P., Connell J., de Mutsert R., Doney A. S. F., Farrall M., Menni C., Morris A. D., Noordam R., Paré G., Poulter N. R., Shields D. C., Stanton A., Thom S., Abecasis G., Amin N., Arking D. E., Ayers K. L., Barbieri C. M., Batini C., Bis J. C., Blake T., Bochud M., Boehnke M., Boerwinkle E., Boomsma D. I., Bottinger E. P., Braund P. S., Brumat M., Campbell A., Campbell H., Chakravarti A., Chambers J. C., Chauhan G., Ciullo M., Cocca M., Collins F., Cordell H. J., Davies G., de Borst M. H., de Geus E. J., Deary I. J., Deelen J., Del Greco M. F., Demirkale C. Y., Dörr M., Ehret G. B., Elosua R., Enroth S., Erzurumluoglu A. M., Ferreira T., Frånberg M., Franco O. H., Gandin I., Gasparini P., Giedraitis V., Gieger C., Girotto G., Goel A., Gow A. J., Gudnason V., Guo X., Gyllensten U., Hamsten A., Harris T. B., Harris S. E., Hartman C. A., Havulinna A. S., Hicks A. A., Hofer E., Hofman A., Hottenga J. J., Huffman J. E., Hwang S. J., Ingelsson E., James A., Jansen R., Jarvelin M. R., Joehanes R., Johansson Å., Johnson A. D., Joshi P. K., Jousilahti P., Jukema J. W., Jula A., Kähönen M., Kathiresan S., Keavney B. D., Khaw K. T., Knekt P., Knight J., Kolcic I., Kooner J. S., Koskinen S., Kristiansson K., Kutalik Z., Laan M., Larson M., Launer L. J., Lehne B., Lehtimäki T., Liewald D. C. M., Lin L., Lind L., Lindgren C. M., Liu Y., Loos R. J. F., Lopez L. M., Lu Y., Lyytikäinen L. P., Mahajan A., Mamasoula C., Marrugat J., Marten J., Milaneschi Y., Morgan A., Morris A. P., Morrison A. C., Munson P. J., Nalls M. A., Nandakumar P., Nelson C. P., Niiranen T., Nolte I. M., Nutile T., Oldehinkel A. J., Oostra B. A., O'Reilly P. F., Org E., Padmanabhan S., Palmas W., Palotie A., Pattie A., Penninx B. W. J. H., Perola M., Peters A., Polasek O., Pramstaller P. P., Nguyen Q. T., Raitakari O. T., Ren M., Rettig R., Rice K., Ridker P. M., Ried J. S., Riese H., Ripatti S., Robino A., Rose L. M., Rotter J. I., Rudan I., Ruggiero D., Saba Y., Sala C. F., Salomaa V., Samani N. J., Sarin A. P., Schmidt R., Schmidt H., Shrine N., Siscovick D., Smith A. V., Snieder H., Sõber S., Sorice R., Starr J. M., Stott D. J., Strachan D. P., Strawbridge R. J., Sundström J., Swertz M. A., Taylor K. D., Teumer A., Tobin M. D., Tomaszewski M., Toniolo D., Traglia M., Trompet S., Tuomilehto J., Tzourio C., Uitterlinden A. G., Vaez A., van der Most P. J., van Duijn C. M., Vergnaud A. C., Verwoert G. C., Vitart V., Völker U., Vollenweider P., Vuckovic D., Watkins H., Wild S. H., Willemsen G., Wilson J. F., Wright A. F., Yao J., Zemunik T., Zhang W., Attia J. R., Butterworth A. S., Chasman D. I., Conen D., Cucca F., Danesh J., Hayward C., Howson J. M. M., Laakso M., Lakatta E. G., Langenberg C., Melander O., Mook-Kanamori D. O., Palmer C. N. A., Risch L., Scott R. A., Scott R. J., Sever P., Spector T. D., van der Harst P., Wareham N. J., Zeggini E., Levy D., Munroe P. B., Newton-Cheh C., Brown M. J., Metspalu A., Hung A. M., O'Donnell C. J., Edwards T. L., Psaty B. M., Tzoulaki I., Barnes M. R., Wain L. V., Elliott .P, Caulfield M. J.; Million Veteran Program. (2018). Genetic analysis of over 1 million people identifies 535 new loci associated with blood pressure traits. *Nature Genetics, 50(10),* 1412–1425. https://doi.org/10.1038/s41588-018-0205-x.

Fakhri, M., Sarokhani, D., Ghiasi, B., & Dehkordi, A. H. (2020). Prevalence of hypertension in cardiovascular disease in Iran: Systematic review and meta-analysis.

International Journal of Preventive Medicine, 11, 56. https://doi.org/10.4103/ijpvm.IJPVM_351_18.

Fang, Y. J., Deng, H. B., Thomas, G. N., Tzang, C. H., Li, C. X., Xu, Z. L., Yang, M., & Tomlinson, B. (2010). Linkage of angiotensinogen gene polymorphisms with hypertension in a sibling study of Hong Kong Chinese. *Journal of Hypertension, 28(6),* 1203–1209. https://doi.org/10.1097/HJH.0b013e3283384b07.

Fardella, C. E., Claverie, X., Vignolo, P., Montero, J., & Villarroel, L. (1998). T235 variant of the angiotensinogen gene and blood pressure in the Chilean population. *Journal of Hypertension, 16(6),* 829–833. https://doi.org/10.1097/00004872-199816060-00014.

Farheen, S., Basu, A., & Majumder, P. P. (2011). Haplotype variation in the ACE gene in global populations, with special reference to India, and an alternative model of evolution of haplotypes. *The HUGO journal, 5(1-4),* 35–45. https://doi.org/10.1007/s11568-011-9153-6.

Fernández-Llama, P., Poch, E., Oriola, J., Botey, A., Rivera, F., & Revert, L. (1998). Angiotensinogen gene M235T and T174M polymorphisms in essential hypertension: relation with target organ damage. *American Journal of Hypertension, 11*(4 Pt 1), 439–444. https://doi.org/10.1016/s0895-7061(97)00483-4.

Filigheddu, F., Reid, J. E., Troffa, C., PinnaParpaglia, P., Argiolas, G., Testa, A., Skolnick, M., & Glorioso, N. (2004). Genetic polymorphisms of the β-adrenergic system: association with essential hypertension and response to β-blockade. *The Pharmacogenomics Journal, 4(3),* 154–160. https://doi.org/10.1038/sj.tpj.6500247.

Fox, E. R., Young, J. H., Li, Y., Dreisbach, A. W., Keating, B. J., Musani, S. K., Liu K., Morrison A. C., Ganesh S., Kutlar A., Ramachandran V. S., Polak J. F., Fabsitz R. R., Dries D. L., Farlow D. N., Redline S., Adeyemo A., Hirschorn J. N., Sun Y. V., Wyatt S. B., Penman A. D., Palmas W., Rotter J. I., Townsend R. R., Doumatey A. P., Tayo B. O., Mosley T. H. Jr., Lyon H. N., Kang S. J., Rotimi C. N., Cooper R. S., Franceschini N., Curb J. D., Martin L. W., Eaton C. B., Kardia S. L., Taylor H. A., Caulfield M. J., Ehret G. B., Johnson T.; International Consortium for Blood Pressure Genome-wide Association Studies (ICBP-GWAS); Chakravarti A, Zhu X, Levy D. (2011). Association of genetic variation with systolic and diastolic blood pressure among African Americans: the Candidate Gene Association Resource study. *Human Molecular Genetics, 20(11),* 2273–2284. https://doi.org/10.1093/hmg/ddr092.

Freitas, S. R. S., Cabello, P. H., Moura-Neto, R. S., Dolinsky, L. C., & Bóia, M. N. (2007). Combined analysis of genetic and environmental factors on essential hypertension in a Brazilian rural population in the Amazon region. *Arquivos Brasileiros de Cardiologia, 88(4),* 447–451. https://doi.org/10.1590/s0066-782x2007000400014.

Fryar, C. D., Ostchega, Y., Hales, C. M., Zhang, G., & Kruszon-Moran, D. (2017). Hypertension prevalence and control among adults: United States, 2015-2016. NCHS data brief, (289), 1–8.

Frossard, P. M., Hill, S. H., Elshahat, Y. I., Obineche, E. N., Bokhari, A. M., Lestringant, G. G., John, A., & Abdulle, A. M. (1998). Associations of angiotensinogen gene mutations with hypertension and myocardial infarction in a gulf population. *Clinical Genetics, 54(4),* 285–293. https://doi.org/10.1034/j.1399-0004.1998.5440405.x.

Garies, S., Hao, S., McBrien, K., Williamson, T., Peng, M., Khan, N. A., Padwal, R. S., Huan, Q., & Leung, A. A. (2019). Prevalence of hypertension, treatment, and blood pressure targets in Canada associated with the 2017 American College of Cardiology and American Heart Association Blood Pressure Guidelines. *JAMA Network Open, 2*(3), e190406. https://doi.org/10.1001/jamanetworkopen.2019.0406.

Ge, D., Huang, J., He, J., Li, B., Duan, X., Chen, R., & Gu, D. (2005). β2-Adrenergic Receptor Gene Variations Associated with Stage-2 Hypertension in Northern Han Chinese. *Annals of Human Genetics, 69(Pt 1),* 36–44. https://doi.org/10.1046/j.1529-8817.2003.00093.x.

Ghafar, M. T. A. (2019). Aldosterone synthase gene (CYP11B2) polymorphisms and enhanced cardiovascular risk. In The recent topics in genetic polymorphisms. *IntechOpen*. https://doi.org/10.5772/intechopen.89133.

Ghazali, D. M., Rehman, A., & Rahman, A. R. A. (2008). Candidate gene polymorphisms and their association with hypertension in Malays. *Clinica Chimica Acta; International Journal of Clinical Chemistry, 388(1-2),* 46–50. https://doi.org/10.1016/j.cca.2007.10.002.

Gong, H. T., Mu, L. Y., Zhang, T., Xu, X. Y., & Du, F. H. (2019). Association of mononucleotide polymorphisms of angiotensinogen gene at promoter region with antihypertensive response to angiotensin receptor blockers in hypertensive Chinese. *Journal of the Renin-Angiotensin-Aldosterone System, 20(1),* 1470320319827205. https://doi.org/10.1177/1470320319827205.

Goode, E. L. (2011). Linkage Disequilibrium. In: Schwab, M. (eds) Encyclopedia of Cancer. Springer, Berlin, Heidelberg. https://doi.org/10.1007/978-3-642-16483-5_3368.

Gorący, I., Peregud-Pogorzelska, M., Safranow, K., & Ciechanowicz, A. (2021). Key genetic variants in the renin-angiotensin system and left ventricular mass in a cohort of Polish patients with heart failure. *Kardiologia polska, 79(7-8),* 765–772. https://doi.org/10.33963/KP.15989.

Gu, D., Ge, D., He, J., Li, B., Chen, J., Liu, D., Chen, J & Chen, R. (2004). Haplotypic analyses of the aldosterone synthase gene CYP11B2 associated with stage-2 hypertension in northern Han Chinese. *Clinical Genetics, 66(5),* 409–416. https://doi.org/10.1111/j.1399-0004.2004.00317.x.

Guo, Y., Tomlinson, B., Chu, T., Fang, Y. J., Gui, H., Tang, C. S., Yip, B. H., Cherny, S. S., Hur, Y. M., Sham, P. C., Lam, T. H., & Thomas, N. G. (2012). A genome-wide linkage and association scan reveals novel loci for hypertension and blood pressure traits. *PloS One, 7(2),* e31489. https://doi.org/10.1371/journal.pone.0031489.

Hata, A., Namikawa, C., Sasaki, M., Sato, K., Nakamura, T., Tamura, K., & Lalouel, J. M. (1994). Angiotensinogen as a risk factor for essential hypertension in Japan. *The Journal of Clinical Investigation, 93(3),* 1285–1287. https://doi.org/10.1172/JCI117083.

Henderson, S. O., Haiman, C. A., & Mack, W. (2004). Multiple polymorphisms in the renin-angiotensin-aldosterone system (ACE, CYP11B2, AGTR1) and their contribution to hypertension in African Americans and Latinos in the multiethnic cohort. *The American Journal of the Medical Sciences, 328(5),* 266–273. https://doi.org/10.1097/00000441-200411000-00006.

Herrmann, S. M., Nicaud, V., Tiret, L., Evans, A., Kee, F., Ruidavets, J. B., Arveiler, D., Luc, G., Morrison, C., Hoehe, M. R., Paul, M., & Cambien, F. (2002). Polymorphisms of the beta2 -adrenoceptor (ADRB2) gene and essential hypertension: the ECTIM and PEGASE studies. *Journal of Hypertension, 20(2),* 229–235. https://doi.org/10.1097/00004872-200202000-00012.

Herrmann, V., Büscher, R., Go, M. M., Ring, K. M., Hofer, J. K., Kailasam, M. T., O'Connor, D. T., Parmer, R. J., & Insel, P. A. (2000). Beta2-adrenergic receptor polymorphisms at codon 16, cardiovascular phenotypes and essential hypertension in whites and African Americans. *American Journal of Hypertension, 13(9),* 1021–1026. https://doi.org/10.1016/s0895-7061(00)01188-2.

Hingorani, A. D., Sharma, P., Jia, H., Hopper, R., & Brown, M. J. (1996). Blood pressure and the M235T polymorphism of the angiotensinogen gene. *Hypertension, 28(5),* 907–911. https://doi.org/10.1161/01.hyp.28.5.907.

Hlubocká, Z., Jáchymová, M., Heller, S., Umnerová, V., Danzig, V., Lánská, V., Horký, K., & Linhart, A. (2009). Association of the -344T/C aldosterone synthase gene variant with essential hypertension. *Physiological Research, 58(6),* 785–792. https://doi.org/10.33549/physiolres.931450.

Hoit, B. D., Suresh, D. P., Craft, L., Walsh, R. A., & Liggett, S. B. (2000). beta2-adrenergic receptor polymorphisms at amino acid 16 differentially influence agonist-stimulated blood pressure and peripheral blood flow in normal individuals. *American Heart Journal, 139(3),* 537–542. https://doi.org/10.1016/s0002-8703(00)90099-1.

Hoh, B. P., Abdul Rahman, T., & Yusoff, K. (2019). Natural selection and local adaptation of blood pressure regulation and their perspectives on precision medicine in hypertension. *Hereditas, 156,* 1. https://doi.org/10.1186/s41065-019-0080-1.

Hong, K. W., Jin, H. S., Lim, J. E., Kim, S., Go, M. J., & Oh, B. (2010). Recapitulation of two genome wide association studies on blood pressure and essential hypertension in the Korean population. *Journal of Human Genetics, 55(6),* 336–341. https://doi.org/10.1038/jhg.2010.31.

Hu, D. C., Zhao, X. L., Shao, J. C., Wang, W., Qian, J., Chen, A. H., Zhang, H. Q., Guo, H., Jiang, J., & Li, H. Y. (2014). Interaction of six candidate genes in essential hypertension. *Genetics and Molecular Research, 13(4),* 8385–8395. https://doi.org/10.4238/2014.October.20.14.

Huang, Y., Guo, P., Karmacharya, B. M., Seeruttun, S. R., Xu, D. R., & Hao, Y. (2019). Prevalence of hypertension and prehypertension in Nepal: a systematic review and meta-analysis. *Global Health Research and Policy, 4,* 11. https://doi.org/10.1186/s41256-019-0102-6.

Inoue, I., Nakajima, T., Williams, C. S., Quackenbush, J., Puryear, R., Powers, M., Cheng, T., Ludwig, E. H., Sharma, A. M., Hata, A., Jeunemaitre, X., & Lalouel, J. M. (1997). A nucleotide substitution in the promoter of human angiotensinogen is associated with essential hypertension and affects basal transcription in vitro. The *Journal of Clinical Investigation, 99(7),* 1786–1797. https://doi.org/10.1172/JCI119343.

Institute for Public Health (IPH) 2008. The Third National Health and Morbidity Survey (NHMS III) 2006. Executive Summary. Ministry of Health, Malaysia. Retrieved on Dec 12, 2022. https://iku.moh.gov.my/images/IKU/Document/REPORT/2006/Asthma.pdf.

Institute for Public Health (IPH) 2011. National Health and Morbidity Survey 2011 (NHMS 2011). Vol. II: Non-Communicable Diseases. Retrieved on Dec 12, 2022. https://iku.moh.gov.my/images/IKU/Document/REPORT/NHMS2011-VolumeII.pdf.

Institute for Public Health (IPH) 2015. National Health and Morbidity Survey 2015 (NHMS 2015). Vol. II: Non-Communicable Diseases, Risk Factors & Other Health Problems. Retrieved on Dec 12, 2022. https://www.moh.gov.my/moh/resources/nhmsreport2015vol2.pdf.

Institute for Public Health (IPH), National Institutes of Health, Ministry of Health Malaysia. 2020. National Health and Morbidity Survey (NHMS) 2019: Vol. I: NCDs – Non-Communicable Diseases: Risk Factors and other Health Problems. Retrieved on Dec 12, 2022. https://iku.moh.gov.my/images/IKU/Document/REPORT/NHMS2019/Report_NHMS2019-NCD_v2.pdf.

Iso, H., Harada, S., Shimamoto, T., Sato, S., Kitamura, A., Sankai, T., Tanigawa, T., Iida, M., & Komachi, Y. (2000). Angiotensinogen T174M and M235T variants, sodium intake and hypertension among non-drinking, lean Japanese men and women. *Journal of Hypertension, 18(9),* 1197–1206. https://doi.org/10.1097/00004872-200018090-00005.

Jeunemaitre, X., Charru, A., Chatellier, G., Dumont, C., Sassano, P., Soubrier, F., Ménard, J., & Corvol, P. (1993). M235T variant of the human angiotensinogen gene in unselected hypertensive patients. *Journal of Hypertension, 11(5),* S80–S81.

Jeunemaitre, X., Inoue, I., Williams, C., Charru, A., Tichet, J., Powers, M., Sharma, A. M., Gimenez-Roqueplo, A. P., Hata, A., Corvol, P., & Lalouel, J. M. (1997). Haplotypes of angiotensinogen in essential hypertension. *American Journal of Human Genetics, 60(6),* 1448–1460. https://doi.org/10.1086/515452.

Jeunemaitre, X., Soubrier, F., Kotelevtsev, Y. V., Lifton, R. P., Williams, C. S., Charru, A., Hunt, S. C., Hopkins, P. N., Williams, R. R., & Lalouel, J. M. (1992). Molecular basis of human hypertension: role of angiotensinogen. *Cell, 71*(1), 169–180. https://doi.org/10.1016/0092-8674(92)90275-h.

Ji, X., Qi, H., Li, D. B., Liu, R. K., Zheng, Y., Chen, H. L., & Guo, J. C. (2015). Associations between human aldosterone synthase CYP11B2 (-344T/C) gene polymorphism and antihypertensive response to valsartan in Chinese patients with essential hypertension. *International Journal of Clinical and Experimental Medicine, 8(1),* 1173–1177.

Jia, H., Sharma, P., Hopper, R., Dickerson, C., Lloyd, D. D., & Brown, M. J. (2000). Beta2-adrenoceptor gene polymorphisms and blood pressure variations in East Anglian Caucasians. *Journal of Hypertension, 18(6),* 687–693. https://doi.org/10.1097/00004872-200018060-00005.

Kamitani, A., Rakugi, H., Higaki, J., Yi, Z., Mikami, H., Miki, T., & Ogihara, T. (1994). Association analysis of a polymorphism of the angiotensinogen gene with essential hypertension in Japanese. *Journal of Human Hypertension, 8(7),* 521–524.

Kang, S. H., Kim, S. H., Cho, J. H., Yoon, C. H., Hwang, S. S., Lee, H. Y., Youn, T. J., Chae, I. H., & Kim, C. H. (2019). Prevalence, Awareness, Treatment, and Control of Hypertension in Korea. *Scientific reports, 9(1),* 10970. https://doi.org/10.1038/s41598-019-46965-4.

Kario, K., Hoshide, S., Umeda, Y., Sato, Y., Ikeda, U., Nishiuma, S., Matsuo, M., & Shimada, K. (1999). Angiotensinogen and angiotensin-converting enzyme genotypes, and day and night blood pressures in elderly Japanese hypertensives. *Hypertension Research, 22(2),* 95–103. https://doi.org/10.1291/hypres.22.95.

Kato, N., Sugiyama, T., Morita, H., Kurihara, H., Sato, T., Yamori, Y., & Yazaki, Y. (2001). Association analysis of beta (2)-adrenergic receptor polymorphisms with hypertension in Japanese. *Hypertension, 37(2),* 286–292. https://doi.org/10.1161/01.hyp.37.2.286.

Kato, N., Sugiyama, T., Morita, H., Kurihara, H., Furukawa, T., Isshiki, T., Sato, T., Yamori, Y., & Yazaki, Y. (2000). Comprehensive analysis of the renin-angiotensin gene polymorphisms with relation to hypertension in the Japanese. *Journal of Hypertension, 18(8),* 1025–1032. https://doi.org/10.1097/00004872-200018080-00006.

Kato, N., Sugiyama, T., Morita, H., Kurihara, H., Yamori, Y., & Yazaki, Y. (1999). Angiotensinogen gene and essential hypertension in the Japanese: extensive association study and meta-analysis on six reported studies. *Journal of Hypertension, 17(6),* 757–763. https://doi.org/10.1097/00004872-199917060-00006.

Kiema, T. R., Kauma, H., Rantala, A. O., Lilja, M., Reunanen, A., Kesäniemi, Y. A., & Savolainen, M. J. (1996). Variation at the angiotensin-converting enzyme gene and angiotensinogen gene loci in relation to blood pressure. *Hypertension, 28(6),* 1070–1075. https://doi.org/10.1161/01.hyp.28.6.1070.

Kishimoto, T., Suyama, A., Osaki, Y., Miyamoto, T., Igarashi, A., Okamoto, M., Kurosawa, Y., & Fukumoto, S. (2001). A molecular variant of the angiotensinogen gene and hypertension in a case-control study in Japanese. *Yonago Acta Medica, 44(1),* 79-83.

Kerna, I., Kisand, K., Tamm, A. E., Kumm, J., & Tamm, A. O. (2013). Two single-nucleotide polymorphisms in ADAM12 gene are associated with early and late radiographic knee osteoarthritis in Estonian population. *Arthritis, 2013,* 878126. https://doi.org/10.1155/2013/878126.

Kohli, S., Kumar, R., Gupta, M., Tyagi, S., & Pasha, M. A. (2016). Impact of interactions between risk alleles on clinical endpoints in hypertension. *Heart Asia, 8(1),* 83–89. https://doi.org/10.1136/heartasia-2016-010723.

Kolifarhood, G., Sabour, S., Akbarzadeh, M., Sedaghati-Khayat, B., Guity, K., Rasekhi Dehkordi, S., Amiri Roudbar, M., Hadacgh, F., Azizi, F., & Daneshpour, M. S. (2021). Genome-wide association study on blood pressure traits in the Iranian population suggests ZBED9 as a new locus for hypertension. *Scientific Reports, 11(1),* 11699. https://doi.org/10.1038/s41598-021-90925-w.

Kolovou, V., Lagou, E., Mihas, C., Vasiliki, G., Katsiki, N., Kollia, A., Triposkiadis, F., Degiannis, D., Mavrogeni, S., & Kolovou, G. (2015). Angiotensinogen (AGT) M235T, AGT T174M and Angiotensin-1-Converting Enzyme (ACE) I/D gene polymorphisms in essential hypertension: effects on ramipril efficacy. *The Open Cardiovascular Medicine Journal, 9,* 118–126. https://doi.org/10.2174/1874192401509010118.

Komiya, I., Yamada, T., Takara, M., Asawa, T., Shimabukuro, M., Nishimori, T., & Takasu, N. (2000). Lys(173)Arg and -344T/C variants of CYP11B2 in Japanese patients with low-renin hypertension. *Hypertension, 35(3),* 699–703. https://doi.org/10.1161/01.hyp.35.3.699.

Krizanová, O., Obdrzálková, D., Poláková, H., Jelok, I., & Hudecová, S. (1997). Molecular variants of the renin-angiotensin system components in the Slovak population. *Physiological Research, 46(5),* 357–361.

Kumar, V., Abbas, A.K., and Fusto, N. (2005). Blood vessels, Robbins and cotran Pathologic Basis. The critical roles of cardiac output and peripheral resistance in blood pressure regulation. (7th ed.). Elsevier Saunders, pg 527 – 9.

Kunz, R., Kreutz, R., Beige, J., Distler, A., & Sharma, A. M. (1997). Association between the angiotensinogen 235T-variant and essential hypertension in whites: a systematic review and methodological appraisal. *Hypertension, 30(6),* 1331–1337. https://doi.org/10.1161/01.hyp.30.6.1331.

Kurtz, T. W., DiCarlo, S. E., Pravenec, M., Schmidlin, O., Tanaka, M., & Morris, R. C., Jr (2016). An alternative hypothesis to the widely held view that renal excretion of sodium accounts for resistance to salt-induced hypertension. *Kidney International, 90(5),* 965–973. https://doi.org/10.1016/j.kint.2016.05.032.

Lang, C. C., Stein, C. M., Brown, R. M., Deegan, R., Nelson, R., He, H. B., Wood, M., & Wood, A. J. (1995). Attenuation of isoproterenol-mediated vasodilatation in blacks. *The New England Journal of Medicine, 333*(3), 155–160. https://doi.org/10.1056/NEJM199507203330304.

Lateshia B. (2016). Hypertension is now more common in poor and middle-income countries than rich ones. https://www.washingtonpost.com/news/to-your-health/wp/2016/08/09/hypertension-is-now-more-common-in-poor-and-middle-income-countries-than-rich-ones/[accessed on 13 August 2022].

Levy, D., Ehret, G. B., Rice, K., Verwoert, G. C., Launer, L. J., Dehghan, A., Glazer, N. L., Morrison, A. C., Johnson, A. D., Aspelund, T., Aulchenko, Y., Lumley, T., Köttgen, A., Vasan, R. S., Rivadeneira, F., Eiriksdottir, G., Guo, X., Arking, D. E., Mitchell, G. F., Mattace-Raso, F. U., Smith A. V., Taylor K., Scharpf R. B., Hwang S. J., Sijbrands E. J., Bis J., Harris T. B., Ganesh S. K., O'Donnell C. J., Hofman A., Rotter J. I., Coresh J., Benjamin E. J., Uitterlinden A. G., Heiss G., Fox C. S., Witteman J. C., Boerwinkle E., Wang T. J., Gudnason V., Larson M. G., Chakravarti A., Psaty B. M., & van Duijn, C. M. (2009). Genome-wide association study of blood pressure and hypertension. *Nature Genetics, 41(6),* 677–687. https://doi.org/10.1038/ng.384.

Levy, D., Larson, M. G., Benjamin, E. J., Newton-Cheh, C., Wang, T. J., Hwang, S. J., Vasan, R. S., & Mitchell, G. F. (2007). Framingham Heart Study 100K Project: genome-wide associations for blood pressure and arterial stiffness. *BMC Medical Genetics, 8*(Suppl 1), S3. https://doi.org/10.1186/1471-2350-8-S1-S3.

Lou, Y., Liu, J., Li, Y., Liu, Y., Wang, Z., Liu, K., Wu, H., Niu, Q., Gu, W., Guo, Y., Li, Z., & Wen, S. (2011). Association study of the β2-adrenergic receptor gene polymorphisms and hypertension in the Northern Han Chinese. *PloS One, 6(4),* e18590. https://doi.org/10.1371/journal.pone.0018590.

Li, H., Du, Z., Zhang, L., Wu, T., Deng, Z., Li, J., Cong, M., Liu, J., & Qiu, C. (2014). The relationship between angiotensinogen gene polymorphisms and essential hypertension in a Northern Han Chinese population. *Angiology, 65(7),* 614–619. https://doi.org/10.1177/0003319713491309.

Li, K., Liang, Y., Sun, Y., Zhang, L. X., Yi, X., Chen, Y., LA Mu, G. S., & Wang, J. (2012). The relationship between polymorphisms at 17 gene sites and hypertension among the Aboriginal Tibetan people. *Biomedical and Environmental Sciences, 25*(5), 526–532. https://doi.org/10.3967/0895-3988.2012.05.005.

Li, Q. X., Gao, H., Xu, F. X., Zhang, Y. Q., Wu, H. Y., Yan, H. B., & Liu, G. Z. (2006). Zhonghua yi xue yi chuan xue za zhi = Zhonghua Yixue Yichuanxue Zazhi, *Chinese Journal of Medical Genetics, 23(3),* 294–297.

Li, X., Xie, P., He, J., Cai, H., Yang, R., Zhang, Q., Li, B., Qi, W., & Ma, H. (2016). CYP11B2 gene polymorphism and essential hypertension among Tibetan, Dongxiang and Han populations from northwest of China. *Clinical and Experimental Hypertension, 38(4),* 375–380. https://doi.org/10.3109/10641963.2015.1131287.

Li, X. M., Ling, Y., Lu, D. R., Lu, Z. Q., Yi, Q. L., Liu, Y., Chen, H. Y., & Gao, X. (2011). Association of the aldosterone synthase gene -344T>C polymorphism with essential hypertension and glucose homeostasis: a case-control study in a Han Chinese population. *Clinical and Experimental Pharmacology & Physiology, 38(9),* 598–604. https://doi.org/10.1111/j.1440-1681.2011.05555.x.

Lu, J., Lu, Y., Wang, X., Li, X., Linderman, G. C., Wu, C., Cheng, X., Mu, L., Zhang, H., Liu, J., Su, M., Zhao, H., Spatz, E. S., Spertus, J. A., Masoudi, F. A., Krumholz, H. M., & Jiang, L. (2017). Prevalence, awareness, treatment, and control of hypertension in China: data from 1·7 million adults in a population-based screening study (China PEACE Million Persons Project). *Lancet, 390(10112),* 2549–2558. https://doi.org/10.1016/S0140-6736(17)32478-9.

Maamor, N. H, Rizal, I. J., Abd Malek, K., Williams, G. H., Yusoff, K., & Boon-Peng, H. (2023a). Genetic variation and the adaptation of AGT, CYP11B2 and ADRB2 to salt sensitivity. *Under review.*

Maamor, N. H., Rizal, I. J., Abd Malek, K., Williams, G. H., Yusoff, K., & Boon-Peng, H. (2023b). AGT, CYP11B2 and ADRB2 genes and susceptibility towards essential hypertension (HT): A meta-analysis. *Under review.*

Maciejewska-Skrendo, A., Cięszczyk, P., Chycki, J., Sawczuk, M., & Smółka, W. (2019). Genetic markers associated with power athlete status. *Journal of Human Kinetics, 68,* 17–36. https://doi.org/10.2478/hukin-2019-0053.

Manosroi, W., & Williams, G. H. (2019). Genetics of human primary hypertension: focus on hormonal mechanisms. *Endocrine Reviews, 40(3),* 825–856. https://doi.org/10.1210/er.2018-00071.

Maranon, R., & Reckelhoff, J. F. (2013). Sex and gender differences in control of blood pressure. *Clinical Science, 125(7),* 311–318. https://doi.org/10.1042/CS20130140.

Martorell-Marugan, J., Toro-Dominguez, D., Alarcon-Riquelme, M.E., & Carmona-Saez, P. (2017). MetaGenyo: a web tool for meta-analysis of genetic association studies. *BMC Bioinformatics, 18(1),* 563. https://doi.org/10.1186/s12859-017-1990-4.

McCorry L. K. (2007). Physiology of the autonomic nervous system. *American Journal of Pharmaceutical Education, 71(4),* 78. https://doi.org/10.5688/aj710478.

Meiqari, L., Essink, D., Wright, P., & Scheele, F. (2019). Prevalence of hypertension in Vietnam: a systematic review and meta-analysis. *Asia-Pacific Journal of Public Health, 31(2),* 101–112. https://doi.org/10.1177/1010539518824810.

Mills, K. T., Bundy, J. D., Kelly, T. N., Reed, J. E., Kearney, P. M., Reynolds, K., Chen, J., & He, J. (2016). Global disparities of hypertension prevalence and control: a systematic analysis of population-based studies from 90 countries. *Circulation, 134(6),* 441–450. https://doi.org/10.1161/CIRCULATIONAHA.115.018912.

Ministry of Health (MOH) Bahrain. 2018. Bahrain National Health Survey 2018. Retrieved on Nov 11, 2022. https://www.data.gov.bh/en/ResourceCenter/Download File?id=3470.

Misono, M., Maeda, S., Iemitsu, M., Nakata, Y., Otsuki, T., Sugawara, J., Zempo, H., Yoshizawa, M., Miyaki, A., Kuno, S., Matsuda, M., & Ajisaka, R. (2009). Combination of polymorphisms in the beta2-adrenergic receptor and nitric oxide synthase 3 genes increases the risk for hypertension. *Journal of Hypertension, 27(7),* 1377–1383. https://doi.org/10.1097/HJH.0b013e32832b7ead.

Mo, W., Zhang, G. G., Yang, T. L., Dai, X. P., Li, H. H., Zeng, H., Liu, J., Tan, Y. M., Zhou, H. H., & Liu, Z. Q. (2007). The genetic polymorphisms of beta3-adrenergic receptor (AR) Trp64Arg and beta2-AR Gln27Glu are associated with obesity in Chinese male hypertensive patients. *Clinical Chemistry and Laboratory Medicine, 45(4),* 493–498. https://doi.org/10.1515/CCLM.2007.089.

MOH. 2018. Clinical practice guideline Management of Hypertension 4th Edition. Retrieved on Nov 13, 2022. https://www.moh.gov.my/moh/resources/Penerbitan/CPG/CPG_Management_of_Hypertension_4th_Edition.pdf.

Mohana, V. U., Swapna, N., Surender, R. S., Vishnupriya, S., & Padma, T. (2012). Gender-related association of AGT gene variants (M235T and T174M) with essential hypertension--a case-control study. *Clinical and Experimental Hypertension, 34(1),* 38–44. https://doi.org/10.3109/10641963.2011.618207.

Mondorf, U. F., Russ, A., Wiesemann, A., Herrero, M., Oremek, G., & Lenz, T. (1998). Contribution of angiotensin I converting enzyme gene polymorphism and angiotensinogen gene polymorphism to blood pressure regulation in essential hypertension. *American Journal of Hypertension, 11(2),* 174–183. https://doi.org/10.1016/s0895-7061(97)00402-0.

Morise, T., Takeuchi, Y., & Takeda, R. (1995). Rapid detection and prevalence of the variants of the angiotensinogen gene in patients with essential hypertension. *Journal of Internal Medicine, 237(2),* 175–180. https://doi.org/10.1111/j.1365-2796.1995.tb01158.x.

Naing, C., Yeoh, P. N., Wai, V. N., Win, N. N., Kuan, L. P., & Aung, K. (2016). Hypertension in Malaysia: an analysis of trends from the national surveys 1996 to 2011. *Medicine, 95(2),* e2417. https://doi.org/10.1097/MD.0000000000002417.

Nakajima, T., Wooding, S., Sakagami, T., Emi, M., Tokunaga, K., Tamiya, G., Ishigami, T., Umemura, S., Munkhbat, B., Jin, F., Guan-Jun, J., Hayasaka, I., Ishida, T., Saitou, N., Pavelka, K., Lalouel, J. M., Jorde, L. B., & Inoue, I. (2004). Natural selection and population history in the human angiotensinogen gene (AGT): 736 complete AGT sequences in chromosomes from around the world. *American Journal of Human Genetics, 74(5),* 898–916. https://doi.org/10.1086/420793.

NCD Risk Factor Collaboration (NCD-RisC) (2017). Worldwide trends in body-mass index, underweight, overweight, and obesity from 1975 to 2016: a pooled analysis of 2416 population-based measurement studies in 128·9 million children, adolescents, and adults. *Lancet, 390*(10113), 2627–2642. https://doi.org/10.1016/S0140-6736(17)32129-3.

Nejatizadeh, A., Kumar, R., Stobdan, T., Goyal, A. K., Gupta, M., Javed, S., & Pasha, M. Q. (2008). Significance of angiotensinogen gene haplotypes and genotypes combinations in hypertension. *Journal of Hypertension, 26(6),* 1094–1101. https://doi.org/10.1097/HJH.0b013e3282fad951.

Nejatizadeh, A., Kumar, R., Stobdan, T., Goyal, A. K., Gupta, M., Tyagi, S., Jain, S. K., & Pasha, M. A. (2010). CYP11B2 gene haplotypes independently and in concurrence with aldosterone and aldosterone to renin ratio increase the risk of hypertension. *Clinical Biochemistry, 43(1-2),* 136–141. https://doi.org/10.1016/j.clinbiochem.2009.09.015.

Niu, W. Q., Guo, S. J., Zhang, Y., Gao, P. J., & Zhu, D. L. (2010). Genetic and functional analyses of aldosterone synthase gene C-344T polymorphism with essential hypertension. *Journal of Human Hypertension, 24(6),* 427–429. https://doi.org/10.1038/jhh.2010.12.

Norat, T., Bowman, R., Luben, R., Welch, A., Khaw, K. T., Wareham, N., & Bingham, S. (2008). Blood pressure and interactions between the angiotensin polymorphism AGT M235T and sodium intake: a cross-sectional population study. *The American Journal of Clinical Nutrition, 88(2),* 392–397. https://doi.org/10.1093/ajcn/88.2.392.

Oparil, S., Acelajado, M. C., Bakris, G. L., Berlowitz, D. R., Cífková, R., Dominiczak, A. F., Grassi, G., Jordan, J., Poulter, N. R., Rodgers, A., & Whelton, P. K. (2018). Hypertension. *Nature reviews. Disease primers, 4,* 18014. https://doi.org/10.1038/nrdp.2018.14.

Pacanowski, M. A., Gong, Y., Cooper-Dehoff, R. M., Schork, N. J., Shriver, M. D., Langaee, T. Y., Pepine, C. J., Johnson, J. A., & INVEST Investigators (2008). beta-adrenergic receptor gene polymorphisms and beta-blocker treatment outcomes in hypertension. *Clinical Pharmacology and Therapeutics, 84(6),* 715–721. https://doi.org/10.1038/clpt.2008.139.

Padma, G., Charita, B., Swapna, N., Mamata, M., & Padma, T. (2015). Novel variants detected in AGT gene among patients with essential hypertension. *Journal of the Renin-Angiotensin-Aldosterone System, 16(3),* 642–646. https://doi.org/10.1177/1470320313513483.

Patel, P. A., & Ali, N. (2017). Mechanisms involved in regulation of systemic blood pressure. *Archives of Clinical Hypertension, 3(1),* 016-020.

Patnaik, M., Pati, P., Swain, S. N., Mohapatra, M. K., Dwibedi, B., Kar, S. K., & Ranjit, M. (2014). Aldosterone synthase C-344T, angiotensin II type 1 receptor A1166C and 11-β hydroxysteroid dehydrogenase G534A gene polymorphisms and essential hypertension in the population of Odisha, India. *Journal of Genetics, 93(3),* 799–808. https://doi.org/10.1007/s12041-014-0464-y.

Pearson, T. A., & Manolio, T. A. (2008). How to interpret a genome-wide association study. *JAMA, 299(11),* 1335–1344. https://doi.org/10.1001/jama.299.11.1335.

Peltzer, K., & Pengpid, S. (2018). The prevalence and social determinants of hypertension among adults in Indonesia: a cross-sectional population-based national survey. *International Journal of Hypertension, 2018,* 5610725. https://doi.org/10.1155/2018/5610725.

Pengpid, S., Vonglokham, M., Kounnavong, S., Sychareun, V., & Peltzer, K. (2019). The prevalence, awareness, treatment, and control of hypertension among adults: the first cross-sectional national population-based survey in Laos. *Vascular Health and Risk Management, 15,* 27–33. https://doi.org/10.2147/VHRM.S199178.

Pojoga, L., Gautier, S., Blanc, H., Guyene, T. T., Poirier, O., Cambien, F., & Benetos, A. (1998). Genetic determination of plasma aldosterone levels in essential hypertension. *American Journal of Hypertension, 11(7),* 856–860. https://doi.org/10.1016/s0895-7061(98)00048-x.

Pojoga, L., Kolatkar, N. S., Williams, J. S., Perlstein, T. S., Jeunemaitre, X., Brown, N. J., Hopkins, P. N., Raby, B. A., & Williams, G. H. (2006). Beta-2 adrenergic receptor diplotype defines a subset of salt-sensitive hypertension. *Hypertension, 48(5),* 892–900. https://doi.org/10.1161/01.HYP.0000244688.45472.95.

Procopciuc, L., Popescu, T., Jebeleanu, G., Pop, D., & Zdrenghea, D. (2002). Essential arterial hypertension and polymorphism of angiotensinogen M235T gene. *Journal of Cellular and Molecular Medicine, 6(2),* 245–250. https://doi.org/10.1111/j.1582-4934.2002.tb00191.x.

Purkait, P., Halder, K., Thakur, S., Ghosh Roy, A., Raychaudhuri, P., Bhattacharya, S., Sarkar, B. N., & Naidu, J. M. (2017). Association of angiotensinogen gene SNPs and haplotypes with risk of hypertension in eastern Indian population. *Clinical Hypertension, 23,* 12. https://doi.org/10.1186/s40885-017-0069-x.

Ramu, P., Umamaheswaran, G., Shewade, D. G., Swaminathan, R. P., Dutta, T. K., Balachander, J., & Adithana, C. (2011). Candidate gene polymorphisms of renin angiotensin system and essential hypertension in a South Indian Tamilian population. *International Journal of Human Genetics, 11(1),* 31-40. https://doi.org/10.1080/09723757.2011.11886120.

Rajput, C., Makhijani, K., Norboo, T., Afrin, F., Sharma, M., Pasha, S. T., & Pasha, M. A. (2005). CYP11B2 gene polymorphisms and hypertension in highlanders accustomed to high salt intake. *Journal of Hypertension, 23(1),* 79–86. https://doi.org/10.1097/00004872-200501000-00016.

Rajan, S., Ramu, P., Umamaheswaran, G., & Adithan, C. (2010). Association of aldosterone synthase (CYP11B2 C-344T) gene polymorphism & susceptibility to essential hypertension in a south Indian Tamil population. *The Indian Journal of Medical Research, 132,* 379–385.

Ram C. V. (2010). Beta-blockers in hypertension. *The American Journal of Cardiology, 106(12),* 1819–1825. https://doi.org/10.1016/j.amjcard.2010.08.023.

Rashid, R. A., Hameed, R., & Hamid, T. (2021). Prevalence of hypertension among the adult population in Qatar: a literature review. *Scholars Journal of Applied Medical Sciences, 12,* 1805-1812. http://doi.org/10.36347/sjams.2021.v09i12.008.

Riedel, K., Deussen, A. J., Tolkmitt, J., Weber, S., Schlinkert, P., Zatschler, B., Friebel, C., Müller, B., El-Armouche, A., Morawietz, H., Matschke, K., & Kopaliani, I. (2019). Estrogen determines sex differences in adrenergic vessel tone by regulation of endothelial β-adrenoceptor expression. *American Journal of Physiology. Heart and Circulatory Physiology, 317(2),* H243–H254. https://doi.org/10.1152/ajpheart.00456.2018.

Rodríguez-Pérez, J. C., Rodríguez-Esparragón, F. J., Hernández-Perera, O., Fiuza-Pérez, M. D., Anabitarte-Prieto, A., & Losada-Cabrera, A. (2000). Effects of the angiotensinogen gene M235T and A(-6)G variants on blood pressure and other vascular risk factors in a Spanish population. *Journal of Human Hypertension, 14(12),* 789–793. https://doi.org/10.1038/sj.jhh.1001110.

Saab, Y. B., Gard, P. R., & Overall, A. D. (2011). The association of hypertension with renin-angiotensin system gene polymorphisms in the Lebanese population. *Journal of the Renin-Angiotensin-Aldosterone System, 12(4),* 588–594. https://doi.org/10.1177/1470320311408465.

Saju, M. D., Allagh, K. P., Scaria, L., Joseph, S., & Thiyagarajan, J. A. (2020). Prevalence, awareness, treatment, and control of hypertension and its associated risk factors: results from baseline survey of SWADES family cohort study. *International Journal of Hypertension, 2020,* 4964835. https://doi.org/10.1155/2020/4964835.

Sarki, A. M., Nduka, C. U., Stranges, S., Kandala, N. B., & Uthman, O. A. (2015). Prevalence of hypertension in low- and middle-income countries: a systematic review and meta-analysis. *Medicine, 94(50),* e1959. https://doi.org/10.1097/MD.0000000000001959.

Sato, N., Katsuya, T., Rakugi, H., Takami, S., Nakata, Y., Miki, T., Higaki, J., & Ogihara, T. (1997). Association of variants in critical core promoter element of angiotensinogen gene with increased risk of essential hypertension in Japanese. *Hypertension, 30(3 Pt 1),* 321–325. https://doi.org/10.1161/01.hyp.30.3.321.

Say, Y. H., Ling, K. H., Duraisamy, G., Isaac, S., & Rosli, R. (2005). Angiotensinogen M235T gene variants and its association with essential hypertension and plasma renin activity in Malaysian subjects: a case control study. *BMC Cardiovascular Disorders, 5(1),* 7. https://doi.org/10.1186/1471-2261-5-7.

Shafi, S. T., & Shafi, T. (2017). A survey of hypertension prevalence, awareness, treatment, and control in health screening camps of rural central Punjab, Pakistan. *Journal of Epidemiology and Global Health, 7(2),* 135–140. https://doi.org/10.1016/j.jegh.2017.01.001.

Yu, S. F., Zhou, W. H., Jiang, K. Y., Gu, G. Z., & Wang, S. (2008). Job stress, gene polymorphism of beta2-AR, and prevalence of hypertension. *Biomedical and Environmental Sciences, 21(3),* 239–246. https://doi.org/10.1016/S0895-3988(08)60036-7.

Shih, P. A., & O'Connor, D. T. (2008). Hereditary determinants of human hypertension: strategies in the setting of genetic complexity. *Hypertension, 51(6),* 1456–1464. https://doi.org/10.1161/HYPERTENSIONAHA.107.090480.

Skrzypecki, J., & Ufnal, M. (2015). Drug resistant hypertension – no simple way out. *Kidney & Blood Pressure Research, 40(1),* 66–76. https://doi.org/10.1159/000368483.

Slatkin M. (2008). Linkage disequilibrium--understanding the evolutionary past and mapping the medical future. *Nature Reviews. Genetics, 9(6),* 477–485. https://doi.org/10.1038/nrg2361.

Sookoian, S., Gianotti, T. F., González, C. D., & Pirola, C. J. (2007). Association of the C-344T aldosterone synthase gene variant with essential hypertension: a meta-analysis. *Journal of Hypertension, 25(1),* 5–13. https://doi.org/10.1097/01.hjh.0000254372.88488.a9.

Srivastava, K., Chandra, S., Bhatia, J., Narang, R., & Saluja, D. (2012). Association of angiotensinogen (M235T) gene polymorphism with blood pressure lowering response to angiotensin converting enzyme inhibitor (Enalapril). *Journal of Pharmacy & Pharmaceutical Sciences, 15(3),* 399–406. https://doi.org/10.18433/j3kw3b.

Staessen, J. A., Wang, J. G., Brand, E., Barlassina, C., Birkenhäger, W. H., Herrmann, S. M., Fagard, R., Tizzoni, L., & Bianchi, G. (2001). Effects of three candidate genes on prevalence and incidence of hypertension in a Caucasian population. *Journal of Hypertension, 19(8),* 1349–1358. https://doi.org/10.1097/00004872-200108000-00002.

Sun, X., Yang, J., Hou, X., Li, J., Shi, Y., & Jing, Y. (2011). Relationship between -344T/C polymorphism in the aldosterone synthase gene and atrial fibrillation in patients with essential hypertension. *Journal of the Renin-Angiotensin-Aldosterone System, 12(4),* 557–563. https://doi.org/10.1177/1470320311417654.

Sun, B., Williams, J. S., Svetkey, L. P., Kolatkar, N. S., & Conlin, P. R. (2010). Beta2-adrenergic receptor genotype affects the renin-angiotensin-aldosterone system response to the Dietary Approaches to Stop Hypertension (DASH) dietary pattern. *The American Journal of Clinical Nutrition, 92(2),* 444–449. https://doi.org/10.3945/ajcn.2009.28924.

Sunder-Plassmann, G., Kittler, H., Eberle, C., Hirschl, M. M., Woisetschläger, C., Derhaschnig, U., Laggner, A. N., Hörl, W. H., & Födinger, M. (2002). Angiotensin converting enzyme DD genotype is associated with hypertensive crisis. *Critical Care Medicine, 30(10),* 2236–2241. https://doi.org/10.1097/00003246-200210000-00010.

Takeuchi, F., Akiyama, M., Matoba, N., Katsuya, T., Nakatochi, M., Tabara, Y., Narita, A., Saw, W. Y., Moon, S., Spracklen, C. N., Chai, J. F., Kim, Y. J., Zhang, L., Wang, C., Li, H., Li, H., Wu, J. Y., Dorajoo, R., Nierenberg, J. L., Wang, Y. X., He J., Bennett D. A., Takahashi A., Momozawa Y., Hirata M., Matsuda K., Rakugi H., Nakashima E., Isono M., Shirota M., Hozawa A., Ichihara S., Matsubara T., Yamamoto K., Kohara K., Igase M., Han S., Gordon-Larsen P., Huang W., Lee N. R., Adair L. S., Hwang M. Y., Lee J., Chee M. L., Sabanayagam C., Zhao W., Liu J., Reilly D. F., Sun L., Huo S., Edwards T. L., Long J., Chang L. C., Chen C. H., Yuan J. M., Koh W. P., Friedlander Y., Kelly T. N., Bin Wei W., Xu L., Cai H., Xiang Y. B., Lin K., Clarke R., Walters R. G., Millwood I. Y., Li L., Chambers J. C., Kooner J. S., Elliott P., van der Harst P.; International Genomics of Blood Pressure (iGEN-BP) Consortium; Chen Z., Sasaki M., Shu X. O., Jonas J. B., He J., Heng C. K., Chen Y. T., Zheng W., Lin X., Teo Y. Y., Tai E. S., Cheng C. Y., Wong T. Y., Sim X., Mohlke K. L., Yamamoto M., Kim B. J., Miki T., Nabika T., Yokota M., Kamatani Y., Kubo M., & Kato, N. (2018). Interethnic analyses of blood pressure loci in populations of East Asian and European descent. *Nature Communications, 9(1),* 5052. https://doi.org/10.1038/s41467-018-07345-0.

Takeuchi, F., Yamamoto, K., Katsuya, T., Sugiyama, T., Nabika, T., Ohnaka, K., Yamaguchi, S., Takayanagi, R., Ogihara, T., & Kato, N. (2012). Reevaluation of the association of seven candidate genes with blood pressure and hypertension: a replication study and meta-analysis with a larger sample size. *Hypertension Research, 35(8),* 825–831. https://doi.org/10.1038/hr.2012.43.

Tang, W., Devereux, R. B., Kitzman, D. W., Province, M. A., Leppert, M., Oberman, A., Hopkins, P. N., & Arnett, D. K. (2003). The Arg16Gly polymorphism of the beta2-adrenergic receptor and left ventricular systolic function. *American Journal of Hypertension, 16(11),* 945–951. https://doi.org/10.1016/s0895-7061(03)01001-x.

Tanira, M. O., & Al Balushi, K. A. (2005). Genetic variations related to hypertension: a review. *Journal of Human Hypertension, 19(1),* 7–19. https://doi.org/10.1038/sj.jhh.1001780.

Tay, J. C., & Teo, B. W. (2020). Asian management of hypertension: current status, home blood pressure, and specific concerns in Singapore. *Journal of Clinical Hypertension, 22(3),* 508–510. https://doi.org/10.1111/jch.13782.

Thomas, G. N., Young, R. P., Tomlinson, B., Woo, K. S., Sanderson, J. E., & Critchley, J. A. (2000). Renin-angiotensin-aldosterone system gene polymorphisms and hypertension in Hong Kong Chinese. *Clinical and Experimental Hypertension,* 22(1), 87–97. https://doi.org/10.1081/ceh-100100064.

Timmermann, B., Mo, R., Luft, F. C., Gerdts, E., Busjahn, A., Omvik, P., Li, G. H., Schuster, H., Wienker, T. F., Hoehe, M. R., & Lund-Johansen, P. (1998). Beta-2 adrenoceptor genetic variation is associated with genetic predisposition to essential hypertension: The Bergen Blood Pressure Study. *Kidney International, 53*(6), 1455–1460. https://doi.org/10.1046/j.1523-1755.1998.00926.x.

Touyz, R. M. (2014). Blood pressure regulation and pathology. *In Cellular and Molecular Pathobiology of Cardiovascular Disease* (pp. 257-275). Academic Press. https://doi.org/10.1016/B978-0-12-405206-2.00014-4.

Tsukada, K., Ishimitsu, T., Teranishi, M., Saitoh, M., Yoshii, M., Inada, H., Ohta, S., Akashi, M., Minami, J., Ono, H., Ohrui, M., & Matsuoka, H. (2002). Positive association of CYP11B2 gene polymorphism with genetic predisposition to essential hypertension. *Journal of Human Hypertension, 16(11),* 789–793. https://doi.org/10.1038/sj.jhh.1001484.

Tsujita, Y., Iwai, N., Katsuya, T., Higaki, J., Ogihara, T., Tamaki, S., Kinoshita, M., Mannami, T., Ogata, J., & Baba, S. (2001). Lack of association between genetic polymorphism of CYP11B2 and hypertension in Japanese: the Suita Study. *Hypertension Research, 24(2),* 105–109. https://doi.org/10.1291/hypres.24.105.

Unger, T., Borghi, C., Charchar, F., Khan, N. A., Poulter, N. R., Prabhakaran, D., Ramirez, A., Schlaich, M., Stergiou, G. S., Tomaszewski, M., Wainford, R. D., Williams, B., & Schutte, A. E. (2020). 2020 International Society of Hypertension global hypertension practice guidelines. *Journal of Hypertension, 38(6),* 982–1004. https://doi.org/10.1097/HJH.0000000000002453.

Vallejos-Vidal, E., Reyes-Cerpa, S., Rivas-Pardo, J. A., Maisey, K., Yáñez, J. M., Valenzuela, H., Cea, P. A., Castro-Fernandez, V., Tort, L., Sandino, A. M., Imarai, M., & Reyes-López, F. E. (2020). Single-Nucleotide Polymorphisms (SNP) mining and their effect on the tridimensional protein structure prediction in a set of immunity-related expressed sequence tags (EST) in atlantic salmon (salmo salar). *Frontiers in Genetics, 10,* 1406. https://doi.org/10.3389/fgene.2019.01406.

Vamsi, U. M., Swapna, N., Padma, G., Vishnupriya, S., & Padma, T. (2016). Haplotype association and synergistic effect of human aldosterone synthase (CYP11B2) gene polymorphisms causing susceptibility to essential hypertension in Indian patients. *Clinical and Experimental Hypertension, 38(8),* 659–665. https://doi.org/10.1080/10641963.2016.1200595.

van Dijk, E. L., Auger, H., Jaszczyszyn, Y., & Thermes, C. (2014). Ten years of next-generation sequencing technology. *Trends in Genetics, 30(9),* 418–426. https://doi.org/10.1016/j.tig.2014.07.001.

Vaskû, A., Soucek, M., Znojil, V., Rihácek, I., Tschöplová, S., Strelcová, L., Cídl, K., Blazková, M., Hájek, D., Hollá, L., & Vácha, J. (1998). Angiotensin I-converting enzyme and angiotensinogen gene interaction and prediction of essential hypertension. *Kidney International, 53(6),* 1479–1482. https://doi.org/10.1046/j.1523-1755.1998.00924.x.

Wang, D. G., Fan, J. B., Siao, C. J., Berno, A., Young, P., Sapolsky, R., Ghandour, G., Perkins, N., Winchester, E., Spencer, J., Kruglyak, L., Stein, L., Hsie, L., Topaloglou, T., Hubbell, E., Robinson, E., Mittmann, M., Morris, M. S., Shen, N., Kilburn, D., Rioux, J., Nusbaum, C., Rozen, S., Hudson, T.J., Lipshutz, R., Chee, M., & Lander, E. S. (1998). Large-scale identification, mapping, and genotyping of single-nucleotide polymorphisms in the human genome. *Science, 280(5366),* 1077–1082. https://doi.org/10.1126/science.280.5366.1077.

Wang, L., Zhang, B., Li, M., Li, C., Liu, J., Liu, Y., Wang, Z., Zhou, J., & Wen, S. (2014). Association between single-nucleotide polymorphisms in six hypertensive candidate genes and hypertension among northern Han Chinese individuals. *Hypertension Research, 37(12),* 1068–1074. https://doi.org/10.1038/hr.2014.124.

Wellcome Trust Case Control Consortium (2007). Genome-wide association study of 14,000 cases of seven common diseases and 3,000 shared controls. *Nature, 447(7145),* 661–678. https://doi.org/10.1038/nature05911.

Wellcome Trust Case Control Consortium (2018). Wellcome Trust Case Control Consortium. https://www.wtccc.org.uk/ [Accessed 11 July 2022].

WHO. (2021). Hypertension. Available from: https://www.who.int/news-room/fact-sheets/detail/hypertension. [Accessed 11 July 2022].

Wu, S. J., Chiang, F. T., Chen, W. J., Liu, P. H., Hsu, K. L., Hwang, J. J., Lai, L. P., Lin, J. L., Tseng, C. D., & Tseng, Y. Z. (2004). Three single-nucleotide polymorphisms of the angiotensinogen gene and susceptibility to hypertension: single locus genotype vs. haplotype analysis. *Physiological Genomics, 17(2),* 79–86. https://doi.org/10.1152/physiolgenomics.00133.2003.

Xie, H. G., Stein, C. M., Kim, R. B., Gainer, J. V., Sofowora, G., Dishy, V., Brown, N. J., Goree, R. E., Haines, J. L., & Wood, A. J. (2000). Human beta2-adrenergic receptor polymorphisms: no association with essential hypertension in black or white Americans. *Clinical Pharmacology and Therapeutics, 67(6),* 670–675. https://doi.org/10.1067/mcp.2000.106293.

Yako, Y. Y., Balti, E. V., Matsha, T. E., Dzudie, A., Kruger, D., Sobngwi, E., Agyemang, C., & Kengne, A. P. (2018). Genetic factors contributing to hypertension in African-based populations: A systematic review and meta-analysis. *Journal of Clinical Hypertension, 20(3),* 485–495. https://doi.org/10.1111/jch.13225.

Zhang, H., Li, X., Zhou, L., Zhang, K., Zhang, Q., Li, J., Wang, N., Jin, M., Wu, N., Cong, M., & Qiu, C. (2017). A novel haplotype of low-frequency variants in the aldosterone synthase gene among northern Han Chinese with essential hypertension. *Medicine, 96(39),* e8150. https://doi.org/10.1097/MD.0000000000008150.

Zhen, Z., Gao, L., Wang, Q., Chen, X., Na, J., Xu, X., & Yuan, Y. (2020). Angiotensinogen M235T polymorphism and susceptibility to hypertrophic cardiomyopathy in Asian population: A meta analysis. *Journal of the Renin-Angiotensin-Aldosterone System, 21(4),* 1470320320978100. https://doi.org/10.1177/1470320320978100.

Zhu, X., Chang, Y. P., Yan, D., Weder, A., Cooper, R., Luke, A., Kan, D., & Chakravarti, A. (2003). Associations between hypertension and genes in the renin-angiotensin system. *Hypertension, 41(5),* 1027–1034. https://doi.org/10.1161/01.HYP.0000068681.69874.CB.

Chapter 11

E3 Ligase and Deubiquitinating Enzyme (DUB) in Reducing Phenylketonuria Severity

Sa'udah Badriah Mohd Sani and Nurulisa Zulkifle*

Department of Biomedical Sciences, Advanced Medical and Dental Institute, Universiti Sains Malaysia, Kepala Batas, Pulau Pinang, Malaysia

Abstract

Inborn errors of metabolism (IEM) are a rare genetic condition that makes the body unable to metabolise certain substances from ingested food as it lacks the enzymes required to utilise those metabolic pathways. This occurs when the genes that are supposed to be coded for those proteins (enzymes) mutate, eventually resulting in abnormal enzymes either in terms of quantity, structure, or function after the transcription and translation processes. These abnormal enzyme conditions obstruct the metabolic pathways, which typically aim to break down molecules so that they can be used by the body. Consequently, this contributes to a variety of effects on the patient's overall health, growth, and development. This chapter focuses on phenylketonuria (PKU), which is listed as one of the 491 Rare Diseases in Malaysia by the Ministry of Health, Malaysia that was updated in 2020. PKU is an inherited autosomal recessive genetic disorder characterised by a deficiency of hepatic phenylalanine-4-hydroxylase (PAH), which is required for phenylalanine catalysis. This resulted in a harmful build-up of phenylalanine in the body, which is toxic to the nervous system and potentially fatal. Subtopics of this chapter include an in-depth discussion on the potential capacity of the ubiquitin-proteasome system (UPS) to

* Corresponding Author's Email: nurulisa@usm.my.

In: Genetic Disorders and Rare Diseases
Editors: Shazlin Shaharudin, Hisham Atan Edinur and Nor Fazila Che Mat
ISBN: 979-8-88697-953-4

control PKU severity. UPS is a protein quality survey mechanism that tags defective proteins with ubiquitin for elimination via proteasomal degradation. The conjugation of ubiquitin to proteins requires the coordinated action of the E1, E2, and E3 enzymes, with E3 serving as the process' playmaker. Interestingly, the ubiquitination process can be reversed by a class of proteins known as deubiquitin enzymes (DUBs), which may allow mutant PAH that could still serve its function to be saved from degradation. From this, it is clear that E3 and DUBs hold a lot of promise as an alternative therapeutic strategy for PKU, and research into manipulating E3 and DUBs to lessen the severity of PKU should be explored.

Keywords: alternative therapeutic strategy, deubiquitin enzymes (DUBs), E3 ligase, phenylketonuria, ubiquitin proteasome system

Introduction

Phenylketonuria, or PKU (OMIM# 261600), is a rare inherited disorder characterised by an inability to metabolise phenylalanine (Phe), an essential amino acid (Kaufman, 1977; van Spronsen et al., 2021). Essential amino acids are those that the body cannot make on its own and must be obtained through diet. PKU can be caused by one of two factors; a lack or reduced level of phenylalanine hydroxylase (PAH), a liver enzyme that converts phenylalanine (Phe) to tyrosine (Tyr), or a deficiency of PAH's co-substrate, tetrahydrobiopterin (BH4), which is required for PAH stabilisation and increasing its steady state level (Kaufman, 1977; Lichter-Konecki & Vockley, 2019). Under normal circumstances, our bodies convert Phe from food into amino acids, and PAH oxidises excess Phe into carbon dioxide and water. People with PKU, on the other hand, lack this enzyme, causing dietary Phe to accumulate in their brain and blood. If not treated, this can lead to mental retardation, epilepsy, microcephaly, brain damage, and death, particularly in children (William et al., 2008).

PKU can be found in varying degrees all over the world. In Europe, PKU is the most common IEM, affecting approximately one in every 10,000 newborns (Blau et al., 2010). Its prevalence ranges from very rare (1:125000) in Japan to very common (1:850) in the Karachay Cherkess Republic of Russia (Okano *et* al., 2011; Gundurova et al., 2018). PKU prevalence was found to be the lowest in Asian countries such as Thailand (1:227,273), Japan (1:125,000), the Philippines (1:116,006), and Singapore (1:83,333) (Hillert et al., 2020). As far as the authors are aware, there is no solid data on the prevalence of PKU in Malaysia, owing to the fact that the disease has not been very well-explored in this country. However, PKU was listed among the 491 Malaysian Rare Disease List by the Malaysian Health Ministry, implying that its prevalence in the country may be low (MOH, 2020). So far, only one case report has been published, involving a six-year-old Malay boy who was referred to Hospital Universiti Sains Malaysia (HUSM) in January 1988, with aggressive behaviour and developmental delays (Karnaneedi et al., 1989).

Patients with PKU cannot be cured; instead, they are managed by restricting foods that are high in protein, such as meat, poultry, seafood, eggs, dairy, and nuts in their diets. Aspartame, a sugar substitute, should also be avoided; hence, PKU patients are not allowed to have chewing gum, squash, cordial or sports drinks as well (MacDonald et al., 2020). However, dietary restrictions have the drawback of possibly resulting in nutrient deficiencies, necessitating the use of medical food as a supplement. This treatment strategy is frequently regarded as inconvenient due to the poor palatability of protein-free and medical foods and the fact that such foods are expensive and not socially friendly. For patients with residual PAH enzyme activity, a synthetic formulation of BH4 is also an option in addition to a Phe-restricted diet. Other treatment options include enzyme replacement therapy that delivers faultless PAH via a liver transplant. It is a challenging procedure that is only beneficial to those who are at a critical stage. Another viable treatment option involves *Pegvaliase* (PALYNZIQTM), an enzyme substitution therapy that was United States Food and Drug Administration (US FDA)-approved since 2018. It is more practical because patients only need one shot per day, but unfortunately, it has been associated with a number of adverse effects including injection site reactions, arthralgia, hypersensitivity reactions, nausea, vomiting, anaphylactic shock and the development of antibodies against its components (Markham, 2018).

In this chapter, alternative approaches to treating PKU will be discussed from the standpoint of protein quality control mechanisms. The cellular protein quality control system will be reviewed, with an emphasis on the ubiquitination-mediated degradation of defective and dysfunctional proteins. The severity of the PAH mutation is then discussed, as is the prospect of rescuing functional mutated PAH by manipulating the ubiquitination system. By doing so, the PAH concentration in cells could be increased and despite being mutants, the PAH can still metabolise Phe, potentially reducing the severity of the disease.

Protein Quality Control

Protein synthesis begins with the transcription process, which converts DNA to mRNA, followed by the translation process, which uses mRNA as a template for recruiting amino acids that are then linearly arranged into polypeptides. The polypeptide then folds, a process that commonly occurs in the endoplasmic reticulum (Afinsen, 1972). Protein folding is an important cellular process because proteins require specific three-dimensional shapes to function properly, and unfolded or misfolded proteins often contribute to the pathology of many diseases. Unfortunately, misfolded proteins are constantly produced in cells due to genetic mutations, translational errors, abnormal protein modifications, thermal or oxidative stress, and incomplete complex formation. PKU is an example of a disease caused by improper protein folding, and there are many others including Alzheimer's and Parkinson's diseases and cystic fibrosis, to name a few (Yadav et al., 2019).

Since misfolded proteins typically lose their native function and tend to aggregate, several cellular mechanisms have been evolved to deal with these potentially toxic conformations (Tyedmers et al., 2010). In eukaryotic cells, the proteome integrity is maintained by the protein quality control system (Pilla et al., 2017). This system keeps check on protein misfolding events through molecular chaperones that refold aggregated protein as well as proteases that degrade misfolded protein. During protein folding, proteins with particularly complex or unstable conformations may have difficulty folding to their native state, typically as a result of crowded cell environment, the presence of numerous biomolecules, and other factors may lead to less-than-ideal folding conditions. In these circumstances, specialised proteins known as "molecular chaperones" play an important role of limiting aggregation of the denatured proteins and refolding them to their native state (Laskey et al., 1978). However, in the worst-case scenario, the proteins misfold anyway and rapidly degraded via two main proteolysis pathways: the autophagy-lysosome pathway and ubiquitin-proteasome system (UPS) (Fredrickson & Gardner, 2012; Tyedmers et al., 2010). The UPS degrades at least four-fifth, if not more, of native and improperly folded intracellular proteins (Wang & Maldonado, 2006). It recycles and degrades soluble proteins in both the nucleus and the cytosol, in contrast to autophagy, which operates only in the cytoplasm to eliminate large and insoluble aggregates that escape from the UPS (Ciechanover & Kwon, 2017).

Ubiquitin-Proteasome System

Prior to protein degradation via UPS, a process called ubiquitination needs to occur in which ubiquitin molecules (Ub) are covalently attached to the substrate. The ubiquitination is accomplished through the coordinated action of three enzyme families: the ubiquitin-activating enzyme (E1), the ubiquitin-binding enzyme (E2) and the ubiquitin-protein ligase (E3). The process starts with the activation of the ubiquitin by E1 in an ATP-dependent reaction to produce a thioester-linked E1~Ub conjugate. The transthiolation reaction then takes place, allowing E2 to take up the activated Ub. The E2 cooperates with E3 to position the target protein and attaches the ubiquitin moiety to its ε-amino group in a lysine residue (Pickart, 2001). Deubiquitinating enzymes (DUBs), a vital group of enzymes, are then responsible for determining the fate of ubiquitinated target proteins because, in the absence of DUB to remove the (poly)ubiquitin chain, the 26S proteasome will recognise and degrade the target protein (Komander & Rape, 2012) (Figure 1).

The E3 ubiquitin ligases, which regulate the final step of the enzymatic cascade, are the most important component of the UPS because they provide regulatory specificity by selectively attaching ubiquitin to lysine, serine, threonine, or cysteine residues on specific substrates. Ubiquitin's attachment to different residues acts as a signal, conferring a different function that the substrate must commit to. To accomplish this task, E3 ligases are equipped with over 600 members with little sequence homology and vastly different compositions, classified into four types: HECT type, U-box type, RING-finger type, and RBR type (Zheng & Shabek, 2017). Meanwhile, DUBs are a group of enzymes with approximately 101 members divided into seven families: USP, OTU, MJD, UCH, JAMM, ZUFSP and MINDY (Zulkifle, 2020). DUBs play specific roles in the ubiquitination pathway, including ubiquitin precursor processing, ubiquitin conjugates editing or rescue, recycling ubiquitin from ubiquitin-substrate degradation targets and disassembly of unanchored ubiquitin oligomers (Amerik & Hochstrasser, 2004). Here, the role of DUBs as rescuers is highlighted, as DUBs can reverse ubiquitination by catalysing the separation between the target protein and the (poly)ubiquitin chain, thereby saving the ubiquitinated substrate proteins from degradation (Nijman et al., 2005). On top of that, DUBs also function as a balance between ubiquitination and deubiquitination, which is necessary to keep the pool of cellular proteins in check. This is critical because if the UPS fails to eliminate the defective protein, the cells will move to the apoptosis process and eventually die (Li et al., 2022).

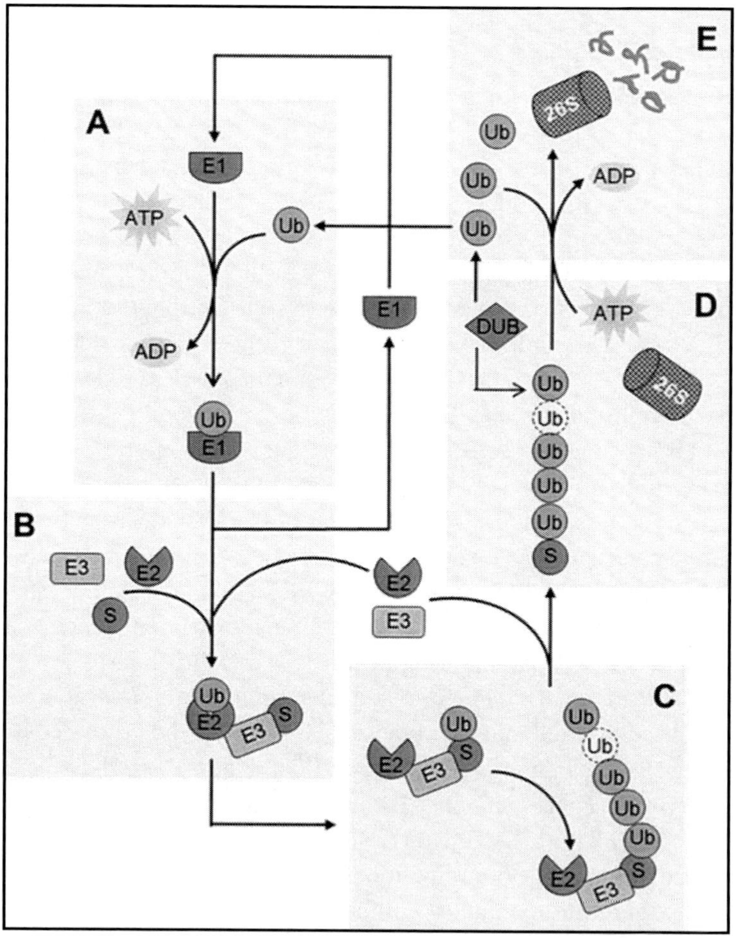

Figure 1. Protein degradation through the UPS: (A) Ubiquitin molecule is activated by E1 in an ATP-dependent manner. (B) E1 delivers the activated ubiquitin to E2, which forms a complex with E3 and the substrate. (C) Generation of polyubiquitin chain. (D) Proteasome recognises the polyubiquitin chain as a signal for degradation. DUBs are capable of removing the polyubiquitin chain here and rescuing the substrate from degradation. (E) The substrate is degraded and released as peptides, while the polyubiquitin chain is processed by DUBs into a monomer and be recycled. Created with Microsoft PowerPoint ver2301.

PAH Mutation and PKU Severity

The wild-type *PAH* gene encodes a homotetrameric protein that has four subunits, each of which has an N-terminal regulatory domain for allosteric activation by Phe, a central catalytic domain, and a C-terminal helix that facilitates tetramer formation (Arturo et al., 2016). The gene is located on chromosome 12, band region q23.2 and is made up of 13 exons and 12 introns, covering approximately 100 kb of genomic DNA (Donlon et al., 2014). As of November 6, 2022, the Database of Phenotypes and Genotypes causing Phenylalanine Hydroxylase Deficiency (PKU) including BH4-responsive HPA/PKU (BIOPKU) (http://www.biopku.org) listed 1,564 *PAH* variants, with approximately half of them being disease-causing mutations. The spectrum of *PAH* mutations ranged from 65.4% missense substitutions to 12.2% splice variants, ~13% deletions, 5.2% nonsense (termination) mutations and a few insertions (Scriver et al., 1999).

The severity of the mutation is determined by its effect on the PAH protein's conformation and function and is correlated with varying degrees of defect. Mutations in the regulatory and catalytic domains typically result in PAH instabilities and folding defects (Sheller et al., 2019). *In vitro* expression analysis of approximately 100 missense mutations revealed at least three enzymatic phenotypes, i.e., (i) structurally stable but with changed kinetic properties; (ii) kinetic properties that are normal or nearly normal, but with decreased stability; and (iii) distorted in both kinetic and stability properties (Waters, 2003). Some of these defective PAHs could still be functional, but they will be degraded rapidly resulting in insufficient amounts of cellular PAH protein (Wettstein et al., 2015). Depending on the spectrum of *PAH* mutations and the protein's concentration level, clinical manifestations of PAH deficiency ranged from mild hyperphenylalaninemia to severe and persistent classic PKU (Guldberg et al., 1998).

Potential Manipulation of UPS-Mediated Degradation of Mutant PAH

Even before the defective protein is subjected to UPS-mediated degradation, the ubiquitination system has played an important role. In other diseases, numerous E3-chaperone complexes work in tandem to target misfolded proteins for autophagy, while DUBs oppose the process. Thus, it is critical to investigate the chaperones, E3s, and DUBs that are involved in the molecular mechanisms of PKU in order to retain the aggregated PAH that confer functional roles.

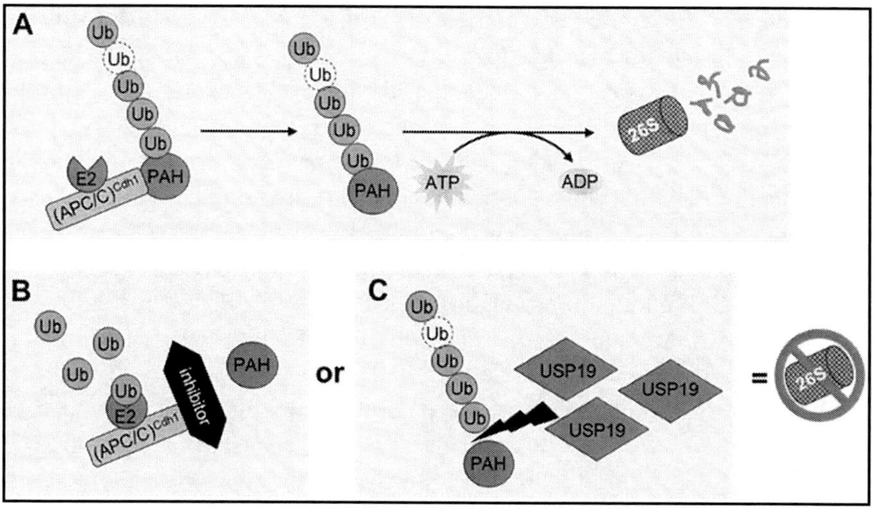

Figure 2. Rescuing functional PAH from UPS-mediated degradation: (A) $(APC/C)^{Cdh1}$ ubiquitinates defective mutant PAH, which is then degraded by the 26S proteasome. (B) The ubiquitination of a functional mutant PAH could be prevented by developing an $(APC/C)^{Cdh1}$ inhibitor. (C) Delivering USP19 to remove polyubiquitin chains could reverse the degradation of functional mutant PAH. Created with Microsoft PowerPoint ver2301.

In regard to UPS-mediated degradation, previous studies have confirmed that the protein quality control system opted for UPS to degrade wild-type and mutant PAH in a rat model (Sarkissian et al., 2012; Døskeland & Flatmark, 2001). The E3 ligase responsible for PAH polyubiquitination and degradation through the 26S proteasomal pathway was later identified as the anaphase-promoting complex/cyclosome-Cdh1 $(APC/C)^{Cdh1}$ (Tyagi et al., 2020). The study also proved that there is indeed a physical interaction between Cdh1 and PAH *in vivo*, which shortens the PAH's half-life and reduces its availability for Phe metabolism. Meanwhile, a genome-wide screening study has discovered that among all DUBs, USP19 is the one that regulates PAH's stability and functionality by reversing the polyubiquitination of PAH (Sarodaya et al., 2022). The study also verified the localisation and interaction between USP19 and PAH in the human liver cell line Huh7. In the presence of USP19, the half-life of the PAH protein was prolonged, implying that

USP19 is protecting PAH from degradation and therefore aiding in the replenishment of the PAH available pool in cells.

Based on this, manipulation of UPS-mediated degradation is viewed as an appealing therapeutic strategy for reducing the severity of PKU. A therapeutic approach could be proposed, such as developing an $(APC/C)^{Cdh1}$ inhibitor to inhibit degradation of Phe or elevating and restoring PAH levels via gene therapy that delivers USP19 to rescue functional PAH (Figure 2). To commit to this, the most crucial step is to find a way to distinguish between lethal defects and negligible defects of PAH. Furthermore, the roles of $(APC/C)^{Cdh1}$ and USP19 in other cellular functions should be carefully examined to avoid disturbing other critical pathways.

Conclusion

PKU is a concerning condition that is caused by a lack or low concentration of PAH, an enzyme that metabolises Phe, as a consequence of multiple types of mutations in the *PAH* gene. Even though some PAH mutants with folding defects are still functional, they are quickly destroyed, primarily by UPS-mediated protein quality control. The severity of PKU is determined by the level of the PAH concentration. Studies have identified $(APC/C)^{Cdh1}$ as the E3 ligase responsible for conjugating ubiquitin molecules to PAH for proteasomal degradation and USP19 as the DUB responsible for removing the ubiquitin link and thus rescuing PAH. Thus, manipulating the UPS system via these two enzymes could be proposed as an attractive therapeutic target in the treatment of PKU, provided that their other roles in the cellular landscape are carefully reviewed in order to avoid perturbation of other vital cellular pathways.

Acknowledgment

This work was supported by Universiti Sains Malaysia through RUI Grant (1001.CIPPT.8012340).

References

Amerik, A. Y., & Hochstrasser, M. (2004). Mechanism and function of deubiquitinating enzymes. *Biochimica et Biophysica Acta*, *1695*(1-3), 189–207. https://doi.org/10.1016/j.bbamcr.2004.10.003.

Anfinsen C. B. (1972). The formation and stabilization of protein structure. *The Biochemical Journal*, *128*(4), 737–749. https://doi.org/10.1042/bj1280737.

Arturo, E. C., Gupta, K., Héroux, A., Stith, L., Cross, P. J., Parker, E. J., Loll, P. J., & Jaffe, E. K. (2016). First structure of full-length mammalian phenylalanine hydroxylase reveals the architecture of an autoinhibited tetramer. *Proceedings of the National Academy of Sciences of the United States of America*, *113*(9), 2394–2399. https://doi.org/10.1073/pnas.1516967113.

Blau, N., van Spronsen, F. J., & Levy, H. L. (2010). Phenylketonuria. *Lancet (London, England)*, *376*(9750), 1417–1427. https://doi.org/10.1016/S0140-6736(10)60961-0.

Ciechanover, A., & Kwon, Y. T. (2017). Protein quality control by molecular chaperones in neurodegeneration. *Frontiers in Neuroscience*, *11*, 185. http://doi.org/10.3389/fnins.2017.00185 Donlon J, & Sarkissian C, & Levy H, & Scriver C. R. (2019). Hyperphenylalaninemia: phenylalanine hydroxylase deficiency. In: Valle D. L., & Antonarakis S, & Ballabio A, & Beaudet A. L., & Mitchell G. A.(Eds.), *The Online Metabolic and Molecular Bases of Inherited Disease*. McGraw Hill. https://ommbid.mhmedical.com/content.aspx?bookid=2709&sectionid=225081923.

Døskeland, A. P., & Flatmark, T. (2001). Conjugation of phenylalanine hydroxylase with polyubiquitin chains catalysed by rat liver enzymes. *Biochimica et Biophysica Acta*, *1547*(2), 379–386. https://doi.org/10.1016/s0167-4838(01)00206-0.

Fredrickson, E. K., & Gardner, R. G. (2012). Selective destruction of abnormal proteins by ubiquitin-mediated protein quality control degradation. *Seminars in Cell & Developmental Biology*, *23*(5), 530–537. http://doi.org/10.1016/j.semcdb.2011.12.006

Guldberg, P., Rey, F., Zschocke, J., Romano, V., François, B., Michiels, L., Ullrich, K., Hoffmann, G. F., Burgard, P., Schmidt, H., Meli, C., Riva, E., Dianzani, I., Ponzone, A., Rey, J., & Güttler, F. (1998). A European multicenter study of phenylalanine hydroxylase deficiency: classification of 105 mutations and a general system for genotype-based prediction of metabolic phenotype. *American Journal of Human Genetics*, *63*(1), 71–79. https://doi.org/10.1086/301920.

Gundorova, P., Zinchenko, R. A., Kuznetsova, I. A., Bliznetz, E. A., Stepanova, A. A., & Polyakov, A. V. (2018). Molecular-genetic causes for the high frequency of phenylketonuria in the population from the North Caucasus. *PloS one*, *13*(8), e0201489. https://doi.org/10.1371/journal.pone.0201489.

Hillert, A., Anikster, Y., Belanger-Quintana, A., Burlina, A., Burton, B. K., Carducci, C., Chiesa, A. E., Christodoulou, J., Đorđević, M., Desviat, L. R., Eliyahu, A., Evers, R. A. F., Fajkusova, L., Feillet, F., Bonfim-Freitas, P. E., Giżewska, M., Gundorova, P., Karall, D., Kneller, K., Kutsev, S. I., Leuzzi, V., Levy, H. L., Lichter-Konecki, U., Muntau, A. C., Namour, F., Oltarzewski, M., Paras, A., Perez, B., Polak, E., Polyakov, A. V., Porta, F., Rohrbach, M., Scholl-Bürgi S, Spécola, N., Stojiljković, M., Shen,

N., Santana-da Silva, L. C., Skouma, A., van Spronsen, F., Stoppioni, V., Thöny, B., Trefz, F. K., Vockley, J., Yu, Y., Zschocke, J., Hoffmann, G. F., Garbade, S. F., & Blau, N. (2020). The Genetic Landscape and Epidemiology of Phenylketonuria. *American Journal of Human Genetics*, *107*(2), 234–250. https://doi.org/10.1016/j.ajhg.2020.06.006.

Karnaneedi, S., Choo, K. E., Ariffin, W. A., & Norimi, M. (1989). Phenylketonuria in a six year old Malay boy--a case report. *The Medical Journal of Malaysia*, *44*(3), 248–251.

Kaufman, S. (1977). Phenylketonuria: Biochemical Mechanisms. In: Agranoff, B. W., Aprison, M. H. (eds) Advances in Neurochemistry. Advances in Neurochemistry, vol 2. Springer, Boston, MA. https://doi.org/10.1007/978-1-4615-8237-3_1.

Komander, D., & Rape, M. (2012). The ubiquitin code. *Annual Review of Biochemistry*, *81*, 203–229. https://doi.org/10.1146/annurev-biochem-060310-170328.

Laskey, R. A., Honda, B. M., Mills, A. D., & Finch, J. T. (1978). Nucleosomes are assembled by an acidic protein which binds histones and transfers them to DNA. *Nature*, *275*(5679), 416–420. https://doi.org/10.1038/275416a0.

Li, Y., Li, S., & Wu, H. (2022). Ubiquitination-Proteasome System (UPS) and autophagy two main protein degradation machineries in response to cell stress. *Cells*, *11*(5), 851. https://doi.org/10.3390/cells11050851.

Lichter-Konecki, U., & Vockley, J. (2019). Phenylketonuria: current treatments and future developments. *Drugs*, *79*(5), 495–500. https://doi.org/10.1007/s40265-019-01079-z.

MacDonald, A., van Wegberg, A. M. J., Ahring, K., Beblo, S., Bélanger-Quintana, A., Burlina, A., Campistol, J., Coşkun, T., Feillet, F., Giżewska, M., Huijbregts, S. C., Leuzzi, V., Maillot, F., Muntau, A. C., Rocha, J. C., Romani, C., Trefz, F., & van Spronsen, F. J. (2020). PKU dietary handbook to accompany PKU guidelines. *Orphanet Journal of Rare Diseases*, *15*(1), 171. https://doi.org/10.1186/s13023-020-01391-y.

Markham A. (2018). Pegvaliase: first global approval. *BioDrugs: Clinical Immunotherapeutics, Biopharmaceuticals and Gene Therapy*, *32*(4), 391–395. https://doi.org/10.1007/s40259-018-0292-3.

Ministry of Health Malaysia (2021). *Malaysian Orphan Medicine Guideline. 1st edition.* Pharmaceutical Services Programme, Ministry of Health, Malaysia.

Nijman, S. M., Luna-Vargas, M. P., Velds, A., Brummelkamp, T. R., Dirac, A. M., Sixma, T. K., & Bernards, R. (2005). A genomic and functional inventory of deubiquitinating enzymes. *Cell*, *123*(5), 773–786.https://doi.org/10.1016/j.cell.2005.11.007

Okano, Y., Kudo, S., Nishi, Y., Sakaguchi, T., & Aso, K. (2011). Molecular characterization of phenylketonuria and tetrahydrobiopterin-responsive phenylalanine hydroxylase deficiency in Japan. *Journal of Human Genetics*, *56*(4), 306–312. https://doi.org/10.1038/jhg.2011.10.

Pickart C. M. (2001). Mechanisms underlying ubiquitination. *Annual Review of Biochemistry*, *70*, 503–533. https://doi.org/10.1146/annurev.biochem.70.1.503.

Pilla, E., Schneider, K., & Bertolotti, A. (2017). Coping with Protein Quality Control Failure. *Annual Review of Cell and Developmental Biology*, *33*, 439–465. https://doi.org/10.1146/annurev-cellbio-111315-125334.

Sarkissian, C. N., Ying, M., Scherer, T., Thöny, B., & Martinez, A. (2012). The mechanism of BH4 -responsive hyperphenylalaninemia--as it occurs in the ENU1/2 genetic mouse model. *Human Mutation*, *33*(10), 1464–1473. https://doi.org/10.1002/humu.22128.

Sarodaya, N., Tyagi, A., Kim, H. J., Colaco, J. C., Kang, J. S., Kim, W. J., Kim, K. S., & Ramakrishna, S. (2022). Deubiquitinase USP19 enhances phenylalanine hydroxylase protein stability and its enzymatic activity. *Cell Biology and Toxicology*, 10.1007/s10565-022-09719-z. Advance online publication. https://doi.org/10.1007/s10565-022-09719-z.

Scheller, R., Stein, A., Nielsen, S. V., Marin, F. I., Gerdes, A. M., Di Marco, M., Papaleo, E., Lindorff-Larsen, K., & Hartmann-Petersen, R. (2019). Toward mechanistic models for genotype-phenotype correlations in phenylketonuria using protein stability calculations. *Human Mutation*, *40*(4), 444–457. https://doi.org/10.1002/humu.23707.

Scriver, C. R., & Waters, P. J. (1999). Monogenic traits are not simple: lessons from phenylketonuria. *Trends in genetics: TIG*, *15*(7), 267–272. https://doi.org/10.1016/s0168-9525(99)01761-8.

Tyagi, A., Sarodaya, N., Kaushal, K., Chandrasekaran, A. P., Antao, A. M., Suresh, B., Rhie, B. H., Kim, K. S., & Ramakrishna, S. (2020). E3 ubiquitin ligase APC/C^{Cdh1} regulation of phenylalanine hydroxylase stability and function. *International Journal of Molecular Sciences*, *21*(23), 9076. https://doi.org/10.3390/ijms21239076.

Tyedmers, J., Mogk, A., & Bukau, B. (2010). Cellular strategies for controlling protein aggregation. *Nature reviews. Molecular Cell Biology*, *11*(11), 777–788. https://doi.org/10.1038/nrm2993.

van Spronsen, F. J., Blau, N., Harding, C., Burlina, A., Longo, N., & Bosch, A. M. (2021). Phenylketonuria. *Nature reviews. Disease Primers*, *7*(1), 36. https://doi.org/10.1038/s41572-021-00267-0.

Waters P. J. (2003). How PAH gene mutations cause hyper-phenylalaninemia and why mechanism matters: insights from in vitro expression. *Human Mutation*, *21*(4), 357–369. https://doi.org/10.1002/humu.10197.

Wang, J., & Maldonado, M. A. (2006). The ubiquitin-proteasome system and its role in inflammatory and autoimmune diseases. *Cellular & Molecular Immunology*, *3*(4), 255–261.

Wettstein, S., Underhaug, J., Perez, B., Marsden, B. D., Yue, W. W., Martinez, A., & Blau, N. (2015). Linking genotypes database with locus-specific database and genotype-phenotype correlation in phenylketonuria. *European Journal of Human Genetics: EJHG*, *23*(3), 302–309. https://doi.org/10.1038/ejhg.2014.114.

Williams, R. A., Mamotte, C. D., & Burnett, J. R. (2008). Phenylketonuria: an inborn error of phenylalanine metabolism. *The Clinical Biochemist. Reviews*, *29*(1), 31–41.

Yadav, K., Yadav, A., Vashistha, P., Pandey, V. P., & Dwivedi, U. N. (2019). Protein misfolding diseases and therapeutic approaches. *Current Protein & Peptide Science*, *20*(12), 1226–1245. https://doi.org/10.2174/1389203720666190610092840.

Zheng, N., & Shabek, N. (2017). Ubiquitin ligases: structure, function, and regulation. *Annual Review of Biochemistry*, *86*, 129–157. https://doi.org/10.1146/annurev-biochem-060815-014922.

Zulkifle, N. (2020). Topological analysis of cancer protein subnetwork in deubiquitinase (DUB) interactome. In: Rojas, I., Valenzuela, O., Rojas, F., Herrera, L., Ortuño, F.

(eds) *Bioinformatics and Biomedical Engineering. IWBBIO 2020. Lecture Notes in Computer Science*, vol 12108. Springer, Cham. https://doi.org/10.1007/978-3-030-45385-5_23.

Chapter 12

Genetic Mutations and Clinical Diagnoses Associated with Increased Risk of Malignancy in Primary Immunodeficiencies

Aminah Suhaila Haron[1]
Saiful E. Syafruddin[2]
Ilie Fadzilah Hashim[3]
Muggunna Balasubramaniam[4]
Saw Keat Chuan[4]
Yasmin Hasnizan[4]
Nurul Syafawani Fizal[4]
Chong Chien Fung[4]
and Ana Masara Ahmad Mokhtar[4,5,*]

[1]Faculty of Dentistry, AIMST University, Bedong, Kedah, Malaysia
[2]UKM Medical Molecular Biology Institute, Universiti Kebangsaan Malaysia, Cheras, Kuala Lumpur, Malaysia
[3]Department of Clinical Medicine, Advanced Medical and Dental Institute, Universiti Sains Malaysia, Kepala Batas, Pulau Pinang, Malaysia
[4]Bioprocess Technology Division, School of Industrial Technology, Universiti Sains Malaysia, Pulau Pinang, Malaysia
[5]Green Biopolymer Coating and Packaging Centre, School of Industrial Technology, Universiti Sains Malaysia, Pulau Pinang, Malaysia

---

[*] Corresponding Author's Email: anamasara@usm.my.

In: Genetic Disorders and Rare Diseases
Editors: Shazlin Shaharudin, Hisham Atan Edinur and Nor Fazila Che Mat
ISBN: 979-8-88697-953-4

Abstract

Primary immunodeficiencies (PIDs) are a group of clinically and genetically diverse disorders characterised by over 400 gene mutations. They impede the function of immune cells, including chemokine-induced motility, receptor signalling, development and maturation. Malaysia has a lower prevalence of PIDs than other countries, occurring at a rate of 0.37 per 100,000 individuals. However, due to the lack of a Malaysian PID registry database, the true prevalence in this nation is unknown and most likely under-reported. In addition to the documented immunological defects, some PID patients also acquire cancer, implying that the immune system plays a role in recognising and eliminating nascent cancer. Over 460 distinct PIDs have been identified, with common variable immunodeficiency (CVID), Wiskott–Aldrich syndrome, ataxia-telangiectasia, and severe combined immunodeficiency serving as the most common clinical diagnoses reported to be associated with cancer. Although the mechanism by which PID patients develop cancer progression is unknown, genomic instability induced by defective DNA repair pathways and increased cancer-related pathways may play a role. Additionally, since cancer phenotypes have been identified in certain PID diagnostic classifications, this suggests that certain mutations or clinical diagnoses are associated with an increased risk of developing cancer, whilst others are not. Thus, the review will discuss the most frequently detected mutations and clinical diagnoses among PID patients diagnosed with cancer.

Keywords: autoimmune, cancer, primary immunodeficiency

Introduction

The integrity of the immune system is essential for defending against harmful organisms and monitoring abnormal cellular changes, such as cancer progression. Primary immunodeficiency diseases (PIDs) are a varied set of inherited genetic illnesses characterised by the absence or malfunctioning of immune system components (Al-Herz et al., 2011). PIDs can be characterised by an increased susceptibility to infections, organ damage, autoimmunity and cancer. More than 400 PID-causing genes have now been identified and categorised into eight categories depending on the impaired immunological function (Bousfiha et al., 2020; Derpoorter et al., 2018).

Over the last two decades, significant effort has been put into determining the genetic modification of PIDs to reduce disease-related mortality and morbidity. A survey in the United States revealed that only 40% of individuals were diagnosed with PIDs until adulthood, although most patients had chronic or severe health problems before their diagnoses. Hospitalisation rates pre- and post-diagnosis highlight the urgency of detecting and controlling PIDs as soon as feasible. Although 70% had been hospitalised prior to diagnosis, nearly half (48%) of them were not hospitalised following their diagnosis (McCusker & Warrington, 2011).

Malignancy is one of the leading causes of death in PIDs following infection, and the most frequent type of cancer observed in patients is haematological malignancies (66.7%), including lymphoma and leukaemia (Maffeis et al., 2019). Unfortunately, there is still a knowledge vacuum on how this illness develops, making treatments ineffective. As a result, it is critical to precisely identify all the possible mutations that may underpin cancer growth in PIDs. This knowledge will aid in developing effective medicines to improve patients' quality of life.

PID Prevalence in Malaysia

Malaysia is a small Southeast Asian country with a population of 33.9 million in 2020 (Unicef, 2020). In the same year, the life expectancy at birth was 75.1 years, with an under-5 mortality rate of 8.6 deaths per 1,000 live births (Department of Statistics Malaysia, 2021; Unicef, 2020).

In comparison to other nations, Malaysia has a low prevalence of PIDs, with 0.37 PID cases per 100,000 people (Abd Hamid et al., 2020). However, due to the lack of a National PID registry, Malaysia's actual number of PID cases is uncertain and most likely under-reported (Abd Hamid et al., 2020).

Abd Hamid et al. (2020) assessed 4,838 papers relevant to PIDs in Malaysia from 1979 to 2019, including 34 publications and 119 PID cases. Interestingly, PIDs were most common in Malays (67%), followed by Indians (17%) and Chinese (14%), respectively. According to the data, Malays are more likely than other races in Malaysia to have PID. Nonetheless, because the patient's race was not available in 35 of the 119 instances studied, the relationship between PIDs and ethnicity cannot be substantiated (Abd Hamid et al., 2020). According to Abd Hamid et al. (2020), a very common form of PID is found to affect humoral and cellular immunity (30.3%) (Abd Hamid et al., 2020), with severe combined immunodeficiency (SCID), constituting the most typical PID diagnosis. SCID patients usually have a defect in T-cell development as well as a functional aberration in the B-cell compartment (Abd Hamid et al., 2020).

T and B cells are the principal cells of the adaptive immune system. B cells produce antibodies and hence play an essential role in antibody-mediated (humoral) immunity. On the other hand, T cells are in charge of cell-mediated immune responses. T-cell (cellular) immunodeficiency disorders are usually caused by defective T-cell development, differentiation, or maturation (Bonilla & Oettgen, 2010). Interestingly, since B-cell-mediated antibody production relies on T-cell function, any T-cells abnormalities may also lead to combined (B- and T-cell) immunodeficiencies (CIDs) (Bonilla & Oettgen, 2010). Meanwhile, B-cell (antibody-deficiency) disorders are mainly caused by impaired B-cell development and/or maturation. In Malaysia, 10 out of 22 SCID-diagnosed individuals had specific genetic abnormalities that caused a malfunction in the production and function of infection-fighting immune cells.

The second most prevalent PID diagnosis was X-linked agammaglobulinemia (XLA), followed by chronic granulomatous disease (CGD), with 17 and 14 cases, respectively. Both PID diagnoses are associated with a reduced ability to fight infections caused by pathogenic bacteria and fungi. XLA is usually caused by Bruton tyrosine kinase (*BTK*) gene mutation, which is essential for B cell development (El-Sayed et al., 2019). GCD, on the other hand, is a genetic disorder commonly associated with impaired NADPH oxidase complex in neutrophilic granulocytes and monocytes, which is necessary for infection resistance (Arnold & Heimall, 2017).

Defence against infections is necessary as some viruses or bacteria are known to promote cancer progression. Furthermore, pathogenic infection is often associated with inflammation, and chronic or prolonged exposure to these inflammatory events may progress to cancer development, as inflammation and cancer are highly related (Goldszmid et al., 2014).

Common PID Clinical Diagnosis Linked to Cancer

The most commonly diagnosed symptoms in PID patients include infections, autoimmunity and malignancies. Malignancy is one of the leading causes of mortality in PIDs (Satgé, 2018). Moreover, the European Society of Immunodeficiencies has acknowledged the existence of cancer phenotypes as one of the diagnostic criteria for some PIDs (Derpoorter et al., 2018). Due to the diverse nature of this illness, assessing the cancer risk linked with PIDs is challenging. Several underlying cancer pathways in PID offer another layer of complexity. Cancer therapy in the setting of PID is particularly complicated by considerable toxicities and long-term repercussions, such as the emergence of secondary malignancies (Derpoorter et al., 2018).

Nonetheless, the link between a weakened immune system and cancer implies that the immune system plays a vital role in recognising and eliminating pre-cancerous cells (Finn, 2012; Satgé, 2018). This is based on the theory that cancer cells express antigens that the immune system can recognise. However, malignant cells may not be removed and may instead enter an equilibrium phase in which the immune system governs tumour cell proliferation. Tumour immunogenicity is altered at this stage and tumour cell growth is restricted. In this stage, cancer cells may not grow or metastasise, but they may eventually be able to evade and fight the antitumor immune response, resulting in the development of the tumour (Finn, 2012; Swann & Smyth, 2007). This is frequently observed in individuals with impaired immune systems as they are unable to eliminate cancer cells efficiently. As a result, these patients have a higher risk of acquiring cancer than healthy persons. Cancer incidence among PIDs has been demonstrated to diminish patients' quality of life and create pressure on medical care, directly related to high expenses.

The most prevalent PID subtype related to cancer is "common variable immunodeficiency" (CVID), in which patients have a high risk of lymphoma, stomach cancer, and skin cancer (Mortaz et al., 2016). This heightened risk seems likely due to a combination of factors, especially bacterial and viral infections. Some pathogens were reported to stimulate cancer-related signalling pathways, such as Wnt, p53, JAK/STAT, PI3K/Akt, MAPK and NF-kB signalling (Kellogg et al., 2021). Furthermore, ~20% of cancer cases are preceded by infection and persistent inflammation in the exact inflammatory areas (Greten & Grivennikov, 2019; Grivennikov et al., 2010). This is supported by several cases in which patients with chronic hepatitis, inflammatory bowel disease (IBD) and *Helicobacter*-induced gastritis were also found to have liver cancer, colorectal cancer (CRC) and stomach cancer, respectively. (Trinchieri, 2012).

Other PID diagnoses related to cancer include selective IgA deficiency, Wiskott-Aldrich Syndrome, X-linked Agammaglobulinemia, Hyper IgM Syndrome, Congenital Neutropenia, and Ataxia Telangiectasia (Table 1). Interestingly, all of these diagnoses increase patient's susceptibility to bacterial infections (Mortaz et al., 2016). The most widely accepted explanation is probably reduced cancer monitoring resulting from PID mutations (Ribatti, 2017). PID genes are known to influence T- and B- cells formation and function, either via somatic hypermutation or impaired class switch recombination and V(D)J recombination, resulting in persistent infections, inflammation and cancer development later in life (Ruffner et al., 2017).

The main immunodeficiency, known as immunoglobulin A (IgA) deficiency, is frequently present and is defined by undetectable blood IgA, concurrently low levels of secretory IgA, and normal levels of other immunoglobulins. It is important to distinguish between IgA deficiency and any other causes of hypogammaglobulinemia or T lymphocyte defects (Rawla et al., 2022). An increased prevalence of malignant lymphoma and of gastric cancer has been observed in large cohorts of patients with common variable immunodeficiency (CVID), the most frequent symptomatic primary immunodeficiency. Based on the high rate of mortality due to gastric cancer in Italian CVID patients, we suggest a strategy aimed at early diagnosis, based on regular upper endoscopy and on Helicobacter pylori infection treatment, and recommend an implementation of national guidelines (Pulvirenti et al., 2018).

Panhypogammaglobulinemia, the absence of B-cells, recurring gastrointestinal and respiratory infections beginning at a young age, as well as other diseases such cellulitis, meningitis, arthritis, and sepsis, are characteristics of X-linked Agammaglobulinemia (XLA). These individuals have had a variety of non-infectious consequences, such as autoimmune disorders and cancer, particularly lymphomas. Solid cancer appears to be linked to persistent infection in XLA and mostly affects the gastrointestinal system. Gastric adenocarcinoma and megaloblastic anaemia brought on by achlorhydria in the context of persistent infection may be traced back naturally (Staines et al., 2014).

Low blood quantities of IgG, IgA and IgE, combined with normal or high serum amounts of IgM, are the hallmarks of X-linked hyper IgM syndrome (HIGM1), a condition of aberrant T- and B-cell activity. Medical repercussions of this condition have been described as autoimmune and/or inflammatory illnesses (such sclerosing cholangitis) and pose an elevated risk for neoplasms. In 5%-15% of afflicted boys, there are significant neurologic problems, frequently brought on by a CNS infection. With proper screening and treatment of Cryptosporidium infection, liver disease, a severe consequence of HIGM1, may be on the decline. HIGM1 was historically associated with liver disease in more than 80% of afflicted males by age 20. In addition to infections, patients with Wiskott-Aldrich syndrome (WAS) are prone to cancer and autoimmune diseases. This research described a case of a boy infant with WAS who had vasculitic skin lesions, dermatitis, thrombocytopenia, autoimmune hemolytic anaemia, and recurring pneumonia (Vignesh et al., 2017).

A mutation in the ataxia telangiectasia mutated (ATM) gene, which codes for a serine/threonine protein kinase, results in ataxia telangiectasia (AT), an autosomal recessive primary immunodeficiency (PID) condition. Progressive cerebellar ataxia, oculocutaneous telangiectasia, variable immunodeficiency, radiosensitivity, susceptibility to malignancies and elevated metabolic disorders are only a few of the clinical symptoms seen in AT patients. In this study, they discussed how ATM acts in the cytoplasm and nucleus as well as how it may contribute to the development of certain disorders, including those involving the nervous system, immune system, vascular system, lungs, and metabolism, and the dermatologic complications that may occur (Amirifar et al., 2019).

RhoH, an unusual small GTPase of the Rho family, has frequent expression in the haematopoietic lineage and only shares less than 50% of its sequence with other Rho family members. RhoH's aberrant protein expression has been linked to immune-related conditions such psoriasis, systemic lupus erythematosus, and primary immunodeficiencies as well as B cell malignancies, suggesting a possible relationship between these conditions and cancer. Other factors involved in the relationship of RhoH with these disorders include its interaction partner ZAP70, activation regulators Vav1 and RhoGDI, and other small GTPases such RhoA, Rac1, and Cdc42. RhoH and its associated proteins are therefore attractive targets, particularly in the therapy of immune- and cancer-related disorders (Ahmad Mokhtar et al., 2021).

Table 1. PID conditions and their cancer risk

Diagnostic Classifications	Cancer types	Ref
Selective IgA deficiency	Gastric cancer, lymphoma	(Shapiro, 2011)
Common variable immune deficiency	Gastric cancer, skin cancers, lymphoma	(Pulvirenti et al., 2018)
X-linked Agammaglobulinemia	Gastric cancer, intestinal carcinoma	(Staines Boone et al., 2014)
Hyper IgM Syndrome	Liver, gallbladder and pancreas cancer	(Nagaraj et al., 2007)
Wiskott-Aldrich Syndrome	Lymphoma, CNS lymphoma	(Vignesh et al., 2017)
Congenital Neutropenia	Acute myeloid leukemia (AML)	(Beekman et al., 2012)
Ataxia Telangiectasia	lymphoma, gastric cancer, skin cancer and/or leukemia	(Amirifar et al., 2019)
Epidermodysplasia Verruciformis	Burkitt lymphoma	(Ahmad Mokhtar et al., 2021)

Nonetheless, discovering the genetic abnormalities prevalent in PIDs that are likely to trigger cancer development is required to decipher the intricate signalling network implicated in PID malignancies. Once the complex signalling network is unravelled, we can identify the most efficacious attack points in tackling PID malignancies.

PID Mutational Defects Associated with Malignancy

Currently, over 400 underlying genetic defects have been discovered. Baleydier et al. (2020) have also listed some genetic mutations and their potential to underpin cancer progression in PIDs (Baleydier et al., 2020). Among the genes are *GATA2* and *BLM*. Both are known as cancer risk genes *GATA2*, where a transcription factor is required to generate and maintain hematopoietic stem cells. *GATA2* mutations have been identified to not only cause MonoMAC syndrome, a type of PID linked with mycobacterial infections but also to promote prostate cancer progression (Rodriguez-Bravo et al., 2017). Meanwhile, the *BLM* gene that encodes a DNA helicase is known to be associated with DNA repair. Since DNA repair is required for the formation of T- and B-cell antigen receptors, deficiencies in *BLM* have been related to cancer susceptibility and immunodeficiency by affecting lymphocyte development (Kaur et al., 2021). *WAS*, *FAS*, *SBDS*, *ATM*, *ITK*, *CDKN2A* and *RECQL4* are also among the other PID-causing genes with high cancer risk (Derpoorter et al., 2018).

Some of the altered genes are also connected to small Rho GTPases. They are known to serve as molecular switches, cycling between active guanosine triphosphate-bound and inactive guanosine diphosphate-bound forms to regulate essential cellular activities, including actin-cytoskeleton reorganisation, cell adhesion, and motility (Hashim & Ahmad Mokhtar, 2021). Interestingly, studies also have associated abnormal Rho GTPase expression or activity with cancer and PIDs (Ahmad Mokhtar et al., 2021; Hashim & Ahmad Mokhtar, 2021). Among the reported small Rho GTPase mutations found in PID patients are RhoH and Cdc42.

RhoH mutations, for example, have been reported in PIDs, most notably in Epidermodysplasia verruciformis. The patient possesses a RhoH mutation at Y38X, which leads to a loss-of-function impact and is associated with a shortage of naïve peripheral T-cells (Crequer et al., 2012). An in vivo investigation using *Rhoh*$^{-/-}$ knockout mice also revealed the same developmental abnormalities (Gu et al., 2006). These phenotypes are likely due to a defect in thymocyte selection and maturation caused by RhoH's inability to mediate TCR-induced ZAP-70 activation and CD3 phosphorylation (Dorn et al., 2007; Gu et al., 2006). RhoH deficiency was also found to affect Lck and ZAP-70 recruitment to CD3 in the immunological synapse (Chae et al., 2010; Gu et al., 2006), suggesting a role for RhoH in pre-TCR and TCR signalling.

Another small Rho GTPase is Cdc42, wherein a patient with Cdc42 C81Y mutation is shown to have immunological defects such as low $CD4^+$ Th cell population and malignancy (Szczawinska-Poplonyk et al., 2020). However, knowledge of the molecular and functional ramifications of this mutation is still limited, rendering treatment ineffective. It also unknown whether the malignancies observed precede or occur concurrently with the immune deficiency. Nonetheless, Guo et al. (2011) discovered that Cdc42 deficiency reduces TCR signalling and T-cell proliferation even upon stimulation with anti-CD3/-CD28, suggesting that Cdc42 is important in maintaining T-cell homeostasis (Guo et al., 2011). This also implies that the C81Y mutation may affect Cdc42 protein expression, activation, and function in T-cells.

Furthermore, a deficiency of T cells is highly associated with viral infections, as was discovered in a Cdc42 C81Y patient, who was found to have cytomegalovirus (CMV) infection (Szczawinska-Poplonyk et al., 2020). This infection will subsequently promote cancer progression since CMV infection has been linked to chromosome damage and genetic instability, both of which are crucial to cancer progression (Rezaei et al., 2011). Furthermore, because small Rho GTPases regulate several cancer-related pathways, including the p38 and NF-KB pathways, decreased Cdc42 functions may promote cancer phenotypes by deregulating TCR signalling (Hashim & Ahmad Mokhtar, 2021) (Figure 1).

Interestingly, some small Rho GTPase regulators, such as Dock8, have also been implicated in both PIDs and cancer development (Hashim & Ahmad Mokhtar, 2021). DOCK8 is an essential modulator of actin cytoskeletal dynamics, and its absence restricts a wide variety of immune cell functions. Initially, DOCK8 mutations were found in 2009 to cause a severe immunological defect in humans and animals. Due to multiple similar traits, including respiratory infections, eosinophilia, and high IgE, the condition was categorized as an autosomal recessive variant of hyper IgE syndrome (AR-HIES) (Engelhardt et al., 2015). DOCK8 deficiency has also been correlated with severe cutaneous viral infections, and the most prevalent viruses are herpes simplex virus, human papillomavirus (HPV), varicella-zoster virus, and molluscum contagiosum virus (Biggs et al., 2017).

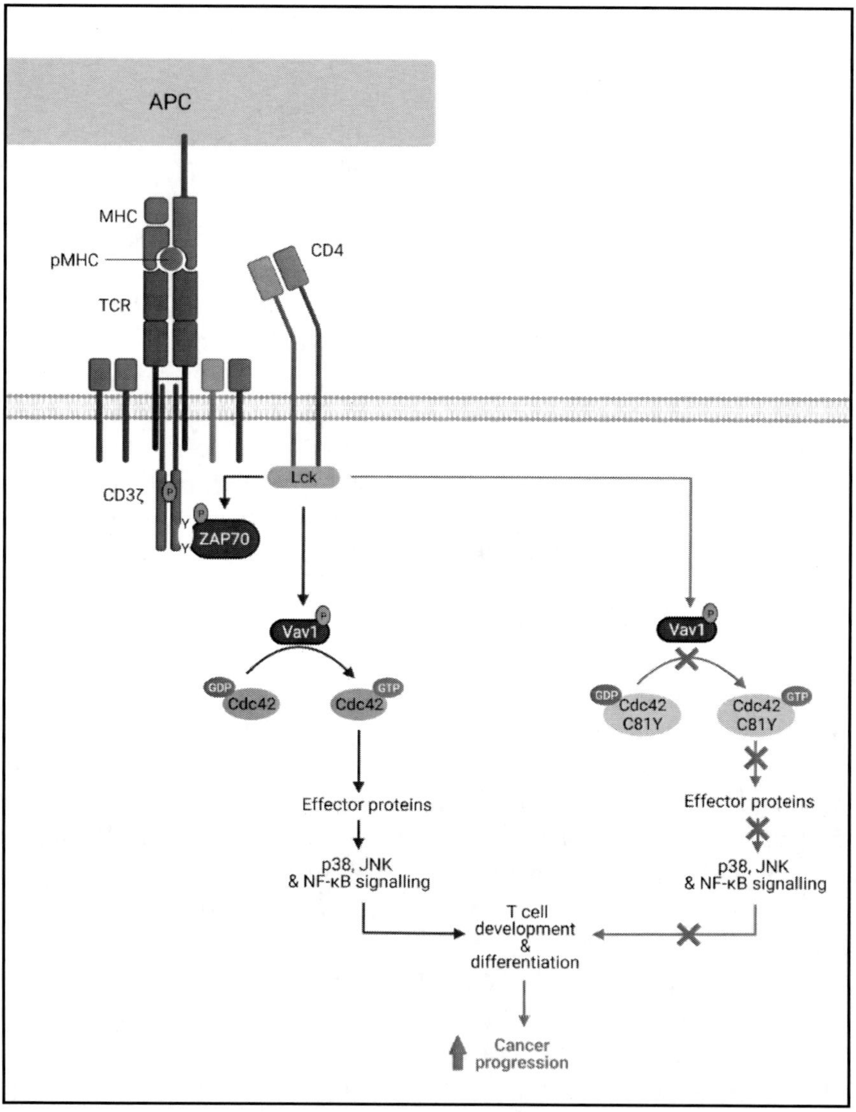

Figure 1. The proposed mechanism of Cdc42 C81Y-induced cancer progression. Cdc42 C81Y mutation may affect the activation status of Cdc42, causing deregulation of the cancer-related pathway such as p38, JNK, and NF-κB signalling. This would later affect T cell development and differentiation. Created with Biorender.com.

Future Direction for Detection of Mutational Defect Associated with PID Malignancy

PIDs were long assumed to be uncommon autosomal recessive diseases that resulted in completely penetrant phenotypes with serious immune system dysfunctions. However, a new paradigm has emerged that views PIDs as a spectrum of illnesses ranging from moderate to severe immunological abnormalities. NGS-based sequencing techniques such as whole genome sequencing (WGS) and whole-exome sequencing (WES) have aided in discovering monogenic illnesses such as PIDs, revealing the underlying mechanism of immune deficiencies (Seleman et al., 2017).

Exome sequencing will detail genomic regions that directly impacting protein structure, which is critical for detecting human illness. Additionally, due to the effectiveness of NGS technologies, interpreting variants and their connection to patient characteristics is becoming a critical practice in clinical and research settings (Vorsteveld et al., 2021). However, the diverse pattern of symptoms shown in PID patients, along with the effect of environmental variables, makes genetic identification complicated, hence necessitating a more advanced detection strategy.

Conclusion

Cancer management in PID patients remains challenging due to a lack of mechanical knowledge of this rare disease and the slow rate of scientific advancement in cancer detection. Thus, treatment and detection procedures should be refined in accordance with current understanding to improve these individuals' prognoses while giving a comprehensive and personalised therapy strategy. Furthermore, efforts should be taken to establish an international and national registry to provide detailed coverage of potential mutational defects associated with cancer progression. This register will also aid in identifying the standard pattern of biological and clinical characteristics, providing practical preventive actions and an early diagnosis.

Acknowledgments

The study is financially supported by the Ministry of Higher Education Malaysia for Fundamental Research Grant Scheme with Project Code: FRGS/1/2022/STG01/USM/03/2 and International Centre for Genetic Engineering & Biotechnology (ICGEB) for the Project No: CRP/MYS21-04_EC.

References

Abd Hamid, I. J., Azman, N. A., Gennery, A. R., Mangantig, E., Hashim, I. F., & Zainudeen, Z. T. (2020). Systematic Review of Primary Immunodeficiency Diseases in Malaysia: 1979–2020. *Frontiers in Immunology*, *11*, 1923. https://doi.org/10.3389/fimmu.2020.01923

Ahmad Mokhtar, A. M., Hashim, I. F., Mohd Zaini Makhtar, M., Salikin, N. H., & Amin-Nordin, S. (2021). The Role of RhoH in TCR Signalling and Its Involvement in Diseases. *Cells*, *10*(4), 950. https://doi.org/10.3390/cells10040950

Al-Herz, W., Bousfiha, A., Casanova, J. L., Chatila, T., Conley, M. E., Cunningham-Rundles, C., Etzioni, A., Franco, J. L., Gaspar, H. B., Holland, S. M., Klein, C., Nonoyama, S., Ochs, H. D., Oksenhendler, E., Picard, C., Puck, J. M., Sullivan, K., & Tang, M. L. (2014). Primary immunodeficiency diseases: an update on the classification from the international union of immunological societies expert committee for primary immunodeficiency. *Frontiers in Immunology*, *5*, 162. https://doi.org/10.3389/fimmu.2014.00162

Amirifar, P., Ranjouri, M. R., Yazdani, R., Abolhassani, H., & Aghamohammadi, A. (2019). Ataxia-telangiectasia: A review of clinical features and molecular pathology. *Pediatric Allergy and Immunology*, *30*(3), 277–288. https://doi.org/10.1111/pai.13020.

Arnold, D. E., & Heimall, J. R. (2017). A Review of Chronic Granulomatous Disease. *Advances in Therapy*, *34*(12), 2543–2557. https://doi.org/10.1007/s12325-017-0636-2.

Baleydier, F., Bernard, F., & Ansari, M. (2020). The Possibilities of Immunotherapy for Children with Primary Immunodeficiencies Associated with Cancers. *Biomolecules*, *10*, 1112. https://doi.org/10.3390/biom10081112.

Beekman, R., Valkhof, M. G., Sanders, M. A., van Strien, P. M. H., Haanstra, J. R., Broeders, L., Geertsma-Kleinekoort, W. M., Veerman, A. J. P., Valk, P. J. M., Verhaak, R. G., Löwenberg, B., & Touw, I. P. (2012). Sequential gain of mutations in severe congenital neutropenia progressing to acute myeloid leukemia. *Blood*, *119*(22), 5071–5077. https://doi.org/https://doi.org/10.1182/blood-2012-01-406116.

Biggs, C. M., Keles, S., & Chatila, T. A. (2017). DOCK8 deficiency: Insights into pathophysiology, clinical features and management. *Clinical Immunology (Orlando, Fla.)*, *181*, 75–82. https://doi.org/10.1016/j.clim.2017.06.003.

Bonilla, F. A., & Oettgen, H. C. (2010). Adaptive immunity. *Journal of Allergy and Clinical Immunology*, *125*(2, Supplement 2), S33–S40. org/10.1016/j.jaci.2009.09.017.

Bousfiha, A., Jeddane, L., Picard, C., Al-Herz, W., Ailal, F., Chatila, T., Cunningham-Rundles, C., Etzioni, A., Franco, J. L., Holland, S. M., Klein, C., Morio, T., Ochs, H. D., Oksenhendler, E., Puck, J., Torgerson, T. R., Casanova, J.-L., Sullivan, K. E., & Tangye, S. G. (2020). Human Inborn Errors of Immunity: 2019 Update of the IUIS Phenotypical Classification. *Journal of Clinical Immunology*, *40*(1), 66–81. https://doi.org/10.1007/s10875-020-00758-x.

Chae, H.-D., Siefring, J. E., Hildeman, D. A., Gu, Y., & Williams, D. A. (2010). RhoH regulates subcellular localization of ZAP-70 and Lck in T cell receptor signaling. *PloS One*, *5*(11), e13970–e13970. https://doi.org/10.1371/journal.pone.0013970.

Crequer, A., Troeger, A., Patin, E., Ma, C. S., Picard, C., Pedergnana, V., Fieschi, C., Lim, A., Abhyankar, A., Gineau, L., Mueller-Fleckenstein, I., Schmidt, M., Taieb, A., Krueger, J., Abel, L., Tangye, S. G., Orth, G., Williams, D. A., Casanova, J.-L., & Jouanguy, E. (2012). Human RHOH deficiency causes T cell defects and susceptibility to EV-HPV infections. *The Journal of Clinical Investigation*, *122*(9), 3239–3247. https://doi.org/10.1172/JCI62949.

Department of Statistics Malaysia. (2021). *Abridged Life Tables, Malaysia, 2019-2021*. Retrieved on August 09, 2022, https://www.dosm.gov.my/v1/index.php?r=column/cthemeByCat&cat=116&bul_id=aHNjSzZadnQ5VHBIeFRiN2dIdnlEQT09&menu_id=L0pheU43NWJwRWVSZklWdzQ4TlhUUT09.

Derpoorter, C., Bordon, V., Laureys, G., Haerynck, F., & Lammens, T. (2018). Genes at the Crossroad of Primary Immunodeficiencies and Cancer. *Frontiers in Immunology*, *9*, 2544. https://doi.org/10.3389/fimmu.2018.02544.

Dorn, T., Kuhn, U., Bungartz, G., Stiller, S., Bauer, M., Ellwart, J., Peters, T., Scharffetter-Kochanek, K., Semmrich, M., Laschinger, M., Holzmann, B., Klinkert, W. E. F., Straten, P. T., Køllgaard, T., Sixt, M., & Brakebusch, C. (2007). RhoH is important for positive thymocyte selection and T-cell receptor signaling. *Blood*, *109*(6), 2346–2355. https://doi.org/10.1182/blood-2006-04-019034.

El-Sayed, Z. A., Abramova, I., Aldave, J. C., Al-Herz, W., Bezrodnik, L., Boukari, R., Bousfiha, A. A., Cancrini, C., Condino-Neto, A., Dbaibo, G., Derfalvi, B., Dogu, F., Edgar, J. D. M., Eley, B., El-Owaidy, R. H., Espinosa-Padilla, S. E., Galal, N., Haerynck, F., Hanna-Wakim, R., Hossny, E., Ikinciogullari, A., Kamal, E., Kanegane, H., Kechout, N., Lau, Y. L., Morio, T., Moschese, V., Neves, J. F., Ouederni, M., Paganelli, R., Paris, K., Pignata, C., Plebani, A., Qamar, F. N., Qureshi, S., Radhakrishnan, N., Rezaei, N., Rosario, N., Routes, J., Sanchez, B., Sediva, A., Seppanen, M. R., Serrano, E. G., Shcherbina, A., Singh, S., Siniah, S., Spadaro, G., Tang, M., Vinet, A. M., Volokha, A., & Sullivan, K. E. (2019). X-linked agammaglobulinemia (XLA): Phenotype, diagnosis, and therapeutic challenges around the world. *World Allergy Organization Journal*, *12*(3), 100018. https://doi.org/10.1016/j.waojou.2019.100018.

Engelhardt, K. R., Gertz, M. E., Keles, S., Schäffer, A. A., Sigmund, E. C., Glocker, C., Saghafi, S., Pourpak, Z., Ceja, R., Sassi, A., Graham, L. E., Massaad, M. J., Mellouli, F., Ben-Mustapha, I., Khemiri, M., Kilic, S. S., Etzioni, A., Freeman, A. F., Thiel, J.,

Schulze, I., Al-Herz, W., Metin, A., Sanal, Ö., Tezcan, I., Yeganeh, M., Niehues, T., Dueckers, G., Weinspach, S., Patiroglu, T., Unal, E., Dasouki, M., Yilmaz, M., Genel, F., Aytekin, C., Kutukculer, N., Somer, A., Kilic, M., Reisli, I., Camcioglu, Y., Gennery, A. R., Cant, A. J., Jones, A., Gaspar, B. H., Arkwright, P. D., Pietrogrande, M. C., Baz, Z., Al-Tamemi, S., Lougaris, V., Lefranc, G., Megarbane, A., Boutros, J., Galal, N., Bejaoui, M., Barbouche, M. R., Geha, R. S., Chatila. T. A., & Grimbacher, B. (2015). The extended clinical phenotype of 64 patients with dedicator of cytokinesis 8 deficiency. *Journal of Allergy and Clinical Immunology*, *136*(2), 402–412. 2014.12.1945.

Finn, O. J. (2012). Immuno-oncology: understanding the function and dysfunction of the immune system in cancer. *Annals of Oncology*, *23*, viii6–viii9. .

Goldszmid, R. S., Dzutsev, A., & Trinchieri, G. (2014). Host Immune Response to Infection and Cancer: Unexpected Commonalities. *Cell Host & Microbe*, *15*(3), 295–305. .

Greten, F. R., & Grivennikov, S. I. (2019). Inflammation and Cancer: Triggers, Mechanisms, and Consequences. *Immunity*, *51*(1), 27–41. org/10.1016/j.immuni.2019.06.025.

Grivennikov, S. I., Greten, F. R., & Karin, M. (2010). Immunity, Inflammation, and Cancer. *Cell*, *140*(6), 883–899. https://doi.org/10.1016/j.cell.2010.01.025.

Gu, Y., Chae, H.-D., Siefring, J. E., Jasti, A. C., Hildeman, D. A., & Williams, D. A. (2006). RhoH GTPase recruits and activates Zap70 required for T cell receptor signaling and thymocyte development. *Nature Immunology*, *7*(11), 1182–1190. https://doi.org/10.1038/ni1396.

Guo, F., Zhang, S., Tripathi, P., Mattner, J., Phelan, J., Sproles, A., Mo, J., Wills-Karp, M., Grimes, H. L., Hildeman, D., & Zheng, Y. (2011). Distinct roles of CDC42 in thymopoiesis and effector and memory T cell differentiation. *PLOS ONE*, *6*(3), e18002-. https://doi.org/10.1371/journal.pone.0018002.

Hashim, I. F., & Ahmad Mokhtar, A. M. (2021). Small Rho GTPases and their associated RhoGEFs mutations promote immunological defects in primary immunodeficiencies. *The International Journal of Biochemistry & Cell Biology*, *137*, 106034. https://doi.org/10.1016/j.biocel.2021.106034.

Kellogg, C., Kouznetsova, V. L., & Tsigelny, I. F. (2021). Implications of viral infection in cancer development. *Biochimica et Biophysica Acta (BBA) - Reviews on Cancer*, *1876*(2), 188622. .

Maffeis, M., Notarangelo, L. D., Schumacher, R. F., Soncini, E., Soresina, A., Lanfranchi, A., & Porta, F. (2019). Primary immunodeficiencies and oncological risk: the experience of the Children's Hospital of Brescia. *Frontiers in Pediatrics*, *7*, 232. https://doi.org/10.3389/fped.2019.00232.

McCusker, C., & Warrington, R. (2011). Primary immunodeficiency. *Allergy, Asthma & Clinical Immunology*, *7*(1), S11. https://doi.org/10.1186/1710-1492-7-S1-S11.

Mortaz, E., Tabarsi, P., Mansouri, D., Khosravi, A., Garssen, J., Velayati, A., & Adcock, I. M. (2016). Cancers related to immunodeficiencies: update and perspectives. *Frontiers in Immunology*, *7*, 365. https://doi.org/10.3389/fimmu.2016.00365.

Nagaraj, N., Egwim, C., & Adler, D. G. (2007). X-linked Hyper-IgM Syndrome associated with poorly differentiated neuroendocrine tumor presenting as obstructive jaundice secondary to extensive adenopathy. *Digestive Diseases and Sciences*, *52*(9), 2312–2316. https://doi.org/10.1007/s10620-006-9702-3.

Pulvirenti, F., Pecoraro, A., Cinetto, F., Milito, C., Valente, M., Santangeli, E., Crescenzi, L., Rizzo, F., Tabolli, S., Spadaro, G., Agostini, C., & Quinti, I. (2018). Gastric Cancer Is the Leading Cause of Death in Italian Adult Patients with Common Variable Immunodeficiency. *Frontiers in Immunology*, *9*, 2546. https://doi.org/10.3389/fimmu.2018.02546.

Rezaei, N., Hedayat, M., Aghamohammadi, A., & Nichols, K. E. (2011). Primary immunodeficiency diseases associated with increased susceptibility to viral infections and malignancies. *Journal of Allergy and Clinical Immunology*, *127*(6), 1329-1341.e2. https://doi.org/10.1016/j.jaci.2011.02.047.

Rodriguez-Bravo, V., Carceles-Cordon, M., Hoshida, Y., Cordon-Cardo, C., Galsky, M. D., & Domingo-Domenech, J. (2017). The role of GATA2 in lethal prostate cancer aggressiveness. *Nature Reviews Urology*, *14*(1), 38–48. https://doi.org/10.1038/nrurol.2016.225.

Ruffner, M. A., Sullivan, K. E., & Henrickson, S. E. (2017). Recurrent and sustained viral infections in primary immunodeficiencies. *Frontiers in Immunology*, *8*, 665. https://doi.org/10.3389/fimmu.2017.00665.

Satgé D. (2018). A tumor profile in primary immune deficiencies challenges the cancer immune surveillance concept. *Frontiers in immunology*, *9*, 1149. https://doi.org/10.3389/fimmu.2018.01149.

Seleman, M., Hoyos-Bachiloglu, R., Geha, R. S., & Chou, J. (2017). Uses of next-generation sequencing technologies for the diagnosis of primary immunodeficiencies. *Frontiers in Immunology*, *8*, 847. https://doi.org/10.3389/fimmu.2017.00847.

Shapiro, R. S. (2011). Malignancies in the setting of primary immunodeficiency: Implications for hematologists/oncologists. *American Journal of Hematology*, *86*(1), 48–55. https://doi.org/https://doi.org/10.1002/ajh.21903.

Staines Boone, A. T., Torres Martínez, M. G., López Herrera, G., de Leija Portilla, J. O., Espinosa Padilla, S. E., Espinosa Rosales, F. J., & Lugo Reyes, S. O. (2014). Gastric adenocarcinoma in the context of X-linked agammaglobulinemia. *Journal of Clinical Immunology*, *34*(2), 134–137. https://doi.org/10.1007/s10875-013-9971-5.

Swann, J. B., & Smyth, M. J. (2007). Immune surveillance of tumors. *The Journal of Clinical Investigation*, *117*(5), 1137–1146. https://doi.org/10.1172/JCI31405.

Szczawinska-Poplonyk, A., Ploski, R., Bernatowska, E., & Pac, M. (2020). A novel *CDC42* Mutation in an 11-Year old child manifesting as syndromic immunodeficiency, autoinflammation, hemophagocytic lymphohistiocytosis, and malignancy: a case report. *Frontiers in Immunology*, *11*, 318. https://doi.org/10.3389/fimmu.2020.00318.

Trinchieri, G. (2012). Cancer and inflammation: an old intuition with rapidly evolving new concepts. *Annual Review of Immunology*, *30*(1), 677–706. https://doi.org/10.1146/annurev-immunol-020711-075008.

UNICEF. (2020). Retrieved on August 09, 2022, *Key demographic indicators*, https://data.unicef.org/country/mys/.

Vignesh, P., Suri, D., Rawat, A., Lau, Y. L., Bhatia, A., Das, A., Srinivasan, A., & Dhandapani, S. (2017). Sclerosing cholangitis and intracranial lymphoma in a child with classical Wiskott–Aldrich syndrome. *Pediatric Blood & Cancer*, *64*(1), 106–109. https://doi.org/https://doi.org/10.1002/pbc.26196.

Vorsteveld, E. E., Hoischen, A., & van der Made, C. I. (2021). Next-Generation Sequencing in the Field of Primary Immunodeficiencies: Current Yield, Challenges, and Future Perspectives. *Clinical Reviews in Allergy & Immunology*, *61*(2), 212–225. https://doi.org/10.1007/s12016-021-08838-5.

Chapter 13

The Genetic Landscape of Hereditary Haemochromatosis

Francis Jatta[1]
Che Ghazali Norul Hajar[1]
Zefarina Zulkafli[2]
Noor Haslina Mohd Noor[2]
Mohd Nazri Hassan[2]
Abd Rashid Nur Haslindawaty[1]
and Hisham Atan Edinur[1,*]
[1]School of Health Sciences, Universiti Sains Malaysia, Kota Bharu, Kelantan, Malaysia
[2]School of Medical Sciences, Universiti Sains Malaysia, Kota Bharu, Kelantan, Malaysia

Abstract

Genetic variants in the haemochromatosis gene (HFE), including C282Y, H63D and S65C polymorphisms, have been associated with an autosomal genetic disorder known as hereditary haemochromatosis (HH). It is a medical condition where iron levels become overloaded in internal organs, such as the heart, liver and pancreas. The C282Y, H63D and S65C single-nucleotide polymorphisms (SNPs) are uniquely distributed in the population and, therefore contribute to different risks of HH profiles. The disease is mainly caused by a homozygous C282Y SNP, while heterozygote genotypes (C282Y/H63D or C282Y/S65C) may cause mild HH in those with existing medical conditions (e.g., viral hepatitis and non-alcohol fatty liver disease). In this book chapter, we

* Corresponding Author's Email: edinur@usm.my.

In: Genetic Disorders and Rare Diseases
Editors: Shazlin Shaharudin, Hisham Atan Edinur and Nor Fazila Che Mat
ISBN: 979-8-88697-953-4

describe allelic variants in HFE that lead to HH and their frequency distributions in the world populations. It is anticipated that C282Y, H63D and S65C frequency data included here can be used for designing appropriate health policies, including population screening programmes for HH.

Keywords: C282Y, H63D, S65C, iron overloaded, disease profile

Introduction

The human genome consists of thousands of polymorphic genes, which include cytokine, human leukocyte antigen (HLA), killer cell immunoglobulin-like receptor (KIR), major histocompatibility complex class I chain- related gene A (MICA) and human homeostatic iron regulator or haemochromatosis gene (*HFE*) (Jin et al. 2004; Kumánovics et al. 2003; Edinur et al. 2015; Reuben et al. 2017). As a consequence, they may confer different individuals with protection or susceptibility towards certain diseases.

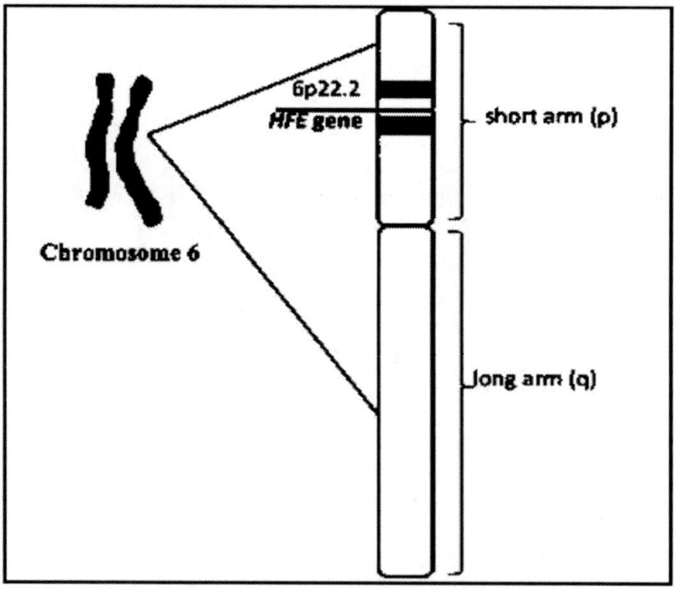

Figure 1. Location of the *HFE* gene on the short arm of chromosome 6.

The *HFE* gene is located on the short arm of chromosome 6 (Figure 1) and encodes a protein that binds with others to regulate iron metabolism in the human body (Barton et al. 2015; Harrison & Bacon 2005). In 1996, Feder et al. identified mutations in *HFE* that contributed to iron overload in the heart, liver and pancreas. Since then, this clinical condition has been known as hereditary haemochromatosis (HH) (Barton & Edwards, 2018; Bellissimo & Agarwal 2016; Milman et al. 2019).

Haemochromatosis Gene Mutations

The HFE protein plays a role in regulating iron intake in the body (Loréal et al. 2018; Nemeth & Ganz 2009). Feder et al. (1996) used a positional cloning technique to examine DNA specimens from a cohort of 178 Caucasian HH patients. The study identified two single-nucleotide polymorphisms (SNPs) in the form of missense mutations in *HFE*; C282Y (rs1800562) and H63D (rs1799945) in exon 4 and 2, respectively. The researchers further observed that most of the patients were homozygous for C282Y, which involved the substitution of guanine at nucleotide 845 to adenine (845G→A). Few other patients were either harbouring a H63D homozygous or C282Y/H63D compound heterozygous. The H63D SNP is due to substitution of cytosine (C) to guanine (G) at position 187 (187C→G) (Feder et al. 1996; Katsarou et al. 2019; Le Gac & Férec 2005). A third mutation (S65C) within *HFE* was later reported in 711 HH patients (Mura et al. 1999). The S65C (rs1800730) SNP is located at nucleotide position 193 of exon 2, which replaces adenine (A) with thymidine (T) (193A→T) (Mura et al. 1999).

Genomic Structure and Function

The *HFE* gene has seven exons, which encodes a predicted 343-amino acid protein. The protein contains peptide-binding domains (α1, α2 and α3), a transmembrane domain (TM) and a small cytoplasmic region that forms a complex with beta 2-microglobulin (β2M) (Barton et al. 2015). β2M is expressed by a separate gene on chromosome 15 (Li et al. 2016). The α1 and α2 domains are the receptor-binding sites of extracellular transferrins that are associated with Transferrin Receptor I (TFRI) (Lebrón et al. 1998). In contrast, the α3 domain binds to Transferrin Receptor 2 (TFR2) (Figure 2), which is a membrane protein homologous to TFR1, but has lower affinity in delivering iron to the plasma compared with TFR2 (Graham et al. 2007). Iron metabolism is regulated by systematic interactions between transferrin, HFE and TFRI (Townsend & Drakesmith 2002). Formation of HFE-TFRI complex will inhibit production of the iron-regulating hormone hepcidin and prevent iron absorption in liver cells (Nemeth & Ganz 2009). In contrast, binding of TFRI to transferrin will allow iron to enter liver cells besides increasing the production of hepcidin (Ganz, 2016). Therefore, defects in the HFE genetic code will lead to increased iron absorption in tissues, as well as decreased production of hepcidin that is important in regulating iron metabolism.

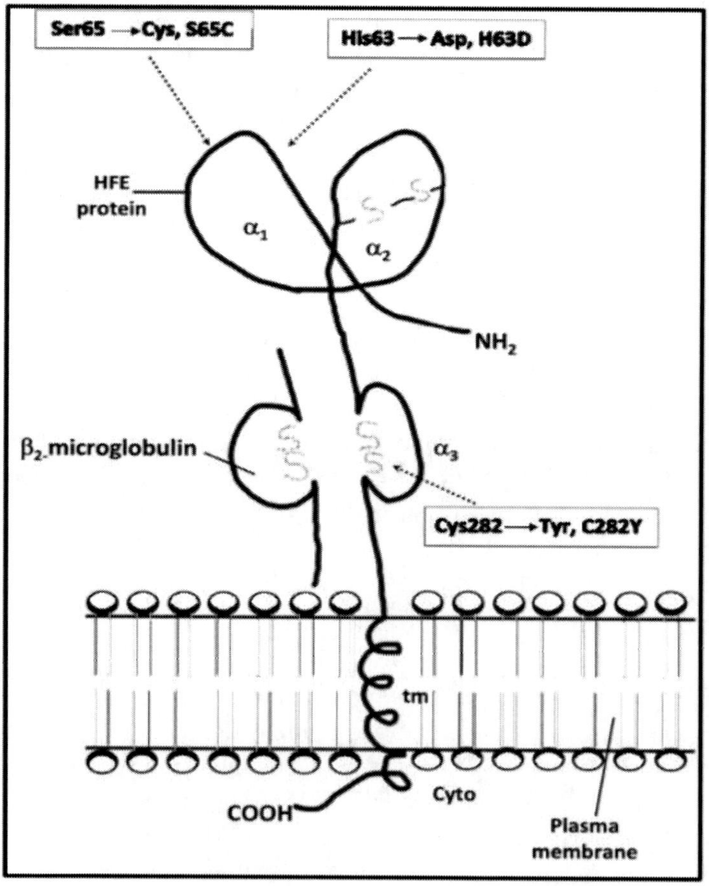

Figure 2. Structure of HFE protein. The three SNPs that affect the protein structure associated with hereditary haemochromatosis are shown in yellow boxes.

Subsequently, the risk of developing severe health complications due to iron overload, such as porphyria cutanea tarda (Barton & Edwards, 2016; Egger et al. 2002), liver cirrhosis (Barton & Edwards 2018), diabetes mellitus (Jennison & Wainwright 2018; Raju & Venkataramappa 2018), cardiac disease (Rasmussen et al. 2001; Sumi et al. 2020), hepatocellular carcinoma and other cancers (Abraham et al. 2005; Jayachandran et al. 2020; Jin et al. 2011; Lv et al. 2016; Robinson et al. 2005) will increase if HH patients are left untreated (Crownover & Covey 2013; Gabriková et al. 2012).

Prevalence of *HFE* SNPs

The most common *HFE* SNP associated with HH is C282Y (Gurrin et al. 2009; Tables 1 and 2). This *HFE* SNP is typically high among Europeans, but is low to absent in populations of non-European descent (Ali et al. 2018; Merryweather-Clarke et al. 1997). For this reason, HH is a genetic disease that mostly affects people of European ancestry, most notably those of Northern European origins (Bacon et al. 2011; Juzėnas et al. 2016; Tsui et al. 2000; Wallace & Subramaniam, 2016, Shiono et al. 2001). The H63D polymorphism, by comparison, is relatively common in populations worldwide, but the highest is still recorded among Europeans (de Juan et al. 2001) compared with Southeast Asian, African, Central and South American populations (Khusainova et al. 2013).

A third polymorphism, S65C, is infrequently linked to severe iron overload and therefore, has not been extensively investigated (Aranda et al. 2010; Brissot et al. 2017; Holmström et al. 2002; Mura et al. 1999; Muro et al. 2007). Individuals who are homozygous for S65C or compound heterozygote (C282Y/S65C) have been associated with mild HH symptoms, such as joint pain, fatigue, unintended weight loss, hepatomegaly and fatigue (Alexander & Kowdley 2009; Ayonrinde et al. 2008; Cheng et al. 2009; Gurrin et al. 2009). The Saami population of Northern Scandinavia has the highest frequency of S65C polymorphism (Beckman et al. 2001), while people of Hispanic, Asian and African descent have the lowest prevalence (Beutler et al. 2000; Barton et al. 1999; Remacha et al. 2000).

Table 1. Genotype frequencies of C282Y, H63D and S65C polymorphisms in the *HFE* gene

Genotype frequencies (%)										
Population	**C282Y/ wt**	**C282Y/ C282Y**	**H63D/ wt**	**H63D/ H63D**	**S65C/ wt**	**S65C/ S65C**	**C282Y/ H63D**	**C282Y/ S65C**	**H63D/ S65C**	**References**
Madeirense (Portugal)	0.00	0.00	32.00	3.90	1.30	0.00	0.65	0.00	0.65	Spínola et al. (2011)
Espírito Santense (Brazil)	3.33	0.00	20.83	0.83	0.83	0.00	0.00	0.00	0.83	Alves et al. (2016)
Chinese Han	0.00	0.00	4.60	0.00	0.00	0.00	0.00	0.00	0.00	Lin et al. (2007)
Dutch	12.70	0.30	23.60	2.20	0.00	0.00	0.00	0.00	0.00	Cobbaert et al. (2012)
Jordanian Arab	0.00	0.00	19.80	1.90	0.00	0.00	0.00	0.00	0.00	Alkhateeb et al. (2013)
Thai	0.00	0.00	20.00	1.00	0.00	0.00	0.00	0.00	0.00	Viprakasit et al. (2004)
Czech	6.86	0.00	26.61	1.67	2.49	0.00	1.87	0.00	0.42	Čimburová et al. (2005
Pakistanis, UK	0.00	0.00	4.00	0.50	0.00	0.00	0.00	0.00	0.00	Ali et al. (2018)
Iranian	1.20	0.00	8.50	0.00	0.00	0.00	0.00	0.00	0.00	Khusainova et al. (2013)
Turkic	0.80	0.00	15.20	1.10	0.00	0.00	0.00	0.00	0.00	Khusainova et al. (2013)
Lithuanian	5.10	0.10	26.70	2.60	3.70	0.00	1.19	0.10	0.40	Kucinskas et al. (2012)
Belarusian	0.00	0.00	25.00	8.30	0.00	0.00	0.00	0.00	0.00	Khusainova et al. (2013)
Northeast Brazilian	3.75	0.00	25.62	1.25	0.62	0.00	0.63	0.00	0.00	Leão et al. (2014)
Ukrainian	0.00	0.00	25.50	2.10	0.00	0.00	0.00	0.00	0.00	Khusainova et al. (2013)
Moldavian	0.00	0.00	19.10	0.00	0.00	0.00	0.00	0.00	0.00	Khusainova et al. (2013)
Karelian (Finland)	0.00	0.00	19.00	1.00	0.00	0.00	0.00	0.00	0.00	Khusainova et al. (2013)

Genotype frequencies (%)										
Population	**C282Y/ wt**	**C282Y/ C282Y**	**H63D/ wt**	**H63D/ H63D**	**S65C/ wt**	**S65C/ S65C**	**C282Y/ H63D**	**C282Y/ S65C**	**H63D/ S65C**	**References**
Volga–Ural (Russia)	0.00	0.00	21.70	1.80	0.00	0.00	0.00	0.00	0.00	Khusainova et al. (2013)
Kazakh	0.00	0.00	15.50	0.00	0.00	0.00	0.00	0.00	0.00	Khusainova et al. (2013)
Uzbek	0.00	0.00	11.10	0.00	0.00	0.00	0.00	0.00	0.00	Khusainova et al. (2013)
Uighur	0.00	0.00	16.40	0.00	0.00	0.00	0.00	0.00	0.00	Khusainova et al. (2013)
Kyrgyz	0.00	0.00	16.10	0.00	0.00	0.00	0.00	0.00	0.00	Khusainova et al. (2013)
Turkmen	0.00	0.00	16.70	5.50	0.00	0.00	0.00	0.00	0.00	Khusainova et al. (2013)
Kurd	0.00	0.00	12.20	0.00	0.00	0.00	0.00	0.00	0.00	Khusainova et al. (2013)
Tajik	0.00	0.00	4.80	0.00	0.00	0.00	0.00	0.00	0.00	Khusainova et al. (2013)

Table 2. The C282Y, H63D and S65C allele frequencies in *HFE* characterized populations

Allele frequencies (%)					
Country	**Population**	**C282Y**	**H63D**	**S65D**	**References**
Myanmar	Burmese	0.00	2.90	NT	Viprakasit et al. (2004)
Indonesia	Indonesian	0.00	2.80	NT	Merryweather-Clarke et al. (1997)
Thailand	Thai	0.00	3.20	NT	Pointon et al. (2003)
Vietnam	Vietnamese	0.00	4.90	0.00	Pointon et al. (2003)
Java	Javanese	0.00	NT	NT	Cullen et al. (1998)
Sri Lanka	Sri Lankan	0.00	9.20	NT	Merryweather-Clarke et al. (1997)

Table 2. (Continued)

Allele frequencies (%)					
Country	**Population**	**C282Y**	**H63D**	**S65D**	**References**
Pakistan	Pakistani	0.00	8.00	NT	Ali et al. (2018)
China	Chinese Han	0.00	2.30	0.00	Lin et al. (2007)
China	Hong Kong Chinese	0.00	2.80	NT	Merryweather-Clarke et al. (1997)
Taiwan	Taiwanese	0.00	1.90	NT	Merryweather-Clarke et al. (1997)
Saudi Arabia	Saudi Arabian	0.00	8.50	NT	Merryweather-Clarke et al. (1997)
Jordan	Jordanian Arab	0.00	11.25	0.11	Alkhateeb et al. (2009)
India	Indian	0.50	7.50	NT	Nadkarni et al. (2017)
Japan	Japanese	0.00	0.99	NT	Sohda et al. (1999)
South Korea	Korean	0.00	3.80	NT	Lee et al. (2000)
Kyrgyzstan	Kyrgyz	NT	8.10	0.00	Khusainova et al. (2013)
Kurdistan	Kurd	NT	6.10	0.00	Khusainova et al. (2013)
Turkmenia	Turkmen	NT	13.90	0.00	Khusainova et al. (2013)
Kazakhstan	Kazakh	NT	7.80	NT	Khusainova et al. (2013)
Uzbekistan	Uzbek	NT	5.60	NT	Khusainova et al. (2013)
Tajikistan	Tajik	NT	2.40	0.00	Khusainova et al. (2013)
Israel	Ashkenazi Jew	1.62	14.08	NT	Reish et al. (2010)
Central Asia	Uighur	0.00	8.20	0.00	Khusainova et al. (2013)
USA	Caucasian	6.30	15.20	1.60	Beutler et al. (2000)
USA	Hispanic	2.70	12.40	0.60	Beutler et al. (2000)
USA	Asian	0.20	3.30	0.00	Beutler et al. (2000)
USA	Black	1.10	5.10	0.70	Beutler et al. (2000)
Brazil	Espiritos- santense	1.67	11.67	0.83	Alves et al. (2016)
Brazil	Brazilian	2.10	13.60	0.60	Santos et al. (2010)
Ecuador	Ecuadorian	0.00	3.50	4.00	Leone et al. (2005)
Mexico	Mexican	0.20	11.50	NT	Avila-Gomez et al. (2008)
Mexico	Mexican	0.00	6.50	NT	Merryweather-Clarke et al. (1997)

Allele frequencies (%)					
Country	**Population**	**C282Y**	**H63D**	**S65D**	**References**
Venezuela	Venezuelan	1.90	11.90	0.90	Avila-Gomez et al. (2008)
Chile	Chilean	1.28	10.58	NT	Avila-Gomez et al. (2008)
Columbia	Columbian	0.00	0.00	NT	Merryweather-Clarke et al. (1997)
Jamaica	Jamaican	1.10	2.20	NT	Merryweather-Clarke et al. (1997)
Uzbekistan	Uzbek	NT	5.60	NT	Khusainova et al. (2013)
Tajikistan	Tajik	NT	2.40	0.00	Khusainova et al. (2013)
Algeria	Mozabite	0.00	8.90	NT	Roth et al. (1997)
Ethiopia	Ethiopian	0.00	9.40	NT	Roth et al. (1997)
Tunisia	Tunisian	0.50	17.50	NT	Zorai et al. (2003)
Gambia	Gambian	0.00	1.30	NT	Merryweather-Clarke et al. (1997)
Ghana	Ghanaian	0.00	1.00	NT	Jeffery et al. (1999)
Kenya	Kenyan	0.00	1.30	NT	Merryweather-Clarke et al. (1997)
Nigeria	Nigerian	0.00	1.90	NT	Merryweather-Clarke et al. (1997)
Senegal	Senegalese	0.00	0.00	NT	Merryweather-Clarke et al. (1997)
South Africa	South African	0.25	0.00	NT	de Villiers et al. (1999)
Zambia	Zambian	0.00	0.70	NT	Merryweather-Clarke et al. (1997)
Australia	Aborigine	0.00	0.00	NT	Merryweather-Clarke et al. (1997)
Australia	Vanuatuan	0.00	0.60	NT	Merryweather-Clarke et al. (1997)
Sweden	Finn, Swede, Swedish Saami	2.00	7.90	3.00	Beckman et al. (2001)
Sweden	Swedish	6.10	12.40	1.60	Milman et al. (2005)
Turkey	Turk	0.00	13.57	NT	Merryweather-Clarke et al. (1997)
Spain	Catalan	3.00	20.00	1.00	Altes et al. (2004)
Spain	Basque	3.60	30.40	NT	Merryweather-Clarke et al. (1997)
Spain	Murcia	0.67	27.02	2.02	Avila-Gomez et al. (2008)
Ireland	Irish	14.00	17.90	NT	Ryan et al. (1998)
Hungary	Hungarian	3.40	14.40	NT	Andrikovics et al. (2001)
Bosnia and Herzegovina	Bosnian and Herzegovinian	2.00	7.90	3.00	Terzić et al. (2006)
Czech Republic	Czech	3.40	16.20	1.25	Čimburová et al. (2005)

Table 2. (Continued)

Allele frequencies (%)					
Country	**Population**	**C282Y**	**H63D**	**S65D**	**References**
Italy	Apulian	1.50	14.00	0.50	Pietrapertosa et al. (2003)
Italy	Italian	3.20	13.40	1.30	Mariani et al. (2003)
Italy	Modena	4.71	14.93	0.74	Salvioni et al. (2003)
Italy	Ossola	1.60	13.30	NT	Cassanelli et al. (2001)
Russia	Russian	3.70	13.30	1.70	Mikhailova et al. (2003)
Serbia and Montenegro	Serbian and Montenegrin	1.60	15.70	1.60	Šarić et al. (2006)
Croatia	Croatian	3.30	14.50	1.80	Ristić et al. (2003)
Slovenia	Slovenian	4.00	14.50	0.50	Ristić et al. (2003)
Slovenia	Slovenian blood donors	3.60	12.80	1.80	Cukjati et al. (2007)
Portugal	Madeirense	0.33	20.50	1.00	Spínola et al. (2011)
Portugal	Portuguese	3.00	23.00	NT	Porto et al. (1998)
Germany	German	3.80	13.20	NT	Merryweather-Clarke et al. (1997)
Germany	German blood donors	4.60	10.80	NT	Raddatz et al. (2003)
Bulgaria	Bulgarian	0.00	23.00	NT	Merryweather-Clarke et al. (1997)
France	North African	1.07	12.23	NT	Aguilar-Martinez et al. (2001)
France	French	7.70	14.00	1.95	Mura et al. (1999)
Finland	Finn	4.60	9.80	2.30	Beckman et al. (2001)
Poland	Polish	3.10	16.20	NT	Moczulski et al. (2001)
Greece	Greek	1.30	13.50	NT	Merryweather-Clarke et al. (1997)
Austria	Austrian	3.70	12.90	NT	Merryweather-Clarke et al. (1997)
Faroe Islands	Faroese	8.00	17.50	1.00	Milman et al. (2005)
UK	British	8.10	15.20	NT	Merryweather-Clarke et al. (1997)

Diagnosis and Treatment

HH is a genetic blood disorder associated with iron metabolism (Pantopoulos 2018). The hereditary disorder causes the body to fail to eliminate excess iron obtained from food due to the inefficiency or defects in its excretory mechanism. Consequently, this excess iron leads to a state of over-accumulation, which is harmful to cells. These clinical disease manifestations are typically associated with C282Y polymorphism in *HFE* and it may lead to severe or fatal consequences if detected late and left untreated (Katsarou et al. 2016). Katsarou et al. (2016) reported that between three to five individuals in every 1,000 people are C282Y homozygous in north western Europe populations.

HH is commonly asymptomatic and primarily affects adult males compared with females. In women, menstruation possibly contributes to the late onset of this disease (Al Wayli et al. 2011; Katsarou et al. 2016). Clinical symptoms usually appear in men at and after age 40 (Puntarulo 2005). Genetic screening of *HFE* gene is thus essential because it will allow for early treatment (Bassett 2010; Brissot et al. 2008). Affected individuals may then be advised to undergo phlebotomy therapy to prevent disease development and normalize their iron level (Asimakopoulou et al. 2017; Koshy et al. 2020; Kowdley et al. 2019; Salgia & Brown 2015).

Conclusion

The distribution of *HFE* C282Y, H63D and S65C polymorphisms has been studied for years. Most of the studies focused on C282Y and H63D variants because both SNPs are the most commonly associated with excessive iron overload. In contrast, S65C polymorphism causes mild iron overload and data are available only from a limited number of populations. Future studies should focus on *HFE* SNP screening in other uncharacterized populations for a better estimating of risk profile to HH.

Acknowledgement

This work was supported by Ministry of Higher Education Malaysia via the Fundamental Research Grant Scheme (FRGS/1/2020/STG03/USM/03/5).

References

Abraham, B. K., Justenhoven, C., Pesch, B., Harth, V., Weirich, G., Baisch, C., Rabstein, S., Ko, Y. D., Brüning, T. & Fischer, H. P. (2005). Investigation of genetic variants of genes of the hemochromatosis pathway and their role in breast cancer. *Cancer Epidemiology and Prevention Biomarkers,* 14(5), 1102-1107. https://doi.org/10.1158/1055-9965.epi-05-0013

Aguilar-Martinez, P., Picot, M. C., Becker, F., Boulot, P., Montoya, F., Mares, P., Bachelard, B., Henry, Y., Delarbre, J. L. & Sarda, P. (2001). Prevalence of HFE mutations in people from North Africa living in southern France. *British Journal of Haematology,* 114(4), 914-916. https://doi.org/10.1046/j.1365-2141.2001.03005.x.

Al Wayli, H., Rastogi, S. & Verma, N. (2011). Hereditary hemochromatosis of tongue. *Oral Surgery, Oral Medicine, Oral Pathology, Oral Radiology, and Endodontology,* 111(1), e1-e5. https://doi.org/10.1016/j.tripleo.2010.09.009.

Alexander, J. & Kowdley, K. V. (2009). HFE-associated hereditary hemochromatosis. *Genetics in Medicine,* 11(5), 307-313. https://doi.org/10.1097/gim.0b013e31819d30f2.

Ali, N., Ahmed, B., Akram, H., Akhtar, J., Williams, R. & Dixon, R. (2018). HFE gene mutations. *The Professional Medical Journal,* 25(1), 129-134. https://doi.org/10.29309/TPMJ/2018.25.01.551.

Alkhateeb, A., Al-khatib, S., Elbetieha, A. & Al-Rashaideh, T. (2013). Clinical characteristics and analysis of HFE gene variants (C282Y and H63D) in Jordanian Arab patients with age-related macular degeneration. *Egyptian Journal of Medical Human Genetics,* 14(2), 177-181. https://doi.org/10.1016/j.ejmhg.2012.10.008.

Alkhateeb, A., Uzrail, A. & Bodoor, K. (2009). Frequency of the hemochromatosis gene (HFE) variants in a Jordanian Arab population and in diabetics from the same region. *Disease Markers,* 27(1), 17-22. https://doi.org/10.3233/dma-2009-0642.

Altes, A., Ruiz, A., Barceló, M. J., Remacha, A. F., Puig, T., Maya, A. J., Castell, C., Amate, J. M., Saz, Z. & Baiget, M. (2004). Prevalence of the C282Y, H63D, and S65C mutations of the HFE gene in 1,146 newborns from a region of Northern Spain. *Genetic Testing,* 8(4), 407-410. https://doi.org/10.1089/gte.2004.8.407.

Alves, L. N., Santos, E. V., Stur, E., Silva Conforti, A. M. & Louro, I. D. (2016). Molecular epidemiology of HFE gene polymorphic variants (C282Y, H63D and S65C) in the population of Espirito Santo, Brazil. *Genetic and Molecular Research:GMR,* 15(2). https://doi.org/10.4238/gmr.15028189.

Andrikovics, H., Kalmár, L., Bors, A., Fandl, B., Petri, I., Kalász, L. & Tordai, A. (2001). Genotype screening for hereditary hemochromatosis among voluntary blood donors in Hungary. *Blood Cells, Molecules, and Diseases,* 27(1), 334-341. https://doi.org/10.1006/bcmd.2001.0384.

Aranda, N., Viteri, F. E., Montserrat, C. & Arija, V. (2010). Effects of C282Y, H63D, and S65C HFE gene mutations, diet, and lifestyle factors on iron status in a general Mediterranean population from Tarragona, Spain. *Annals of Hematology,* 89(8), 767-773. https://doi.org/10.1007/s00277-010-0901-9.

Asimakopoulou, A., Weiskirchen, S. & Weiskirchen, R. (2017). Pathogenesis, Diagnostics, and treatment of hereditary haemochromatosis: A 150-year-long understanding of an iron overload disorder. *EMJ,* 2, 122-133. https://doi.org/10.33590/emj/10310080.

Avila-Gomez, I. C., Aristizabal-Bernal, B., Jimenez-Del-Rio, M. & Velez-Pardo, C. (2008). Prevalence of H63D, S65C and C282Y mutations of the HFE gene in 1120 voluntary blood donors from Antioquia region of northwest Colombia. *Blood Cells, Molecules & Diseases,* 40(3), 449-451. https://doi.org/10.1016/j.bcmd.2008.01.003.

Ayonrinde, O. T., Milward, E. A., Chua, A. C., Trinder, D. & Olynyk, J. K. (2008). Clinical perspectives on hereditary hemochromatosis. *Critical Reviews in Clinical Laboratory Sciences,* 45(5), 451-484. https://doi.org/10.1080/10408360802335716.

Bacon, B. R., Adams, P. C., Kowdley, K. V., Powell, L. W. & Tavill, A. S. (2011). Diagnosis and management of hemochromatosis: 2011 practice guideline by the American Association for the Study of Liver Diseases. *Hepatology,* 54(1), 328-343. https://doi.org/10.1002/hep.24330.

Barton, J. C. & Edwards, C. Q. (2016). Porphyria cutanea tarda associated with HFE C282Y homozygosity, iron overload, and use of a contraceptive vaginal ring. *Journal of Community Hospital Internal Medicine Perspectives,* 6(1), 30380. https://doi.org/10.3402/jchimp.v6.30380.

Barton, J. C. & Edwards, C. Q. (2018). HFE hemochromatosis. In, *GeneReviews®[Internet]*: University of Washington, Seattle.

Barton, J. C., Edwards, C. Q. & Acton, R. T. (2015). HFE gene: structure, function, mutations, and associated iron abnormalities. *Gene,* 574(2), 179-192. https://doi.org/10.1016/j.gene.2015.10.009.

Barton J. C, Sawada-Hirai R, Rothenberg B. E. & Acton, R. T. (1999). Two novel missense mutations of the HFE gene (I105T and G93R) and identification of the S65C mutation in Alabama hemochromatosis probands. *Blood Cell, Molecules and Diseases*, 25(3-4), 147–155. https://doi.org/10.1006/bcmd.1999.0240.

Bassett, M.L. (2010). HFE genotyping: maximising the value for hemochromatosis patients and families. *Journal of Gastroenterology Hepatology*, 25(7), 1186-8. https://doi.org/10.1111/j.1440-1746.2010.06387.x.

Beckman, L., Sjöberg, K., Eriksson, S. & Beckman, L. (2001). Haemochromatosis gene mutations in Finns, Swedes and Swedish Saamis. *Human Heredity,* 52(2), 110-112. https://doi.org/10.1159/000053362.

Bellissimo, D. B. & Agarwal, A. (2016). Hematologic Disorders: Hemochromatosis, Hemoglobinopathies, and Rh Incompatibility. In, *Molecular Pathology in Clinical Practice*: Springer, Cham, Switzerland. https://doi.org/10.1007/978-3-319-19674-9_16.

Beutler, E., Felitti, V., Gelbart, T. & Ho, N. (2000). The effect of HFE genotypes on measurements of iron overload in patients attending a health appraisal clinic. *Annals of Internal Medicine,* 133(5):329-37. https://doi.org/10.7326/0003-4819-133-5-200009050-00008.

Brissot, P., Loréal, O. & Jouanolle, A.-M. (2017). Molecular Testing in Hemochromatosis. In, *Diagnostic Molecular Pathology*: Elsevier, pp 245-253.

Brissot, P., Troadec, M.-B., Bardou-Jacquet, E., Le Lan, C., Jouanolle, A.M., Deugnier, Y. & Loreal, O. (2008). Current approach to hemochromatosis. *Blood Reviews,* 22(4), 195-210. https://doi.org/10.1016/j.blre.2008.03.001.

Cassanelli, S., Pignatti, E., Montosi, G., Garuti, C., Mariano, M., Campioli, D., Carbonieri, A., Baldini, E. & Pietrangelo, A. (2001). Frequency and biochemical expression of C282Y/H63D hemochromatosis (HFE) gene mutations in the healthy adult population in Italy. *Journal of Hepatology,* 34(4), 523-528. https://doi.org/10.1016/s0168-8278(01)00035-6.

Cheng, R., Barton, J. C., Morrison, E. D., Phatak, P. D., Krawitt, E. L., Gordon, S. C. & Kowdley, K. V. (2009). Differences in hepatic phenotype between hemochromatosis patients with HFE C282Y homozygosity and other HFE genotypes. *Journal of Clinical Gastroenterology,* 43(6), 569-573. https://doi.org/10.1097/mcg.0b013e3181919a33.

Čimburová, M., Půtová, I., Provaznikova, H., Pinterova, D. & Horak, J. (2005). S65C and other mutations in the haemochromatosis gene in the Czech population. *Folia Biologica (Praha),* 51(6), 172-176.

Cobbaert, C. M., Delanghe, J., Boer, J. M. & Feskens, E. J. (2012). Regional differences of HFE (C282Y, H63D) allele frequencies in the Netherlands A model case illustrating the significance of genographics and prehistorical population migration. *Acta Clinical Belgia,* 67(6), 430-435. https://doi.org/10.2143/acb.67.6.2062708.

Crownover, B. K. & Covey, C. J. (2013). Hereditary hemochromatosis. *American Family Physician,* 87(3), 183-190.

Cukjati, M., Vaupotič, T., Rupreht, R. & Čurin-Šerbec, V. (2007). Prevalence of H63D, S65C and C282Y hereditary hemochromatosis gene mutations in Slovenian population by an improved high-throughput genotyping assay. *BMC Medical Genetics,* 8, 69. https://doi.org/10.1186/1471-2350-8-69.

Cullen, L. M., Gao, X., Easteal, S. & Jazwinska, E. C. (1998). The hemochromatosis 845 G→ A and 187 C→ G mutations: prevalence in non-Caucasian populations. *The American Journal of Human Genetics,* 62(6), 1403-1407. https://doi.org/10.1086/301878.

de Juan, M., Reta, A., Castiella, A., Pozueta, J., Prada, A. & Cuadrado, E. (2001). HFE gene mutations analysis in Basque hereditary haemochromatosis patients and controls. *European Journal of Human Genetics,* 9(12), 961-964. https://doi.org/10.1038/sj.ejhg.5200731.

de Villiers, J. N. P., Hillermann, R., Loubser, L. & Kotze, M. J. (1999). Spectrum of mutations in the HFE gene implicated in haemochromatosis and porphyria. *Human Molecular Genetics,* 8(8), 1517-1522. https://doi.org/10.1093/hmg/8.8.1517.

Edinur, H. A., Chambers, G. K. & Dunn, P. P. (2015). Recent Developments in Transplantation and Transfusion Medicine. *Annals of Transplantation*, 20, 424-429. https://doi.org/10.12659/aot.894003.

Egger, N. G., Goeger, D. E., Payne, D. A., Miskovsky, E. P., Weinman, S. A. & Anderson, K. E. (2002). Porphyria cutanea tarda: multiplicity of risk factors including HFE mutations, hepatitis C, and inherited uroporphyrinogen decarboxylase deficiency. *Digestive Diseases and Sciences,* 47(2), 419-426. https://doi.org/10.1023/a:1013746828074.

Feder, J., Gnirke, A., Thomas, W., Tsuchihashi, Z., Ruddy, D., Basava, A., Dormishian, F., Domingo, R., Ellis, M. & Fullan, A. (1996). A novel MHC class I–like gene is mutated in patients with hereditary haemochromatosis. *Nature Genetics,* 13, 399-408. https://doi.org/10.1038/ng0896-399.

Gabriková, D., Bernasovská, J., Mačeková, S., Bôžiková, A., Bernasovský, I., Barlišinová, A., Sovičová, A., Behulová, R., Petrejčíková, E. & Soták, M. (2012). Unique frequencies of HFE gene variants in Roma/Gypsies. *Journal of Applied Genetics,* 53(2), 183-187. https://doi.org/10.1007/s13353-012-0088.

Ganz, T. (2016). Hepcidin. *Rinsho Ketsueki*, 57(10):1913-1917. https://doi.org/10.11406/ rinketsu.57.1913.

Graham, R. M., Chua, A. C., Herbison, C. E., Olynyk, J. K., & Trinder, D. Liver iron transport (2007). *World Journal of Gastroenterol,* 13(35): 4725– 4736. https://doi.org/10.3748/wjg.v13.i35.4725.

Gurrin, L. C., Bertalli, N. A., Dalton, G. W., Osborne, N. J., Constantine, C. C., McLaren, C. E., English, D. R., Gertig, D. M., Delatycki, M. B. & Nicoll, A. J. (2009). HFE C282Y/H63D compound heterozygotes are at low risk of hemochromatosis-related morbidity. *Hepatology*, 50(1), 94-101. https://doi.org/10.1002/hep.22972.

Harrison, S. A. & Bacon, B. R. (2005). Relation of hemochromatosis with hepatocellular carcinoma: epidemiology, natural history, pathophysiology, screening, treatment, and prevention. *Medical Clinics,* 89, 391-409. https://doi.org/10.1016/j.mcna.2004.08.005.

Holmström, P., Marmur, J., Eggertsen, G., Gåfvels, M. & Stål, P. (2002). Mild iron overload in patients carrying the HFE S65C gene mutation: a retrospective study in patients with suspected iron overload and healthy controls. *Gut,* 51(5), 723-730. https://doi.org/10.1136/gut.51.5.723.

Jayachandran, A., Shrestha, R., Bridle, K. R. & Crawford, D. H. (2020). Association between hereditary hemochromatosis and hepatocellular carcinoma: a comprehensive review. *Hepatoma Research,* 6, 8. https://doi.org/10.1097/01.mog.0000218955.55688.af.

Jeffery, S., Crosby, A., Plange-Rhule, J., Amoah-Danquah, J., Acheampong, J., Eastwood, J. & Malik, A. S. (1999). Evidence from a Ghanaian population of known African descent to support the proposition that hemochromatosis is a Caucasian disorder. *Genetic Testing,* 3(4), 375-377. https://doi.org/10.1089/gte.1999.3.375.

Jennison, E. & Wainwright, P. (2018). Hereditary haemochromatosis and diabetes. *Journal of Diabetes Nursing,* 22(4).

Jin, P., Panelli, M. C., Marincola, F. M., & Wang, E. (2004). Cytokine polymorphism and its possible impact on cancer. *Immunologic Research,* 30, 181-190. https://doi.org/10.1385/ir:30:2:181.

Jin, F., Xiong, W.-J., Jing, J.-C., Feng, Z., Qu, L.-S. & Shen, X.-Z. (2011). Evaluation of the association studies of single nucleotide polymorphisms and hepatocellular carcinoma: a systematic review. *Journal of Cancer Research and Clinical Oncology,* 137(7), 1095-1104. https://doi.org/10.1007/s00432-010-0970-0.

Juzėnas, S., Kupčinskas, J., Valantienė, I., Šumskienė, J., Petrenkienė, V., Kondrackienė, J., Kučinskas, L., Kiudelis, G., Skiecevičienė, J. & Kupčinskas, L. (2016). Association of HFE gene C282Y and H63D mutations with liver cirrhosis in the Lithuanian population. *Medicina,* 52(5), 269-275. https://doi.org/10.1016/j.medici.2016.09.004.

Katsarou, M. S., Latsi, R., Papasavva, M., Demertzis, N., Kalogridis, T., Tsatsakis, A. M., Spandidos, D. A. & Drakoulis, N. (2016). Population-based analysis of the frequency of HFE gene polymorphisms: Correlation with the susceptibility to develop hereditary hemochromatosis. *Molecular Medicine Reports,* 14(1), 630-636. https://doi.org/10.3892/mmr.2016.5317.

Katsarou, M.-S., Papasavva, M., Latsi, R. & Drakoulis, N. (2019). Hemochromatosis: hereditary hemochromatosis and HFE gene. *Vitamins and Hormones,* 110, 201-222. https://doi.org/10.1016/bs.vh.2019.01.010.

Khusainova, R., Khusnutdinova, N., Litvinov, S. & Khusnutdinova, E. (2013). Analysis of H63D mutation in hemochromatosis (HFE) gene in populations of central Eurasia. *Russian Journal of Genetics,* 49(2), 237-245. https://doi.org/10.7868/s0016675812120041.

Koshy, A., Mukkada, R. J., Chettupuzha, A. P., Francis, J. V., Kandathil, J. C. & Mahadevan, P. (2020). Hemochromatosis in India: first report of whole exome sequencing with review of the literature. *Journal of Clinical Experimental Hepatology,* 10(2), 163-169. https://doi.org/10.1016/j.jceh.2019.04.051.

Kowdley, K. V., Brown, K. E., Ahn, J. & Sundaram, V. (2019). ACG Clinical Guideline: Hereditary Hemochromatosis. *American Journal of Gastroenterology,* 114(8), 1202-1218. https://doi.org/10.14309/ajg.0000000000000315.

Kucinskas, L., Juzenas, S., Sventoraityte, J., Cedaviciute, R., Vitkauskiene, A., Kalibatas, V., Kondrackiene, J. & Kupcinskas, L. (2012). Prevalence ofnC282Y, H63D, and S65C mutations in hereditary HFE-hemochromatosis gene in Lithuanian population. *Annals of Hematology,* 91(4), 491-495. https://doi.org/10.1007/s00277-011-1338-5.

Kumánovics, A., Takada, T. & Lindahl, K. F. (2003). Genomic organisation of the mammalian MHC. *Annual Review of Immunology,* 21, 629-657. https://doi.org/10.1146/annurev.immunol.21.090501.080116.

Le Gac, G. & Férec, C. (2005). The molecular genetics of haemochromatosis. *European Journal of Human Genetics,* 13(11), 1172-1185. https://doi.org/10.1038/sj.ejhg.5201490.

Leão, G. D. R., Freire, J. M., Cunha Fernandes, A. L. A., Moura de Oliveira, T. M., Leão, N. D., Gil, E. A., de Vasconcelos, R. C., Azevedo, J. P. d. S., de Farias Sales, V. S. & de Araújo Moura Lemos, T. M. (2014). Analysis of HFE genes C282Y, H63D, and S65D in patients with hyperferritinemia from northeastern Brazil. *Journal of Clinical Laboratory Analysis,* 28(3), 178-185. https://doi.org/10.1002/jcla.21663.

Lebrón, J. A., Bennett, M. J., Vaughn, D. E., Chirino, A. J., Snow, P. M., Mintier, G. A., Feder, J. N. & Bjorkman, P. J. (1998). Crystal structure of the hemochromatosis protein HFE and characterisation of its interaction with transferrin receptor. *Cell,* 93(1), 111-123. https://doi.org/10.1016/s0092-8674(00)81151-4.

Lee, J. Y., Yoo, K. H. & Hahn, S. H. (2000). HFE gene mutation, C282Y causing hereditary hemochromatosis in Caucasian is extremely rare in Korean population. *Journal of Korean Medical Science,* 15(2), 179-182. https://doi.org/10.3346/jkms.2000.15.2.179.

Leone, P. E., Gimenez, P., Collantes, J. C. & Paz-y-Mino, C. (2005). Analysis of HFE gene mutations (C282Y, H63D, and S65C) in the Ecuadorian population. *Annals of Hematology,* 84(2), 103-105. https://doi.org/10.1007/s00277-004-0966-4.

Li, L., Dong, M. & Wang, X.G., 2016. The implication and significance of beta 2 microglobulin: a conservative multifunctional regulator. *Chinese Medical Journal*, 129(4), 448-455. https://doi.org/10.4103/0366-6999.176084.

Lin, A., Yan, W., Xu, H., Zhu, M. & Zhou, M. (2007). Analysis of the HFE gene (C282Y, H63D and S65C) mutations in a general Chinese Han population. *Tissue Antigens,* 70(3), 252-255. https://doi.org/10.1111/j.1399-0039.2007.00877.x.

Loréal, O., Cavey, T., Robin, F., Kenawi, M., Guggenbuhl, P. & Brissot, P. (2018). Iron as a therapeutic target in HFE-related hemochromatosis: usual and novel aspects. *Pharmaceuticals,* 11(4), 131. https://doi.org/10.3390/ph11040131.

Lv, Y. F., Chang, X., Hua, R. X., Yan, G. N., Meng, G., Liao, X. Y., Zhang, X. & Guo, Q. N. (2016). The risk of new-onset cancer associated with HFE C282Y and H63D mutations: evidence from 87,028 participants. *Journal of Cellular and Molecular Medicine,* 20(7), 1219-1233. https://doi.org/10.1111/jcmm.12764.

Mariani, R., Salvioni, A., Corengia, C., Erba, N., Lanzafame, C., De Micheli, V., Baldini, V., Arosio, C., Fossati, L. & Trombini, P. (2003). Prevalence of HFE mutations in upper Northern Italy: study of 1132 unrelated blood donors. *Digestive and Liver Disease,* 35(7), 479-481. https://doi.org/10.1016/s1590-8658(03)00220-2.

Merryweather-Clarke, A. T., Pointon, J. J., Shearman, J. D. & Robson, K. (1997). Global prevalence of putative haemochromatosis mutations. *Journal of Medical Genetics*, 34(4), 275-278. https://doi.org/10.1136/jmg.34.4.275.

Mikhailova, S., Kobzev, V., Kulikov, I., Romaschenko, A., Khasnulin, V. & Voevoda, M. (2003). Polymorphism of the HFE gene associated with hereditary hemochromatosis in populations of Russia. *Russian Journal of Genetics,* 39(7), 828-835. https://doi.org/10.1023/A:3A1024765406867.

Milman, N., á Steig, T., Koefoed, P., Pedersen, P., Fenger, K. & Nielsen, F. C. (2005). Frequency of the hemochromatosis HFE mutations C282Y, H63D, and S65C in blood donors in the Faroe Islands. *Annals of Hematology,* 84(3), 146-149. https://doi.org/10.1007/s00277-004-0865-8.

Milman, N. T., Schioedt, F. V., Junker, A. E. & Magnussen, K. (2019). Diagnosis and treatment of genetic HFE-hemochromatosis: the Danish aspect. *Gastroenterology Research*, 12(5), 221. https://doi.org/10.14740/gr1206.

Moczulski, D. K., Grzeszczak, W. & Gawlik, B. (2001). Role of hemochromatosis C282Y and H63D mutations in HFE gene in development of type 2 diabetes and diabetic nephropathy. *Diabetes Care,* 24(7), 1187-1191. https://doi.org/10.2337/diacare.24.7.1187.

Mura, C., Raguenes, O. & Férec, C. (1999). HFE mutations analysis in 711 hemochromatosis probands: evidence for S65C implication in mild form of hemochromatosis. *Blood,* 93(8), 2502-2505. https://doi.org/10.1182/blood.V93.8.2502.

Muro, M., Moya-Quiles, M. R., Botella, C., García, I., Minguela, A. & Álvarez-López, M. R. (2007). Genetic relationship between Murcia Region (SE Spain) and other populations in the Iberian Peninsula and Mediterranean area with respect to HFE gene mutations distribution. *Annals of Hematology,* 86(6), 455-457. https://doi.org/10.1007/s00277-006-0242-x.

Nadkarni, A. H., Singh, A. A., Colaco, S., Hariharan, P., Colah, R. B. & Ghosh, K. (2017). Effect of the Hemochromatosis Mutations on Iron Overload among the Indian β Thalassemia Carriers. *Journal of Clinical Laboratory Analysis,* 31(3), e22054. https://doi.org/10.1002/jcla.22054.

Nemeth, E. & Ganz, T. (2009). The role of hepcidin in iron metabolism. *Acta Haematologica,* 122(2-3), 78-86. https://doi.org/10.1159%2F000243791.

Pantopoulos, K. (2018). Inherited disorders of iron overload. *Frontiers in Nutrition,* 5, 103. https://doi.org/10.3389/fnut.2018.00103.

Pietrapertosa, A., Vitucci, A., Campanale, D., Palma, A., Renni, R., Delios, G. & Tannoia, N. (2003). HFE gene mutations an Apulian population: allele frequencies. *European Journal of Epidemiology,* 18(7), 685-690. https://doi.org/10.1023/a:1024844906872.

Pointon, J. J., Viprakasit, V., Miles, K. L., Livesey, K. J., Steiner, M., O'Riordan, S., Hien, T. T., Merryweather-Clarke, A. T. & Robson, K. J. (2003). Hemochromatosis gene (HFE) mutations in South East Asia: a potential for iron overload. *Blood Cells, Molecules, and Diseases,* 30(3), 302-306. https://doi.org/10.1016/s1079-9796(03)00041-x.

Porto, G., Alves, H., Rodrigues, P., Cabeda, J. M., Portal, C., Ruivo, A., Justiça, B., Wolff, R. & De Sousa, M. (1998). Major histocompatibility complex class I associations in iron overload: evidence for a new link between the HFE H63D mutation, HLA-A29, and non-classical forms of hemochromatosis. *Immunogenetics,* 47(5), 404-410. https://doi.org/10.1007/s002510050376.

Puntarulo, S. (2005). Iron, oxidative stress and human health. *Molecular Aspects of Medicine,* 26(4-5), 299-312. https://doi.org/10.1016/j.mam.2005.07.001.

Raddatz, D., Legler, T., Lynen, R., Addicks, N. & Ramadori, G. (2003). HFE genotype and parameters of iron metabolism in german first-time blood donors. *Zeitschrift für Gastroenterologie*, 41(11), 1069-1076. https://doi.org/10.1055/s-2003-44299.

Raju, K. & Venkataramappa, S. M. (2018). Primary hemochromatosis presenting as Type 2 diabetes mellitus: A case report with review of literature. *International Journal of Applied and Basic Medical Research,* 8(1), 57-60. https://doi.org/10.4103/ijabmr.ijabmr_402_16.

Rasmussen, M. L., Folsom, A. R., Catellier, D. J., Tsai, M. Y., Garg, U. & Eckfeldt, J. H. (2001). A prospective study of coronary heart disease and the hemochromatosis gene (HFE) C282Y mutation: the Atherosclerosis Risk in Communities (ARIC) study. *Atherosclerosis,* 154(3), 739-746. https://doi.org/10.1016/s0021-9150(00)00623-7.

Reish, O., Shefer-Kaufmann, N., Shimshoni, D. C., Renbaum, P., Orr-Urtreger, A., Steiner, H., Rapoport, M., Levy-Lahad, E. & Altarescu, G. (2010). Frequencies of C282Y and H63D alleles in the HFE gene among various Jewish ethnic groups in Israel: A change of concept required. *Genetics in Medicine,* 12(2), 122-125. https://doi.org/10.1097/gim.0b013e3181cb78d6.

Remacha, A. F., Barcelo, M. J., Sarda, M. P., Blesa, I., Altés, A. & Baiget M. (2000). The S65C mutation in Spain. Implications for iron overload screening. *Haematologica,* 85(12), 1324-1325.

Reuben, A., Chung, J. W., Lapointe, R. & Santos, M. M. (2017). The hemochromatosis protein HFE 20 years later: An emerging role in antigen presentation and in the immune system. *Immunity, Inflammation and Disease,* 5, 218-232. https://doi.org/10.1002/iid3.158.

Ristić, S., Makuc, J., Starčević, N., Logar, N., Brajenović-Milić, B., Stepec, S., Pleša, I., Kapović, M., Milić, S. & Štimac, D. (2003). Hemochromatosis gene mutations in the Croatian and Slovenian populations. *Clinical Genetics,* 64(5), 444-446. https://doi.org/10.1034/j.1399-0004.2003.00169.x.

Robinson, J. P., Johnson, V. L., Rogers, P. A., Houlston, R. S., Maher, E. R., Bishop, D. T., Evans, D. G. R., Thomas, H. J., Tomlinson, I. P. & Silver, A. R. (2005). Evidence for an association between compound heterozygosity for germ line mutations in the hemochromatosis (HFE) gene and increased risk of colorectal cancer. *Cancer Epidemiology and Prevention Biomarkers,* 14(6), 1460-1463. https://doi.org/10.1158/1055-9965.epi-04-0672.

Roth, M.-P., Giraldo, P., Hariti, G., Poloni, E. S., Sanchez-Mazas, A., De Stefano, G. F., Dugoujon, J.-M. & Coppin, H. (1997). Absence of the hemochromatosis gene Cys282Tyr mutation in three ethnic groups from Algeria (Mzab), Ethiopia, and Senegal. *Immunogenetics,* 46(3), 222-225. https://doi.org/10.1007/s002510050265.

Ryan, E., O'Keane, C. & Crowe, J. (1998). Hemochromatosis in Ireland and HFE. *Blood Cells, Molecules, and Diseases,* 24(4), 428-432. https://doi.org/10.1006/bcmd.1998.0211.

Salgia, R. J. & Brown, K. (2015). Diagnosis and management of hereditary hemochromatosis. *Clinics in Liver Disease,* 19(1), 187-198. https://doi.org/10.1016/j.cld.2014.09.011.

Salvioni, A., Mariani, R., Oberkanins, C., Moritz, A., Mauri, V., Pelucchi, S., Riva, A., Arosio, C., Cerutti, P. & Piperno, A. (2003). Prevalence of C282Y and E168X HFE mutations in an Italian population of Northern European ancestry. *Haematologica,* 88(3), 250-255. https://doi.org/10.3324/%25X.

Santos, P., Cancado, R., Terada, C., Rostelato, S., Gonzales, I., Hirata, R., Hirata, M., Chiattone, C. & Guerra-Shinohara, E. (2010). HFE gene mutations and iron status of Brazilian blood donors. *Brazilian Journal of Medical and Biological Research,* 43(1), 107-114. https://doi.org/10.1590/s0100-879x2009007500031.

Šarić, M., Zamurović, L., Keckarević-Marković, M., Keckarević, D., Stevanović, M., Savić-Pavićević, D., Jović, J. & Romac, S. (2006). Frequency of the hemochromatosis gene mutations in the population of Serbia and Montenegro. *Clinical Genetics,* 70(2), 170-172. https://doi.org/10.1111/j.1399-0004.2006.00655.x.

Shiono, Y., Ikeda, R., Hayashi, H., Wakusawa, S., Sanae, F., Takikawa, T., Imaizumi, Y., Yano, M., Yoshioka, K. & Kawanaka, M. (2001). C282Y and H63D mutations in the HFE gene have no effect on iron overload disorders in Japan. *Internal medicine,* 40(8), 852-856. https://doi.org/10.2169/internalmedicine.40.852.

Sohda, T., Yanai, J., Soejima, H. & Tamura, K. (1999). Frequencies in the Japanese population of HFE gene mutations. *Biochemical Genetics,* 37(1-2), 63-68. https://doi.org/10.1023/a.1018718101579.

Spínola, C., Brehm, A. & Spínola, H. (2011). Prevalence of H63D, S65C, and C282Y hereditary hemochromatosis gene variants in Madeira Island (Portugal). *Annals of Hematology,* 90(1), 29-32. https://doi.org/10.1007/s00277-010-1034-x.

Sumi, M. P., Guru, S. A., Sahu, S., Khan, B., Mp, G. & Saxena, A. (2020). "Role of HFE gene in coronary artery disease"–A study from India. *Clinical Epidemiology and Global Health,* 8(2), 469-472. https://doi.org/10.1016/j.cegh.2019.10.011.

Terzić, R., Šehić, A., Teran, N., Terzić, I. & Peterlin, B. (2006). Frequency of HFE gene mutations C282Y and H63D in Bosnia and Herzegovina. *Collegium Antropologicum,* 30(3), 555-557.

Townsend, A. & Drakesmith, H. 2002. Role of HFE in iron metabolism, hereditary haemochromatosis, anaemia of chronic disease, and secondary iron overload. *The Lancet*, 359(9308), 786-790. https://doi.org/10.1016/s0140-6736(02)07885-6.

Tsui, W., Lam, P., Lee, K., Ma, K., Chan, Y., Wong, M., Yip, S., Wong, C., Chow, A. & Lo, S. (2000). The C282Y mutation of the HFE gene is not found in Chinese haemochromatotic patients: multicentre retrospective study. *Hong Kong Medical Journal,* 6(2), 153-158.

Viprakasit, V., Vathesathokit, P., Chinchang, W., Tachavanich, K., Pung-Amritt, P., Wimhurst, V. L., Yenchitsomanus, P. T., Merryweather-Clarke, A. T. & Tanphaichitr, V. S. (2004). Prevalence of HFE mutations among the Thai population and correlation with iron loading in haemoglobin E disorder. *European Journal of Haematology,* 73(1), 43-49. https://doi.org/10.1111/j.1600-0609.2004.00246.x.

Wallace, D. F. & Subramaniam, V. N. (2016). The global prevalence of HFE and non-HFE hemochromatosis estimated from analysis of next-generation sequencing data. *Genetics in Medicine,* 18(6), 618-626. https://doi.org/10.1038/gim.2015.140.

Zorai, A., Harteveld, C. L., Rachdi, R., Dellagi, K., Abbes, S., Delbini, P. & Giordano, P. C. (2003). Frequency and spectrum of hemochromatosis mutations in Tunisia. *The Hematology Journal,* 4(6), 433-435. https://doi.org/10.1038/sj.thj.6200337.

Index

D

E

F

G

H

I

T

U

V

X

α

About the Editors

Shazlin Shaharudin is an Associate Professor at the School of Health Sciences at Universiti Sains Malaysia's health campus in Kelantan, Malaysia. As an alumna of the university, she graduated with a BHSc (Hons) in biomedicine and obtained an MSc in sports science before pursuing a PhD in biomechanics and movement science at the University of Delaware in the United States. Her main research is in biomechanics and its application in sports and clinical populations. She has received about RM2 million in research funds, whereby she is the principal investigator in 80% of the projects. Together with her team, they have published 39 academic papers, two books, one book chapter and two massive open online courses (MOOCs). She has won the Gold Editor award under The Cochrane Collaboration Malay Language PLS translation initiative for three consecutive years. She is a volunteer academic editor in renowned journals of her field, including *Sports Biomechanics, BMC Sports Science, Medicine and Rehabilitation* and *PLOS ONE*.

Email: shazlin@usm.my

Hisham Atan Edinur is an Associate Professor at School of Health Sciences, Universiti Sains Malaysia. Another bright alumnus of USM, he graduated with a BSc in forensic science in 2006, followed by an MSc in the same field in 2010. He then pursued and obtained his PhD in cell and molecular bioscience at Victoria University, New Zealand, in 2013. As a dynamic researcher, he is affiliated to various higher-learning institutions besides USM. They include the Environmental Futures Research Institute at Griffith University in Nathan, Queensland, Australia. Human genomics is the core element of his research programmes, with the aim of improving medical outcomes and for forensic and ancestry studies. He has published more than 100 articles in journals indexed by Web of Science and/or Scopus.

Email: edinur@usm.my

Nor Fazila Che Mat is a lecturer in the School of Health Sciences, Universiti Sains Malaysia. She graduated with a BSc in biomedical science and received her MSc in health sciences (Biomedicine) from Universiti Kebangsaan Malaysia in 2004 and 2007, respectively. She obtained her PhD in immunology and virology from Queen's University, Canada, in 2011. Since 2012, she has been studying the potential of the Indian trumpet tree (*Oroxylum indicum*) in combating cancer and viral infections. Her research mainly involves molecular experiments on cervical cancer cells. One of her most significant achievements is the discovery of a potential treatment for cervical cancer using *Oroxylum indicum* extracts. As a result, she was awarded several external grants by the prestigious Malaysia National Cancer Council (MAKNA) in 2015 to further her research. Currently she is collaborating with different universities and the industry, including Universitas Airlangga in Indonesia, Bharati Vidyapeeth's College of Pharmacy in India and Sabinsa Corporation in the United States. She believes that the best way of contributing to the development and enhancement of knowledge is to publish her work so that other researchers could use it as a reference. She has more than 30 indexed journals under her belt and is actively writing books on immunology and infectious viral diseases.

Email: fazilacm@usm.my